Developing Clinical Judgment

for Professional Nursing and the Next-Generation **NCLEX-RN**® Examination

DONNA D. IGNATAVICIUS, MS, RN, CNE, ANEF

Speaker and Curriculum Consultant for Academic
Nursing Programs;
Founder, Boot Camp for Nurse Educators;
President, DI Associates, Inc.
Littleton, Colorado

ELSEVIER

Elsevier
3251 Riverport Lane
St. Louis, Missouri 63043

DEVELOPING CLINICAL JUDGMENT FOR PROFESSIONAL NURSING AND THE NEXT-GENERATION NCLEX-RN® EXAMINATION

ISBN: 978-0-323-71858-5

Notice

Practitioners and researchers must always rely on their own experience and knowledge in evaluating and using any information, methods, compounds or experiments described herein. Because of rapid advances in the medical sciences, in particular, independent verification of diagnoses and drug dosages should be made. To the fullest extent of the law, no responsibility is assumed by Elsevier, authors, editors or contributors for any injury and/or damage to persons or property as a matter of products liability, negligence or otherwise, or from any use or operation of any methods, products, instructions, or ideas contained in the material herein.

International Standard Book Number: 978-0-323-71858-5

Executive Content Strategist: Lee Henderson
Director, Content Development: Laurie Gower
Senior Content Development Specialist: Laura Goodrich
Publishing Services Manager: Julie Eddy
Senior Project Manager: Jodi M. Willard
Design Direction: Amy Buxton

Printed in China

Last digit is the print number: 9 8 7 6 5 4 3 2

Contributors

Jessica Hoy, RN, MSNE, PCCN-K
Assistant Professor of Nursing
College of Saint Scholastica
Duluth, Minnesota

Tami Little, DNP, RN, CNE
Corporate Director of Nursing
Vista College
Richardson, Texas

Sabrina Olson, MSN, RN
Professor
Butler Community College
El Dorado, Kansas

Janet Schueller, MSN, RN
Curriculum Chairperson
Professor
Butler Community College
El Dorado, Kansas

Reviewers

Kitty Cashion, RN-BC, MSN
Clinical Nurse Specialist
Department of Obstetrics and Gynecology
Division of Maternal-Fetal Medicine
University of Tennessee Health Science Center
Memphis, Tennessee

Brigid Chvilicek, MSN, RN, CPNP
Faculty of Nursing
Wenatchee Valley College
Wenatchee, Washington

Monica Dobbins, RN
Nursing Instructor
Butler Community College
El Dorado, Kansas

Jessica Hoy, RN, MSNE, PCCN-K
Assistant Professor of Nursing
College of Saint Scholastica
Duluth, Minnesota

Kay R. Jansen, DNP, RN
Undergraduate Program Director
University of Wisconsin—Milwaukee
College of Nursing
Milwaukee, Wisconsin

Tami Little, DNP, MSN, BSN
Corporate Director of Nursing
Vista College
Richardson, Texas

Lisa M. Pugsley, MSN, RN, CNE, CPN
Instructor of Nursing
Georgia Gwinnett College
Lawrenceville, Georgia

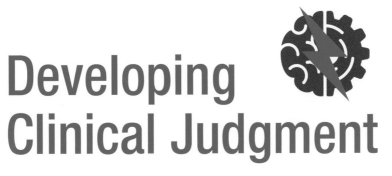

Developing Clinical Judgment

for Professional Nursing and
the Next-Generation **NCLEX-RN**® Examination

Purpose of This Workbook

In just a few years, the National Council of State Boards of Nursing (NCSBN) is expected to begin using the Next-Generation NCLEX® Examination for nursing licensure based on its new model of clinical judgment. This one-of-a-kind workbook is designed for students enrolled in prelicensure programs in preparation for registered nursing (RN) practice to help:

- Develop clinical judgment skills for professional nursing practice to ensure patient safety and quality of care.
- Prepare for success on the Next-Generation NCLEX® Examination (NGN) through practical thinking exercises in which students apply clinical reasoning skills to make appropriate clinical judgments.

This book is intended for students to use throughout their nursing program. Thinking exercises are available for all major areas of clinical specialty practice and are leveled from basic and foundational to more complex and multisystem. Each exercise provides challenging client situations with multiple NGN-style test items. For many thinking exercises, the clinical situation evolves into continuing care requiring the student to address changing client conditions.

Organization of This Workbook

This student-friendly workbook is organized by nursing concepts but is easy to use in any type of prelicensure RN nursing program. It is divided into five distinct parts for a total of 30 chapters. Each health problem throughout the book consists of between 4 and 7 thinking exercises for student practice:

Part 1 (Chapters 1 and 2). Chapter 1 provides an introduction to clinical judgment as a primary skill needed by practicing nurses. Chapter 2 offers tips for answering the practical thinking exercises in the workbook.

Part 2 (Chapters 3 to 17). This section focuses on thinking exercises that address nursing care for clients experiencing commonly occurring medical-surgical, pediatric, and mental health problems across the life span.

Part 3 (Chapter 18). This chapter provides multiple opportunities for students to address the care of childbearing women with uncomplicated and complicated clinical situations. Care of the normal newborn is also included.

Part 4 (Chapters 19 to 28). This section includes thinking exercises that address nursing care for clients experiencing complex multisystem medical-surgical, pediatric, and mental health problems across the life span.

Part 5 (Chapter 29 and 30). Although many pharmacology thinking exercises are integrated throughout Chapters 3 to 28, Chapters 29 and 30 are dedicated solely to the nurse's role in administering commonly used drugs for adult and pediatric clients who have commonly occurring and complex health problems.

Answer Key. The last section of this workbook presents the answers and rationales for each thinking exercise. In addition, the student is provided with reference pages where they can read more about each health problem.

References. At the end of the book is the list of textbook citations that are used for reference for the thinking exercises.

In summary, *Developing Clinical Judgment for Professional Nursing and the Next-Generation NCLEX-RN® Examination* is the first product focused exclusively on developing the clinical judgment skills needed for student success on the NGN and in clinical practice.

Donna D. "Iggy" Ignatavicius

*To all the nursing educators who are passionate about teaching, and
to all the nursing students who are passionate about learning.*

Donna D. Ignatavicius received her diploma in nursing from the Peninsula General School of Nursing in Salisbury, Maryland. After working as a charge nurse in medical-surgical nursing, she became an instructor in staff development at the University of Maryland Medical Center. She then received her BSN from the University of Maryland School of Nursing. For 5 years she taught in several schools of nursing while working toward her MS in Nursing, which she received in 1981. Donna then taught in the BSN program at the University of Maryland, after which she continued to pursue her interest in gerontology and accepted the position of Director of Nursing of a major skilled-nursing facility in her home state of Maryland. Since that time, she has served as an instructor in several associate degree nursing programs. Through her consulting activities, faculty development workshops, and international nursing education conferences (such as Boot Camp for Nurse Educators®), Donna is nationally recognized as an expert in nursing education. She is currently the President of DI Associates, Inc. (http://www.diassociates.com/), a company dedicated to improving health care through education and consultation for faculty. In recognition of her contributions to the field, she was inducted as a charter Fellow of the prestigious Academy of Nursing Education in 2007 and received her Certified Nurse Educator credential in 2016.

Acknowledgments

Publishing a textbook would not be possible without the combined efforts of many people. With that in mind, I would like to extend my deepest gratitude to many people who were such an integral part of this journey.

My contributing authors provided excellent manuscripts to underscore the clinical relevancy of this publication. I give special gratitude to Meg Blair, who was extremely valuable as a project resource from beginning to end. The reviewers—expert clinicians and instructors from around the United States—provided invaluable suggestions and encouragement throughout the development of this book.

The staff of Elsevier has, as always, provided us with meaningful guidance and support throughout every step of the planning, writing, revision, and production of this new title. Executive Content Strategist Lee Henderson worked closely with me from the early stages of this title to help me hone and focus the project from start to finish. Senior Content Development Specialist Laura Goodrich then worked with me from vision to publication.

Senior Project Manager Jodi Willard was, as always, an absolute joy with whom to work. Her unwavering attention to detail, flexibility, and conscientiousness helped to make this title consistently readable while making the production process incredibly smooth. Also, a special thanks to Publishing Services Manager Julie Eddy. Designer Amy Buxton is responsible for the beautiful cover and the interior design.

My acknowledgments would not be complete without recognizing the dedicated team of Educational Solutions Consultants and other key members of the Sales and Marketing staff who helped to put this book into your hands.

Contents

Exemplars

PART 1

Introduction: Developing Clinical Judgment

Transitioning From the Nursing Process to Clinical Judgment

Learning Outcomes

1. Review the evolution of the nursing process and its emphasis on the current NCLEX®.
2. Explain why the National Council of State Boards of Nursing (NCSBN) is planning to add a focus on clinical judgment for the Next Generation NCLEX® (NGN).
3. Identify the six cognitive skills of the NCSBN Clinical Judgment Measurement Model (CJMM).
4. Compare the steps of the nursing process, stages of Tanner's Model of Clinical Judgment, and the six cognitive skills of the NCSBN CJMM.

Key Terms

ADPIE A five-step problem-solving approach that includes assessment, diagnosis, planning, implementation, and evaluation.

clinical judgment The observed outcome of critical thinking and decision making. It is an iterative process that uses nursing knowledge to observe and access presenting situations, identify a prioritized client concern, and generate the best possible evidence-based solutions in order to deliver safe client care (NCSBN, 2019).

clinical reasoning The process of thinking about a client situation in a specific context while considering client and family concerns.

nursing diagnosis A clinical judgment concerning a human response to health conditions or life processes, or a vulnerability for that response, by an individual, family, group, or community (www.nanda.org).

nursing process A scientific, clinical reasoning approach to client care that includes assessment, analysis, planning, implementation, and evaluation (NCSBN, 2018b).

At this point in your nursing program, you have likely learned about the nursing process. This chapter will help you build on what you know about the nursing process and explain why the nursing profession currently supports clinical judgment as the best standard for making evidence-based clinical decisions. This workbook focuses on helping you learn how to use clinical reasoning and critical thinking to make sound clinical judgments in a variety of clinical client situations to keep clients safe.

This chapter begins with a review of the nursing process from a historical perspective. Several models of clinical judgment for nursing practice are presented and compared with the steps of the nursing process. Cognitive skills needed to make sound clinical judgments are then described. End-of-chapter questions encourage you to reflect on the chapter's content.

Review of the Nursing Process and Critical Thinking

Depending on the U.S. state or Canadian province, nursing programs may be expected to teach students how to use the nursing process as part of their prelicensure curriculum. Both U.S. and Canadian practices often include the need to use the nursing process as a basis for professional nursing care to ensure client safety (Doane & Varcoe, 2015).

The nursing process is a systematic method for problem solving to make safe, client-centered care decisions. It has been used since the 1960s as the gold standard to guide professional nursing practice and measured on the NCLEX® for many years. Some authors believe that the nursing process is the universal intellectual standard by which client problems are identified and resolved (Black, 2017; Masters, 2017). The American Nurses Association asserts that the "common thread uniting different types of nurses who work in varied areas is the nursing process" (American Nurses Association, 2020, p. 1).

The original four steps of the nursing process in the late 1960s were:

- Assessment
- Planning
- Implementation
- Evaluation

In the early 1970s a new organization called the North American Nursing Diagnosis Association (NANDA) was formed in an attempt to develop a common nursing language (nursing diagnoses) based on nurses' interpretation of assessment data. This additional step of Diagnosis modified the nursing process to **ADPIE**, a five-step approach to problem solving:

- *Assessment*
- *Diagnosis*
- *Planning*
- *Implementation*
- *Evaluation*

You may have learned the ADPIE method for the nursing process and are required to include NANDA nursing diagnoses in the plan of care for your clients.

The accepted definition of a nursing diagnosis (ND) in the 1970s and 1980s was a statement that described a specific response to a client's actual or potential health condition or needs. The current organization (called *NANDA-International [NANDA-I]*) later amended the definition of **nursing diagnosis** to "a clinical judgment concerning a human response to health conditions/life processes, or a vulnerability for that response, by an individual, family, group or community" (NANDA, 2020, p. 1).

As you might expect, using a problem-solving approach for the nursing process requires thinking and reasoning. In the 1990s the concept of critical thinking was introduced in nursing practice and nursing education. Since that time, experts have agreed that nurses use many types of thinking to make the best evidence-based decisions for their clients.

Clinical reasoning is also an important concept for the nursing process. In their landmark nursing education study, Benner et al. (2010) stated that **clinical reasoning** is the process of thinking about a client situation *in a specific context* while considering client and family concerns. The National Council of State Boards of Nursing (NCSBN) combined these concepts and defined the **nursing process** as "a scientific, *clinical reasoning* approach to client care that includes assessment, analysis, planning, implementation and evaluation" (NCSBN, 2018b, p. 5). This definition is currently an Integrated Process for the NCLEX-RN® and incorporates the concept of clinical reasoning or "thinking like a nurse."

As a result of interprofessional research in 1999 that was published in 2003, the Institute of Medicine (IOM) (now called the *National Academy of Medicine*) developed five competencies that graduates of health profession education programs need to achieve. Based on this work, the Quality and Safety Education (QSEN) initiative to determine the competencies for nursing education programs was created. Six competencies that incorporate the IOM work were identified (QSEN, 2020) (Table 1.1).

The QSEN competencies emphasize that health care decisions are often collaborative; incorporate the client's beliefs, values, and preferences; and are based on the best and most current evidence. The call for collaboration with health care team members led to a movement to use common language that all professions can understand. Since that time, nursing practice and educational programs have

Table 1.1 Quality and Safety Education for Nurses (QSEN) Competencies for Generalist Nursing Practice

Competency Component	Competency Statement
[Client]-Centered Care	Recognize the client or designee as the source of control and full partner in providing compassionate and coordinated care based on respect for client's preferences, values, and needs.
Teamwork and Collaboration	Function effectively within nursing and interprofessional teams, fostering open communication, mutual respect, and shared decision making to achieve quality client care.
Safety	Minimize risk of harm to clients and providers through both system effectiveness and individual performance.
Evidence-Based Practice	Integrate best current evidence with clinical expertise and client/family preferences and values for delivery of optimal health care.
Informatics	Use information and technology to communicate, manage knowledge, mitigate error, and support decision making.
Quality Improvement	Use data to monitor the outcomes of care processes and use improvement methods to design and test changes to continuously improve the quality and safety of health care systems.

Data from www.qsen.org.

decreased emphasis on or minimized the use of NANDA-I nursing diagnoses as a "unique" nursing language. Instead, more common client problem language (often signs and symptoms or client condition) that all health care team members can understand is used in most clinical practice settings.

Many established nursing diagnoses (NDs) are easily understood by other health team members. Examples from the latest edition of the NANDA-I official list of ND labels include (Herdman & Kamitsuru, 2017):

- Anxiety
- Acute Pain
- Hypothermia
- Risk for Infection

Other NDs use language that may not be as familiar to nurses or other health care team members. For example, one NANDA-I nursing diagnosis label is Deficient Fluid Volume. Nurses in practice may not use this terminology and instead communicate that a client is dehydrated. Another example is Impaired Skin Integrity. If the client has a stage 2 sacral pressure injury, nurses typically document the pressure injury rather than the broader NANDA nursing diagnosis terminology. Whatever terminology you use, be sure it is understood by all members of the health care team and is consistent with your agency's policies and practices.

Expanding From the Nursing Process to Clinical Judgment

In 2006 Tanner presented findings from her classic meta-analysis research that examined how practicing nurses actually think and make clinical decisions. She found that nurses use clinical judgment skills more than the nursing process, and become more competent in these skills with experience and confidence. Tanner found that clinical judgment involves specific reasoning and critical thinking skills. These skills include:

- *Noticing* a situation or changes in a client situation triggers the nurse to collect more data for an accurate and thorough assessment. Noticing is affected by what the nurse brings to the situation, such as knowledge, ethical perspective, and expectations. These factors are part of professional relational practice (Doane & Varcoe, 2015).
- *Interpreting* requires clinical reasoning to analyze the data to determine the client's problem(s).

Table 1.2 Comparison of the Nursing Process and Tanner's Clinical Judgment Model

Tanner's Clinical Judgment Model	Nursing Process (AAPIE)
Noticing	Assessment
Interpreting	Analysis
Responding	Planning Implementation
Reflecting	Evaluation

- *Responding* is taking action or monitoring the client based on current evidence to prevent, detect early, or resolve client problem(s).
- *Reflecting* allows the nurse to determine the client's status and think about what he or she learned from the situation that can be used in another similar situation.

As you might expect, Tanner's Model of Clinical Judgment can be aligned with the steps of the nursing process (Table 1.2). However, in some ways, Tanner's components are distinctly different from the nursing process steps. For example, *Noticing* is the trigger that informs the nurse to perform the Assessment. The *Interpreting* component does not require the identification of a NANDA-I nursing diagnosis, but encourages the nurse to communicate effectively with appropriate health care team members using SBAR or another common communication method. *Responding* may require implementing one or more specific actions or frequently monitoring a client's clinical situation. *Reflecting* not only includes evaluating the results of client care, but allows the nurse to examine his or her actions in addressing the clinical situation.

The National League for Nursing (NLN) included nursing judgment as one of its four differentiated new nursing graduate competencies for all types of nursing programs. The NLN states that nursing judgment encompasses three processes: critical thinking, clinical judgment, and integration of best evidence into practice. Nurses use these processes when they make sound decisions about client care. More specifically, the use of nursing judgment involves these specific skills (NLN, 2012).

- Processing of information
- Thinking critically
- Evaluating the evidence
- Applying relevant knowledge
- Using problem-solving skills
- Reflecting on the situation

New Nursing Graduates and Clinical Judgment

A large study of 5000 novice nurses by Kavanaugh and Szweda (2017) found that new nursing graduates are not competent in *basic* clinical reasoning and judgment skills. Although many graduates could *recognize cues* to identify changes in a client's clinical condition, most new nurses did not know what *actions to take* and *why*. The authors concluded that nursing education programs need to focus more on helping students learn how to think like nurses and use clinical reasoning to make prompt evidence-based decisions (clinical judgments) to keep clients and families safe.

The findings of the Kavanaugh and Szweda study are consistent with the classic rights of clinical reasoning identified by Levett-Jones et al. (2010). The rights include:

- Right client
- Right time
- Right reason
- Right cues
- Right action

These rights help guide your ability to notice and recognize relevant data or cues in a client situation to direct your nursing actions based on data analysis. They do not emphasize the need to name a specific nursing diagnostic label, but rather focus on cues and resulting actions.

One of the recommendations from a large study of nursing education (Benner et al., 2010) was to revise the nursing licensure examination to ensure that new graduates are competent in clinical reasoning and decision making. The 2013–2014 NCSBN Strategic Practice Analysis highlighted the increasingly complex decisions that newly licensed nurses make during the course of client care. A thorough literature review by NCSBN on critical thinking and clinical judgment/decision making found that 50% of client errors involved nurses and 65% of those errors were due to poor clinical judgment. Another study found that 80% of nursing employers are not satisfied with the ability of new nurse graduates to make evidence-based clinical decisions (NCSBN, 2018a).

The National Council of State Boards of Nursing Clinical Judgment Measurement Model

The National Council of State Boards of Nursing (NCSBN) is responsible for the design and content of the nursing licensure examination known as the NCLEX®. As a result of the findings regarding new graduates, the NCSBN conducted its own study to determine if the current nursing licensure examination for entry into professional nursing is adequate to ensure that new nurses are competent in clinical judgment skills to protect the public. Current NCLEX® test items do not measure all layers or cognitive skills of clinical judgment, but rather focus more on the nursing process (Dickison et al., 2019). Multiple-choice and SATA (Select All That Apply) questions are not currently presented in a complex clinical situation context and tend to primarily measure content knowledge as right or wrong. The current test items, such as the examples in Box 1.1, measure only whether new graduates are *minimally safe* to practice. The NCSBN study showed that although knowledge is essential, it is not enough to ensure appropriate clinical judgment. Put another way, having content knowledge doesn't translate to having good clinical judgment skills. However, making good clinical judgments requires adequate content knowledge (Dickison et al., 2019).

As a result of the study, NCSBN is planning a major change in the nursing licensure examination, called the Next Generation NCLEX® (NGN), that will include *measuring* new graduates' competence

---

Box 1.1 Examples of Current NCLEX-RN® Test Item Formats

Multiple-Choice Test Item
A client is admitted to the memory care unit with a diagnosis of Alzheimer disease. What **priority** action by the nurse is the most important when caring for the client?
A. Be sure that the client receives environmental stimulation.
B. Reorient the client every time the nurse enters the room.
C. Protect the client and keep him or her safe.
D. Use validation therapy when communicating with the client.

To answer this test item, the student or graduate only needs to know that ensuring safety is essential when caring for a client with dementia. Choice C is the best response. Content knowledge does not guarantee clinical judgment ability.

Select All That Apply Item
A home care nurse is visiting a client who has advanced rheumatoid arthritis. Which findings will the nurse expect when assessing the client? **Select all that apply.**
A. Bony nodes on the client's finger joints
B. Joint inflammation and pain
C. Subcutaneous nodules on the arm(s)
D. Joint deformities in the hands and feet
E. Ulnar deviation of the wrist

To answer this test item, the student or graduate only needs to know the common assessment findings for a client who has late-stage rheumatoid arthritis. Choices C, D, and E are the correct responses. Choice A is common in clients who have osteoarthritis. Content knowledge does not guarantee clinical judgment ability.

in clinical judgment. In one of their first steps toward meeting that outcome and based on an extensive literature review, the NCSBN defines clinical judgment as the observed outcome of critical thinking and decision making. It is "an iterative [repeating] process that uses nursing knowledge to observe and access presenting situations, identify a prioritized client concern, and generate the best possible evidence-based solutions in order to deliver safe client care" (NCSBN, 2018a, p. 12).

In the near future, the NCLEX® is expected to measure the ability of students to use clinical reasoning skills based on the NCSBN Clinical Judgment Measurement Model (CJMM) (Dickison et al., 2019; NCSBN, 2019). Using case scenarios that are somewhat complex in situated contexts, the six cognitive skills in the model that you will need to use to make sound clinical judgments include:

- *Recognize Cues*
   Cues are elements of assessment data that provide important information for the nurse as a basis for making client decisions. In a clinical situation, determine which data are *relevant* (directly related to client outcomes or the priority of care) versus *irrelevant* (unrelated to client outcomes or priority of care). Decide which assessment data are the *most* important and of *immediate* concern to the nurse.
- *Analyze Cues*
   Consider the cues in the context of the client history and situation. Think about how the identified relevant cues relate to the client's condition or history. Identify cues that support and contradict a particular cue in the situation and determine why certain cues are more concerning to the nurse than others.
- *Prioritize Hypotheses*
   Consider all possibilities about what is occurring in the client situation. Consider their urgency and risk for the client. Determine which explanations are *most likely* and *most serious,* and why.
- *Generate Solutions*
   Identify expected client outcomes. Using the prioritized hypotheses, plan specific actions that would achieve the desirable outcomes. Consider which actual or potential evidence-based actions should be *avoided* or are *contraindicated.* Remember that some actions could be harmful for the client a given situation.
- *Take Action*
   Decide which nursing actions will address the highest priorities of care and determine in what priority these actions will be implemented. Actions can include, but are not limited to, additional assessment, health teaching, documentation, requested primary health care provider prescriptions, performance of nursing skills, and consultation with health care team members.
- *Evaluate Outcomes*
   Evaluate the actual client outcomes in the situation and compare with expected outcomes. Determine what client assessment findings indicate improvement, decline, or no change in the client's condition. Decide if the selected nursing actions were effective, ineffective, or made no difference.

The NCSBN CJMM incorporates the nursing process and Tanner's Clinical Judgment Model. Table 1.3 shows the alignment of these three models or processes. Chapter 2 in this workbook presents examples

Table 1.3 **Comparison of the Nursing Process, Tanner's Clinical Judgment Model, and the NCSBN Clinical Judgment Measurement Model (CJMM) Cognitive Skills**

Nursing Process (AAPIE)	Tanner's Clinical Judgment Model	NCSBN CJMM Cognitive Skills
Assessment	Noticing	Recognize Cues
Analysis	Interpreting	Analyze Cues
Analysis	Interpreting	Prioritize Hypotheses
Planning	Responding	Generate Solutions
Implementation	Responding	Take Action
Evaluation	Reflecting	Evaluate Outcomes

of the thinking exercises used in this book and how to approach them to determine the best responses using the cognitive skills of the NCSBN CJMM. When possible they are similar to the proposed test item formats that may be used in the future on the NGN.

Thinking and Discussion Questions

1. Do you think that the NANDA-I nursing diagnosis list helps you in planning nursing care using the nursing process or clinical judgment model? Why or why not?

2. Consider the information in this chapter about the lack of clinical judgment skills of nursing graduates. Why do you think that new nurses lack these essential skills? Consider all factors in your response.

3. Review all three models of clinical decision making as presented in Table 1.3. What are the advantages and disadvantages of each model? Which model do you think is most useful in nursing practice and why?

References

Asterisk (*) denotes classic reference.

American Nurses Association. (2020). *The nursing process.* https://www.nursingworld.org/practice-policy/workforce/what-is-nursing/the-nursing-process/.

*Benner, P., Sutphen, M., Leonard, V., & Day, L. (2010). *Educating nurses: A call for radical transformation.* San Francisco, CA: Jossey-Bass.

Black, B. P. (2017). *Professional nursing: Concepts and challenges* (8th ed.). St. Louis: Elsevier.

Dickison, P., Haerling, K. A., & Lasater, K. (2019). Integrating the National Council of State Boards of Nursing Clinical Judgment Model into nursing educational frameworks. *Journal of Nursing Education, 58*(2), 72–78.

Doane, G. H., & Varcoe, C. (2015). *How to nurse: Relational inquiry with individuals and families in changing health and health care contexts.* Philadelphia: Wolters Kluwer.

Herdman, T. H., & Kamitsuru, S. (2017). *Nursing diagnoses: Definitions and classification. 2018–2020* (11th ed.). New York, NY: Thieme Medical Publishers.

*Institute of Medicine (IOM). (2003). *Health professions education: A bridge to quality.* Washington, DC: National Academies Press.

Kavanaugh, J. M., & Szweda, C. (2017). A crisis in competency: The strategic and ethical imperative to assessing new graduate nurses' clinical reasoning. *Nursing Education Perspectives, 38,* 57–62.

*Levett-Jones, T., Hoffman, K., Dempsey, J., Jeong, S.Y., Noble, D., et al. (2010). The "five rights" of clinical reasoning: An educational model to enhance nursing students' ability to identify and manage clinically "at risk" patients. *Nurse Education Today, 30,* 515–520.

Masters, K. (2017). *Role development in professional nursing practice* (4th ed.). Burlington, MA: Jones & Bartlett Learning.

National Council of State Boards of Nursing. (2018a). Measuring the right things: NCSBN's Next Generation NCLEX® endeavors to go beyond the leading edge. In *Focus. (Winter.)* Chicago, IL: Author.

National Council of State Boards of Nursing (NCSBN). (2018b). *NCLEX-RN® Examination: Test plan for the National Council Licensure Examination for Registered Nurses.* Chicago, IL: Author.

National Council of State Boards of Nursing (NCSBN). (2019). The clinical judgment model. *Next Generation NCLEX News,* (Winter), 1–6.

National League for Nursing (NLN). (2012). *Outcomes and competencies for graduates of practical/vocational, diploma, baccalaureate, master's, practice doctorate, and research doctorate programs in nursing.* Washington, D.C.: Author.

North American Nursing Diagnosis Association International (NANDA-I). (2020). *Glossary of terms.* https://kbnanda.org/article/AA-00226/0/Glossary-of-Terms.html

Quality and Safety Education for Nurses (QSEN). (2019). Competency KSAs (pre-licensure). Retrieved from www.qsen.org.

*Tanner, C. A. (2006). Thinking like a nurse: A research-based model of clinical judgment. *Journal of Nursing Education, 45,* 204–211.

2 Applying the NCSBN Clinical Judgment Measurement Model to Ensure Client Safety

Learning Outcomes

1. Discuss the layers of the National Council of State Boards of Nursing (NCSBN) Clinical Judgment Measurement Model (CJMM).
2. Describe how to apply the six cognitive skills to simulated thinking exercises to make sound clinical judgments.
3. Identify tips for success when using the six cognitive skills to make clinical decisions to answer various types of thinking exercises.

Key Terms

cognitive skills Mental (thinking) processes that are required for appropriate and sound clinical judgment.

National Council of State Boards of Nursing (NCSBN) Clinical Judgment Measurement Model (CJMM) A multilayered model that is based on nursing observation, cognitive skills, and contextual factors.

Nurses need sound clinical judgment to provide competent and safe client care. As introduced in Chapter 1, the National Council of State Boards of Nursing (NCSBN) developed a clinical judgment model consistent with well-respected existing models. This new model was the basis for a major NCSBN study on how to measure the clinical judgment ability of new nursing graduates to protect the public. After a brief review of the model, this chapter will help you learn how to apply it and "think like a nurse" using a variety of thinking exercises. Tips for applying the model to derive the correct responses to these thinking exercises will be outlined. These Tips for Success strategies will assist you when working on the thinking exercises used in this workbook at different points in your program.

Overview of the NCSBN CJMM

The **National Council of State Boards of Nursing (NCSBN) Clinical Judgment Measurement Model (CJMM)** is a multilayered model that is based on Dickison et al. (2019):

- Nursing observation
- Cognitive skills
- Contextual factors

Observation is the first layer of clinical judgment. In practice, nurses observe many client situations in which they need to make sound decisions. Many of these situations are complex and occur in a variety of contexts. Layers 2 and 3 are the most important layers of the model and emphasize the six *cognitive skills* used by nurses in client situations based on those observations. **Cognitive skills** are mental (thinking) processes that are required for appropriate and sound clinical judgment. As introduced in Chapter 1, these skills include:

- Recognize Cues
- Analyze Cues

Table 2.1 Examples of Contextual Factors That Influence Clinical Judgment

Individual Factors (for Nurse)	Environmental Factors (for Client Situation)
• Knowledge • Skills • Level of experience • Confidence • Specialty background • Personal characteristics • Prior experience	• Client observation • Physical environment • Resources • Health/medical records • Time pressure/urgency • Task complexity • Consequences and risks • Cultural considerations

Data adapted from NCSBN CJMM (Dickison et al., 2019).

- Generate Solutions
- Prioritize Hypotheses
- Take Action
- Evaluate Outcomes

Layer 4 consists of *contextual factors,* which include both individual and environmental factors that can affect a nurse's ability to effectively make clinical judgments (Dickison et al., 2019). Examples of these factors are listed in Table 2.1.

Applying the Cognitive Skills of the NCSBN CJMM

Clinical judgment can be learned through simulated thinking exercises to translate knowledge into clinical practice using a variety of complex client contexts. Consider the case study in Box 2.1.

Box 2.1 Case Study

An 82-year-old female client was admitted with a fractured right femoral neck (hip) and a closed nondisplaced left tibial fracture as a result of a fall. According to her daughter, she has a history of osteoporosis, for which she takes a bisphosphonate; controlled diabetes mellitus type 2, for which she takes an oral hypoglycemic agent; and controlled hypertension, for which she takes a diuretic. The client quit smoking 10 years ago but enjoys an occasional glass of wine to help her sleep. She lives alone in a senior housing apartment and depends on her daughter for appointments, food shopping, and other errands. Prior to her fall, she was ADL independent.

Yesterday afternoon she underwent a right open reduction and internal fixation (ORIF) of the hip and had a splint placed on her lower left leg to immobilize the tibial fracture. When entering the client's room, the nurse notes that the abduction device is on the floor. Initial nursing shift assessment findings include:
- Is alert but does not respond verbally to questions
- Apical pulse = 92 beats/min and irregular
- Blood pressure = 166/90 mm Hg
- Breath sounds clear in all lung fields
- Hypoactive bowel sounds $\times$ 4
- Restless and "picking at" bedcovers
- Right hip surgical dressing dry and intact
- Left lower leg splint intact
- Right lower leg externally rotated and shorter than left leg
- Yells when right leg is touched
- No palpable left pedal pulse; right pedal pulse 1+
- Left foot cooler and paler than right foot
- Oxygen saturation = 95% (on 2 L/min via nasal cannula)
- Finger stick blood glucose (FSBG) = 288 mg/dL (16 mmol/L)

Based on the assessment findings in the sample case study, determine which data are relevant or important to the nurse in the situation. To *Recognize Cues* as the first cognitive skill of the NCSBN CJMM for this thinking exercise, you need knowledge of:

- Normal physiologic and psychosocial changes associated with aging
- Adult normal range for vital signs
- Signs and symptoms of adequate perfusion
- Normal ranges for laboratory values
- Time pressure cues
- Environmental cues

Tip for Success

To determine the cues that are of most concern to the nurse, examine those assessment data and other cues that are unusual or abnormal for the client or clinical situation.

To apply that knowledge, you likely selected the following *relevant* cues from the case study that are most concerning to the nurse:

- Abduction device is on the floor
- Apical pulse = 92 beats/min and irregular
- Blood pressure = 166/90 mm Hg
- Restless and "picking at" bedcovers
- Right lower leg externally rotated and shorter than left leg
- Yells when right leg is touched
- No palpable left pedal pulse; right pedal pulse 1+
- Left foot cooler, swollen, and paler than right foot
- FSBG = 288 mg/dL (16 mmol/L)

The next cognitive skill is *Analyze Cues.* Analyzing cues in this case requires you to have knowledge of:

- Postoperative complications of hip ORIF
- Complications of lower extremity musculoskeletal injury
- Normal range for FSBG

Based on your analysis, you then need to *Prioritize Hypotheses.* For this cognitive skill, consider all possibilities about what is happening in the case and then determine the *most likely* explanations. The cues in the case study reveal that the client is *most likely* experiencing two musculoskeletal complications: (1) subluxation or total dislocation of the operative hip as evidenced by right leg shortening, right leg rotation, and acute pain (the abduction device is not in place to help prevent this complication), and (2) possible neurovascular compromise in the left foot as evidenced by the left foot being cooler and paler than the right foot and absence of a pedal pulse in the left foot (and presence of a 1+ pedal pulse in the right foot, which is typical for an older adult). The client's elevated vital signs and restlessness are most likely due to acute pain. In addition, her FSBG value is above the normal range because surgery and trauma are stressors, especially for a client who is a diabetic.

The fourth skill is to *Generate Solutions* that will meet expected client outcomes. The desired outcomes in this situation are that the client will:

- Have adequate perfusion in both lower extremities
- Re-establish proper positioning of the right surgical hip
- Have adequate pain control (2 or 3 on a scale of 0 to 10)
- Have vital signs within usual parameters
- Have an FSBG within normal limits

Consider which actual or potential evidence-based actions will meet these outcomes. Consider which ones should be *avoided* or are *contraindicated.* Remember that some actions could be harmful for the client in the given situation. This cognitive skill requires you to have knowledge of how to manage the musculoskeletal complications and with which members of the health care team you will need to collaborate.

Tip for Success

To effectively *Generate Solutions,* first determine what expected outcomes are essential for the client. Then plan solutions or actions that will meet these outcomes.

When considering possible solutions, recall that neurovascular compromise is a perfusion problem. That means that elevating the client's left leg will *decrease* perfusion and can potentially cause harm. Possible nursing actions based on best practice include:

- Notify the surgeon regarding the musculoskeletal changes.
- Check left pedal pulse with a Doppler ultrasound device.
- Maintain the current position of the lower extremities.
- Loosen the left leg splint to make sure it is not too tight.
- Administer an analgesic to manage pain.
- Administer regular insulin to decrease her blood glucose.

The fifth cognitive skill is to *Take Action.* Determine the priority order of actions that you want to take in the list of possible solutions. Priorities are determined by factors such as urgency, difficulty, or complexity of the client's situation. Therefore the two priority problems at this time are (1) neurovascular compromise of the left leg, possibly due to a tight splint and/or tissue swelling, and (2) acute pain due to probable right hip dislocation or subluxation. Based on these priorities, the nurse's actions would include:

- Check for a left pedal pulse using Doppler.
- Check the left leg splint and loosen if it is too tight.
- Do not elevate the left leg.
- Maintain position of lower extremities.
- Notify the surgeon regarding the client's musculoskeletal changes.
- Administer an analgesic as prescribed.

Tip for Success

When deciding on actions to take and in what order of priority, determine which client problems are potentially life or limb threatening and the urgency of each problem. Notifying the primary health care provider is not usually the first priority because there are always actions that you can take *first* as a nurse.

The last cognitive skill is to *Evaluate Outcomes* by reassessing the client after nursing actions have been implemented. Remember that the desired outcomes are that the client will:

- Have adequate perfusion in both lower extremities
- Achieve proper position of the right hip
- Have adequate pain control (2 or 3 on a scale of 0 to 10)
- Have vital signs within usual parameters for the client
- Have FSBG within normal range

When reassessing the client, if these outcomes have been met, the nursing actions were *effective.* If the outcomes were not met, then the nursing actions were *ineffective* or *not related.*

Applying the NCSBN CJMM for Thinking Exercises in This Workbook

The thinking exercises in this workbook will help you apply the six cognitive skills of the NCSBN CJMM using a variety of formats. Examples of these formats are described in this section with the cognitive skill that is being assessed. Although the following examples are focused on adult medical-surgical nursing, this workbook presents thinking exercises across the life span and across specialties.

The answers and rationales for the correct responses to the thinking exercises are provided in the last part of this workbook. Please note that the reference pages provided for each thinking exercise do not necessarily contain the answers, but rather provide the knowledge that is needed as a basis for answering the exercises.

The five types of thinking exercises in this workbook are similar to the new formats on the Next Generation NCLEX® (NGN) that will measure the cognitive skills of clinical judgment, and include:

- Enhanced Hot Spot
- Cloze
- Extended Drag and Drop
- Extended Multiple Response
- Matrix

Enhanced Hot Spot Thinking Exercises

The case study presented earlier in this chapter can be used as a Enhanced Hot Spot Thinking Exercise as shown in the example below to measure the cognitive skill of *Recognize Cues.* Most of these exercises in this book will ask you to select the most important or relevant information in a client scenario.

Enhanced Hot Spot Thinking Exercise: Example 1

An 82-year-old female client was admitted with a right fractured femoral neck (hip) and a left closed nondisplaced tibial fracture as a result of a fall. According to her daughter, she has a history of osteoporosis, for which she takes a bisphosphonate; controlled diabetes mellitus type 2, for which she takes an oral hypoglycemic agent; and controlled hypertension, for which she takes a diuretic. The client quit smoking 10 years ago but enjoys an occasional glass of wine to help her sleep. She lives alone in a senior housing apartment and depends on her daughter for appointments, food shopping, and other errands. Prior to her fall, she was ADL independent.

Yesterday afternoon she underwent right open reduction and internal fixation (ORIF) of the hip and had a splint placed on her lower left leg to immobilize the tibial fracture. When entering the client's room, the nurse notes that the abduction device is on the floor. Initial nursing shift assessment findings include:

- Is alert but does not respond verbally to questions
- Apical pulse = 92 beats/min and irregular
- Blood pressure = 166/90 mm Hg
- Breath sounds clear in all lung fields
- Hypoactive bowel sounds × 4
- Restless and "picking at" bedcovers
- Right hip surgical dressing dry and intact
- Left lower leg splint intact
- Right lower leg externally rotated and shorter than left leg
- Yells when right leg is touched
- No palpable left pedal pulse; right pedal pulse 1+
- Left foot cooler and paler than right foot
- Oxygen saturation = 95% (on 2 L/min via nasal cannula)
- Finger stick blood glucose (FSBG) = 288 mg/dL (16 mmol/L)

Highlight or place a check mark next to the assessment findings that require follow-up by the nurse.

Answers

- Abduction device is on the floor
- Apical pulse = 92 beats/min and irregular
- Blood pressure = 166/90 mm Hg
- Restless and "picking at" bedcovers

- Right lower leg externally rotated and shorter than left leg
- Yells when right leg is touched
- No palpable left pedal pulse; right pedal pulse 1+
- Left foot cooler, swollen, and paler than right foot
- FSBG = 285 mg/dL (16 mmol/L)

Rationales

The nurse's assessment indicates that the client's surgical hip may be dislocated as evidenced by hip rotation and shortening, yelling when the right hip is touched, and restlessness that could indicate acute pain from subluxation or total hip dislocation. The abduction device was found on the floor, which means that the client may have adducted her right leg. Hip dislocation is a potential complication when a hip prosthesis is used to replace the client's fractured femoral neck. The elevated vital signs could be caused by acute pain. The oxygen saturation is within normal limits and needs to be monitored rather than followed up as an immediate concern for the nurse at this time. The findings indicate that the left leg may have neurovascular compromise due to absent pulse, pallor, and coolness. In addition, the finger stick blood glucose (FSBG) value is above normal and needs to be improved. Therefore these findings should concern the nurse and indicate an urgent need to follow up.

References

Ignatavicius et al., 2018, pp. 1047–1048; 1042–1045

A few of the thinking exercises in this book present a client situation and ask you to select or highlight the information that indicates that the client is not progressing as expected. This variation of the highlighting exercise measures your ability to *Evaluate Outcomes*. For example, consider the thinking exercise below about a postoperative young adult who underwent a laparoscopic cholecystectomy.

Enhanced Hot Spot Thinking Exercise: Example 2

Nurses' Notes
10/12/20 11:30 a.m. (1130) Alert and oriented. Returned from surgery to PACU with report of 7/10 pain with nausea. Vomited × 2 small amount greenish liquid. Wound closures intact and abdomen soft. Apical pulse 100 and B/P 122/82. Placed in semi-Fowler position and taking small sips of ginger ale. ————————————————————————— D. L. Jones, RNC
Highlight the findings in the Nurses' Notes above that would indicate that the client is *not* progressing as expected.

Answers

Nurses' Notes
10/12/20 11:30 a.m. (1130) Alert and oriented. Returned from surgery to PACU with report of 7/10 pain with nausea. Vomited × 2 small amount greenish liquid. Wound closures intact and abdomen soft. Apical pulse 100 and B/P 122/82. Placed in semi-Fowler position and taking small sips of ginger ale. ————————————————————————— D. L. Jones, RNC

Rationales

In the Nurses' Notes, the client is alert and oriented but has more pain than expected, and has nausea and vomiting most likely due to general anesthesia. The expected findings would be that the client's pain and nausea are under control.

Reference

Ignatavicius et al., 2018, Chapter 19.

Cloze Thinking Exercises

Cloze Thinking Exercises will ask you to complete statements about a presented client scenario. For each blank, you will have one or more lists of options from which to select. Consider the example below, which requires you to *Analyze Cues* and *Prioritize Hypotheses*.

Cloze Thinking Exercise: Example 1

An 82-year-old female client is admitted with a fractured left hip. She is scheduled for open reduction and internal fixation (ORIF) of the hip. Her history reveals a diagnosis of osteoporosis, for which she takes a bisphosphonate; diabetes mellitus type 2, for which she takes an oral hypoglycemic agent; and hypertension, for which she takes a diuretic. The client quit smoking 10 years ago but enjoys an occasional glass of wine to help her sleep. **Complete the following sentences by choosing the *most likely* options for the missing information from the lists of options provided.**

The nurse should recognize that after hip surgery the client will be at a high risk for _____1_____ because of _____2_____ and _____3_____ because of her _____4_____. The overall goals for her postoperative care will be to prevent _____5_____ and manage her _____6_____.

Options for 1	Options for 2	Options for 3
Dementia	History of smoking	Delirium
Infection	Alcoholism	Urinary incontinence
Stroke	Osteoporosis	Bowel obstruction
Dysreflexia	Hypertension	Alcohol withdrawal
Myocardial infarction	Diabetes mellitus	Nausea and vomiting
Depression	Dehydration	Persistent pain

Options for 4	Options for 5	Options for 6
History of smoking and drinking	Fat embolism syndrome	Blood pressure
Advanced age and hip fracture	Diabetic ketoacidosis	Serum glucose levels
Multiple medications	Skin breakdown from traction	Emotional behaviors
Persistent pain	Immobility complications	Persistent pain
High blood pressure	Lung congestion	Alcohol withdrawal
Hypoxia	Vertebral compression fractures	Hypothermia

Answers

The nurse should recognize that after hip surgery the client will be at a high risk for infection because of diabetes mellitus and delirium because of her advanced age and hip fracture. The overall goals for her postoperative care will be to prevent immobility complications and manage her serum glucose levels.

Rationales

Clients who have diabetes are always at risk for acquiring an infection after surgery. Even for clients who are alert and oriented, those of advanced age who experience a hip fracture are at a very high risk for delirium (acute confusion). A large number of clients who have a hip fracture die from complications of immobility, and therefore preventing those complications is a desired postoperative outcome. Surgery is a trauma to the body and affects the ability for most clients to have stable serum glucose levels. These clients are often placed on sliding scale insulin during their hospital stay.

References

Ignatavicius et al., 2018, pp. 1042–1045; 1047–1048; also see Chapter 64 on Diabetes Mellitus

Another use of the Cloze Thinking Exercises in this book relates to pharmacology content, which is a major focus for the current and future NCLEX-RN®. These exercises require you to select the correct answer from one or more lists of choices for each blank space, as shown below.

Cloze Thinking Exercise: Example 2

The nurse is admitting a 64-year-old male client with a long-term diagnosis of Parkinson disease. The client provides the nurse with a partial list of the medications he has been taking at home, but some of the information is missing because of his early dementia. **Choose the *most likely* options for the information missing from the table below by selecting from the lists of options provided.**

Medication	Dose, Route, Frequency	Drug Class	Indication
Ropinirole	16 mg orally once daily	1	Management of Parkinson disease
Paroxetine	20 mg orally once daily	Selective serotonin reuptake inhibitor	2
Clopidogrel	75 mg orally once daily	3	History of transient ischemic attack with atrial fibrillation
Hydrochlorothiazide	4	Thiazide diuretic	Management of mild hypertension
5	650 mg orally every 4 hours as needed for back pain	Nonopioid analgesic	Relief of pain

Options for 1	Options for 2	Options for 3
Cephalosporin	Control of hallucinations	Antiviral agent
Calcium channel blocker	Pain management	Antibacterial agent
Antispasmotic agent	Muscle spasticity	Loop diuretic
Immune modifier	Treatment of depression	COMT inhibitor
Dopamine agonist	Anxiety management	Anxiolytic agent
Sedative	Treatment of infection	Antiplatelet agent

Options for 4	Options for 5
250 mg orally before bedtime	Oxycodone
10 mg orally 3 times daily	Acetaminophen
25 mg orally every morning	Ibuprofen
5 mg orally 3 times daily	Oxybutynin
100 mg orally twice daily	Naloxone
125 mg orally 4 times daily	Lorazepam

Answers

Medication	Dose, Route, Frequency	Drug Class	Indication
Ropinirole	16 mg orally once daily	**Dopamine agonist**	Management of Parkinson disease
Paroxetine	20 mg orally once daily	Selective serotonin reuptake inhibitor	**Treatment of depression**
Clopidogrel	75 mg orally once daily	**Antiplatelet drug**	History of transient ischemic attack with atrial fibrillation
Hydrochlorothiazide	**25 mg orally every morning**	Thiazide diuretic	Management of mild hypertension
Acetaminophen	650 mg orally every 4 hours as needed for back pain	Nonopioid analgesic	Relief of pain

References

Burchum & Rosenthal, 2019, pp. 188–192, 360, 464–465, 622–623, 864–866.

Extended Drag and Drop Thinking Exercises

Extended Drag and Drop Thinking Exercises are used in this workbook to help you learn to apply the cognitive skills of *Generate Solutions* or *Take Action*. If this type of item was presented electronically, you could "drag and drop" the actions on the left to the column on the right using a computer mouse. An example of this type of thinking exercise is presented below. In this exercise a list of nursing actions is provided from which you will choose to match with actual or potential client problems.

Enhanced Drag and Drop Thinking Exercise Example

The nurse is planning care to prevent or detect early complications for a 65-year-old male client who underwent a right total knee arthroplasty (TKA) today under epidural anesthesia for severe osteoarthritis. **Indicate which nursing action listed in the far-left column is appropriate for each potential TKA complication. Note that not all actions will be used.**

Nursing Action	Potential TKA Complication	Appropriate Nursing Action for Each TKA Complication
1 Maintain sequential or pneumatic compression stockings/devices while client in bed.	Surgical site infection	
2 Provide cold application to the surgical area.	Venous thromboembolism (VTE)	
3 Monitor the client's temperature and white blood cell count.	Epidural hematoma	
4 Assess the client's ability to move her legs and void.	Pressure injury	
5 Maintain client's right leg in a neutral position while in bed.	Surgical site hematoma	
6 Keep the client's heels off of the bed.		
7 Monitor oxygen saturation every 4 hours.		

Answers

Nursing Action	Potential TKA Complication	Appropriate Nursing Action for Each TKA Complication
1 Maintain sequential or pneumatic compression stockings/devices while client in bed.	Surgical site infection	3 Monitor the client's temperature and white blood cell count.
2 Provide cold application to the surgical area.	Venous thromboembolism (VTE)	1 Maintain sequential or pneumatic compression stockings/devices while client in bed.
3 Monitor the client's temperature and white blood cell count.	Epidural hematoma	4 Assess the client's ability to move her legs and void.
4 Assess the client's ability to move her legs and void.	Pressure injury	6 Keep the client's heels off of the bed.
5 Maintain client's right leg in a neutral position while in bed.	Surgical site hematoma	2 Provide cold application to the surgical area.
6 Keep the client's heels off of the bed.		
7 Monitor oxygen saturation every 4 hours.		

Rationales

To detect surgical infection early, the nurse should carefully monitor the client's temperature and white blood cell count (Action #3). To help prevent VTE from venous stasis and decreased mobility, venous return from the lower extremities is assisted by using sequential or pneumatic compression stockings/devices (Action #1). The client had epidural anesthesia during surgery. To assess whether the spine or its adjacent structures were damaged, the nurse should perform frequent neurologic assessments, which includes the ability of the client to move his legs and ability to void. If spinal impairment occurs, the client may have difficulty with motor and voiding ability (Action #4). The client will be in bed immediately after surgery, so he is at risk for heel breakdown (pressure injury). Therefore the nurse should position his heels such that they are not on the bed by using pillows or other devices (Action #6). The client is expected to have right knee swelling and is at risk for a surgical site hematoma. Frequent cold applications can help decrease swelling and decrease the risk for a hematoma (Action #2).

References

Ignatavicius et al., 2018, pp. 275, 315

Extended Multiple Response Thinking Exercises

Extended Multiple Response Thinking Exercises may be used to measure one of several cognitive skills. For this type of exercise you will need to select the correct responses from a list of choices to answer the question. The example below assesses the cognitive skill of *Take Action.*

Extended Multiple Response Thinking Exercise Example

The nurse is assessing a 37-year-old female client who underwent a total thyroidectomy yesterday afternoon.

Vital Signs	
Temperature	98°F (36.7°C)
Heart rate	84 beats/min
Respirations	22 breaths/min
Blood pressure	108/68 mm Hg
Oxygen saturation	100% (on oxygen via nasal cannula 2 L/min)

Laboratory Test Results This Morning	
Hematocrit	35% (0.35)
Serum sodium	141 mEq/L (141 mmol/L)
Serum potassium	3.9 mEq/L (3.9 mmol/L)
Serum calcium	8.5 mg/dL (2.12 mmol/L)

Physical Assessment Findings
- Reports throat pain as a 7 on a scale of 0 (no pain) to 10 (severe pain)
- Reports hoarseness at times
- Breath sounds clear in all lung fields
- No respiratory distress
- Bowel sounds active × 4
- Throat surgical dressing intact

Which of the following actions should the nurse take? **Select all that apply.**

_____ A. Administer an analgesic as soon as possible.

_____ B. Check the client for muscle twitching and tingling.

_____ C. Request a prescription for oral potassium.

_____ D. Check the client behind her neck for bleeding.

_____ E. Compare the client's preoperative and current hematocrit values.

_____ F. Place the client in a flat position to increase blood pressure.

_____ G. Teach the client that hoarseness is usually temporary.

_____ H. Perform orthostatic blood pressure checks.

Answers

A, B, D, E, G

Rationales

Choice A is an appropriate action for the nurse to take because the client reports a pain level of 7, indicating uncontrolled surgical pain. The desired pain level for most clients is 2 or 3. The client's most current serum calcium level is below the normal range of 9 to 10.5 mg/dL (2.25 to 2.62 mmol/L). Hypocalcemia may occur following thyroid removal due to injury to one or both parathyroid glands. Therefore the nurse should assess for signs of low calcium, including tetany (muscle twitching) and tingling, especially around the mouth (Choice B). The client's hematocrit is a low normal and she could be experiencing bleeding. Therefore the nurse should check for active bleeding by inspecting and feeling behind her neck and determining if the current hematocrit level is significantly different from her preoperative laboratory value (Choices D and E). Temporary hoarseness is not unusual for clients undergoing thyroid removal because the laryngeal nerve can become injured or irritated (Choice G).

References

Ignatavicius et al., 2018, pp. 1269–1270; Pagana & Pagana, 2018, pp. 120, 248

Matrix Thinking Exercises

In this workbook, Matrix Thinking Exercises may be used to assess one of several cognitive skills. To measure *Generate Solutions,* you will be given a list of nursing actions and asked to determine if each action would be ***Anticipated, Contraindicated,*** or ***Non-Essential*** for the client situation presented. The Matrix Thinking Exercise below is used to *Evaluate Outcomes* as to whether the implemented nurse's actions were ***Effective, Ineffective,*** or ***Unrelated.***

Matrix Thinking Exercise Example

The nurse is assessing an 75-year-old female client after implementing interventions to manage delirium. **For each assessment finding, use an X to indicate whether the implemented interventions were** **Effective** **(helped to meet expected outcomes),** **Ineffective** **(did not help to meet expected outcomes), or** **Unrelated** **(not related to the expected outcomes).**

Assessment Finding	Effective	Ineffective	Unrelated
Oriented to person and place			
Becomes combative when touched			
Recognizes her visiting daughter			
Uses her call light appropriately			
Awake all night but sleeps all day			
States she has no pain			

Answers

Assessment Finding	Effective	Ineffective	Unrelated
Oriented to person and place	X		
Becomes combative when touched		X	
Recognizes her visiting daughter	X		
Uses her call light appropriately	X		
Awake all night but sleeps all day		X	
States she has no pain			X

Rationales

Delirium is acute confusion that commonly occurs in older adults and clients who have substance use disorder. In addition to confusion, the client often has problems with his or her sleep-wake cycle and behavioral or emotional manifestations, such as yelling, agitation, and aggression. Being oriented, recognizing her daughter, and using her call light appropriately indicate that her delirium is resolving as a result of appropriate nursing and interprofessional collaborative actions.

Reference

Halter, 2018, pp. 431–435

Thinking and Discussion Questions

1. Which of the six cognitive skills in the NCSBN CJMM do you think will be the least difficult for you to apply in the Thinking Exercises and why? Which one(s) will be the most difficult to apply and why?

2. For those cognitive skills that you think are most difficult, what strategies might you need to develop or what resources might you need to use to help improve your thinking?

Bibliography

Dickison, P., Haerling, K.A., & Lasater, K. (2019). Integrating the National Council of State Boards of Nursing Clinical Judgment Model into nursing educational frameworks. *Journal of Nursing Education, 58*(2), 72–78.

Clinical Judgment for Clients Across the Life Span Experiencing Commonly Occurring Health Problems

Perfusion
Common Health Problems

Exemplar 3A. Heart Failure (Medical-Surgical Nursing: Older Adult)

Thinking Exercise 3A-1

An 89-year-old female client is admitted to a telemetry unit with a diagnosis of heart failure exacerbation. She reports a medical history of osteoarthritis, chronic lymphocytic leukemia, and coronary artery disease including a myocardial infarction and coronary artery bypass surgery 22 years ago. She is alert and her daughter is at her bedside. The nurse's initial client assessment findings include:

- Oriented to person only
- Clear speech
- Follows simple commands
- Has sinus tachycardia
- Respirations = 26 breaths/min
- Oxygen saturation = 90% (on room air)
- Breathing labored with use of accessory muscles
- Has productive cough with pink frothy sputum
- Crepitus in bilateral knee joints
- Enlarged bony nodes on hands
- Hemoglobin = 12.4 g/dL (124 g/L)
- Hematocrit = 39% (0.39)
- White blood cell count = 12,000 mm³ (12 × 10⁹/L)

Highlight or place a check mark next to the assessment findings that require follow-up by the nurse.

Thinking Exercise 3A-2

An 80-year-old female client is admitted to a telemetry unit with an exacerbation of heart failure. She reports a medical history of osteoarthritis, chronic renal insufficiency, and coronary artery disease including a myocardial infarction and coronary artery bypass surgery 22 years ago. She is alert and her daughter is at her bedside. **Indicate which nursing action listed in the far-left column is appropriate for each potential heart failure complication. Note that not all actions will be used.**

Nursing Action	Potential Heart Failure Complication	Appropriate Nursing Action for Each Potential Heart Failure Complication
1 Reduce sodium intake to 1 g daily.	Acute pulmonary edema	
2 Administer oxygen therapy.	Fatigue	
3 Weigh the client each morning on the same scale.	Hypokalemia	
4 Administer furosemide 20 mg intravenous push.	Cardiac dysrhythmias	
5 Encourage the client to drink at least 3 L of fluid daily.	Hypoxemia	
6 Teach the client pursed-lip breathing techniques.		
7 Administer potassium supplements.		
8 Monitor electrocardiogram, oxygen saturation, and serum electrolyte levels.		
9 Reposition every 2 hours while in bed.		
10 Consult a cardiac rehabilitation specialist.		

Thinking Exercise 3A-3

An 80-year-old female client was admitted to a telemetry unit with an exacerbation of heart failure. She has a medical history of osteoarthritis, chronic renal insufficiency, and coronary artery disease including a myocardial infarction and coronary artery bypass surgery 22 years ago. The client is scheduled to be discharged today and will move in with her daughter until she feels well enough to go home alone. Which of the following discharge instructions will the nurse provide the client and her daughter? **Select all that apply.**

_____ A. "Weigh yourself each day at the same time on the same scale to monitor for fluid retention."

_____ B. "Contact your primary health care provider if you experience cold symptoms lasting more than 3 days."

_____ C. "Exertion can cause another episode of heart failure, so help your mother by performing daily activities for her."

_____ D. "Notify your primary health care provider if you experience shortness of breath or chest pain while resting."

_____ E. "Do not use table salt, avoid salty foods, and read labels on all food items to ensure your diet is low in sodium."

_____ F. "Do not take metoprolol if your heart rate is less than 60 beats per minute."

_____ G. "Heart failure is a chronic condition, so you don't need to be alarmed when you experience heart palpitations."

Thinking Exercise 3A-4

An 80-year-old female client was admitted to a telemetry unit with an exacerbation of heart failure. She has a medical history of osteoarthritis, chronic renal insufficiency, and coronary artery disease including a myocardial infarction and coronary artery bypass surgery 22 years ago. The client was discharged 2 weeks ago and is with her daughter for her follow-up primary health care provider visit. **For each assessment finding, use an X to indicate whether the interventions were <u>Effective</u> (helped to meet expected outcomes), <u>Ineffective</u> (did not help to meet expected outcomes), or <u>Unrelated</u> (not related to the expected outcomes).**

Assessment Finding	Effective	Ineffective	Unrelated
States she has had no shortness of breath since hospital discharge			
Has 2+ pitting edema in both ankles and feet			
Blood pressure = 134/76 mm Hg			
Has had no chest pain since hospital discharge			
Reports feeling like she has more energy now when compared with before her hospital stay			
Has new-onset fungal skin infection			

Thinking Exercise 3A-5

A 72-year-old male client is admitted to a telemetry unit after a fall at home. The client is experiencing severe weakness in his extremities and states, "I got out of bed at 4:30 (0430) this morning, my legs gave out on my way to the bathroom, and I was unable to get back up." Emergency medical services transported the client to the hospital. Past medical history provided by the client includes high cholesterol, aortic valve stenosis, and poliomyelitis when he was 2 years old. He saw his cardiologist and had an echocardiogram completed 3 weeks ago. He also received influenza and pneumococcal vaccines this year. The client is married and has two adult children and five grandchildren. He lives in a single-story home, ambulates with a cane, and completes ADLs independently. His echocardiogram results indicate moderate heart failure with an ejection fraction (EF) of 38%. The client's wife provides a list of his current medications, but the list is not complete. **Choose the *most likely* options for the information missing from the table below by selecting from the lists of options provided.**

Medication	Dose, Route, Frequency	Drug Class	Indication
aspirin	**1**	Salicylate	Prevention of platelet aggregation
atorvastatin	20 mg orally once a day	HMG-CoA reductase inhibitor	**2**
3	12.5 mg orally twice a day	Beta-adrenergic blocker	Management of hypertension and heart failure
ibuprofen	400 mg orally every 6-8 hr as needed	Nonsteroidal anti-inflammatory drug	**4**
5	0.125 mg orally once a day	Cardiac glycoside	Increase myocardial contractile force
lisinopril	2.5 mg orally once a day	**6**	Management of heart failure

Options for 1	Options for 2	Options for 3
0.25 mg orally twice a day	Management of angina	carvedilol
81 mg orally every 4–5 hr as needed for pain	Treatment of bronchospasm	hydrochlorothiazide
200 mg subcutaneously every 8 hours	Management of heart failure	furosemide
325 mg orally once a day	Management of hyperlipidemia	nesiritide
1000 mg as a transdermal patch every 2 days	Prevention of pulmonary hypertension	verapamil

Options for 4	Options for 5	Options for 6
Treatment for decreased cardiac output	enalapril	Aldosterone antagonist
Prevention of dyspnea	eplerenone	Angiotensin-converting enzyme inhibitor
Management of extremity pain	digoxin	Calcium channel blocker
Treatment of pyrexia	losartan	Histamine blocker
Prevention of tachycardia	metoprolol	Thiazide diuretic

Thinking Exercise 3A-6

A 72-year-old male client is admitted to a telemetry unit after a fall at home secondary to severe weakness in his lower extremities. Past medical history provided by the client includes hyperlipidemia, aortic valve stenosis, and poliomyelitis when he was 2 years old. His most recent echocardiogram indicates moderate heart failure with an ejection fraction (EF) of 38%. He is prescribed aspirin and a variety of cardiac medications. The nurse's initial client assessment findings include:

- Alert and oriented
- Blurred vision
- Reports lower extremity stiffness
- Ambulates with crutches
- Sinus rhythm with preventricular contractions
- Cardiac murmur
- Reports dyspnea with exertion
- Bilateral basilar crackles
- Blood urea nitrogen (BUN) =11 mg/dL (4.0 mmol/L)
- Creatinine kinase 1200 U/L (1200 IU/L)
- Potassium 5.2 mg/dL (5.2 mmol/L)

Highlight or place a check mark next to the assessment findings that require follow-up by the nurse.

Thinking Exercise 3A-7

A 72-year-old male client is admitted to a telemetry unit after a fall at home secondary to severe weakness in his lower extremities. Past medical history provided by the client includes high cholesterol, aortic valve stenosis, and residual lower extremity muscle pain and weakness secondary to poliomyelitis as a child. His most recent echocardiogram reports moderate heart failure with an ejection fraction (EF) of 38%. He is prescribed aspirin and a variety of cardiac medications. The client is diagnosed with rhabdomyolysis. Prescriptions to place a large-bore intravenous catheter and administer normal saline 0.9% at 125 mL/hr are received. **Choose the *most likely* options for the information missing from the paragraph below by selecting from the lists of options provided.**

When caring for a client who has left ventricular dysfunction, the nurse assesses for _____1_____ related to inadequate cerebral perfusion, _____2_____ related to inadequate myocardium perfusion, and _____3_____ related to inadequate renal perfusion. The nurse monitors a client who has heart failure closely for complications of pulmonary congestion when administering intravenous fluids. Manifestations of pulmonary congestion include _____4_____, _____5_____, and _____6_____. If the client experiences acute pulmonary edema, the nurse would place the client in a sitting position and administer _____7_____ and _____8_____.

Options for 1, 2, and 3	Options for 4, 5, and 6	Options for 7 and 8
Confusion	Crackles	Albuterol nebulizer
Chest pain	Dyspnea	Chest percussion
Nausea	Fatigue	Lorazepam orally
Oliguria	Jugular vein distention	Morphine intravenous push
Orthopnea	Stridor	Nitroglycerin sublingual
Pallor	Tachypnea	Supplemental oxygen
Polyuria	Weight gain	Furosemide intravenous push

Exemplar 3B. Sickle Cell Disease (Pediatric Nursing: Adolescent)

Thinking Exercise 3B-1

An 18-year-old African-American female client is admitted to the emergency department with report of shortness of breath, chest discomfort, fatigue, and fever for the past 3 days. Additional assessment findings include:

- Both parents are sickle cell disease carriers, but the client has had no symptoms of the disease
- No cyanosis of lips, nail beds, or palms
- Reports feeling "lightheaded" at times
- Hemoglobin = 11.4 g/dL (114 g/L)
- Hematocrit = 36% (0.36)
- Red blood cell (RBC) count = 3.2 × 10^6/μL (3.2 × 10^{12}/L)
- White blood cell (WBC) count = 15,500/mm^3 (15.5 × 10^9/L)
- Serum bilirubin = 1.8 mg/dL (30.4 mcmol/L)
- Oral temperature = 101.6°F (38.7°C)
- Pulse = 89 beats/min
- Respirations = 20 breaths/min
- Blood pressure = 98/48 mm Hg

Highlight or place a check mark next to the assessment findings that require follow-up by the nurse.

Thinking Exercise 3B-2

An 18-year-old African-American female client reports shortness of breath, chest discomfort, fatigue, and fever for the past 3 days. She is admitted to the medical-surgical nursing unit with pneumonia and probable sickle cell disease (SCD). **Use an X to indicate whether the nursing actions listed below are <u>Indicated</u> (appropriate or necessary), <u>Contraindicated</u> (could be harmful), or <u>Non-Essential</u> (makes no difference or not necessary) for the client's care at this time.**

Nursing Action	Indicated	Contraindicated	Non-Essential
Initiate oxygen therapy.			
Prepare to give several units of packed red blood cells stat.			
Administer IV antibiotic therapy.			
Refer the client to a social worker to discuss end-of-life care.			
Withhold pain medication until she has a drug screening.			
Keep the head of the client's bed up to at least 30 degrees.			

Thinking Exercise 3B-3

An 18-year-old African-American female client reports shortness of breath, chest discomfort, fatigue, and fever for the past 3 days. She is admitted to the medical-surgical nursing unit with pneumonia and sickle cell disease (SCD). **Choose the *most likely* options for the information missing from the table below by selecting from the list of options provided.**

As a result of the client's diagnosis of sickle cell disease, the nurse is aware that she could have multiple complications including acute severe pain periods known as _____.
The nurse also monitors for other major SCD complications such as _____, _____, and _____.

Options
Seizure episodes
Leukemia
Stroke
Peptic ulcer disease
Acute vaso-occlusive episodes
Pancreatitis
Acute kidney injury
Cholelithiasis
Sepsis
Acute chest syndrome

Thinking Exercise 3B-4

An 18-year-old African-American female client reports shortness of breath, chest discomfort, fatigue, and fever for the past 3 days. She is admitted to the medical-surgical nursing unit with pneumonia and sickle cell disease (SCD). The primary health care provider prescribes hydroxyurea to prevent or reduce sickling or painful events caused by SCD. Which health teaching by the nurse about hydroxyurea is important to include? **Select all that apply.**

_____ A. "Be sure to follow up on all lab testing because the drug can lower your red blood cell and platelet count."

_____ B. "Because the drug can cause birth defects, be sure to use contraception to prevent pregnancy."

_____ C. "After your blood counts improve, you can discontinue the drug."

_____ D. "Try to avoid people with infection and public places where there are large crowds."

_____ E. "Hydroxyurea has been known to cause several types of cancer, so be sure to follow up with your medical appointments."

_____ F. "This drug can cause diabetes mellitus, so report any increased thirst or urination to your primary health care provider."

_____ G. Hydroxyurea can cure your sickle cell disease, but you still need to follow healthy lifestyle habits."

Thinking Exercise 3B-5

An 18-year-old African-American female with a new diagnosis of sickle cell disease is preparing for discharge to home with her parents. The nurse is planning health teaching to help the client prevent a sickle cell crisis event, which could be life threatening. What health teaching will the nurse include? **Select all that apply.**

_____ A. "Decrease your alcohol intake to one drink a day."

_____ B. "Avoid overly strenuous physical activities."

_____ C. "Avoid temperatures that are extremely hot or cold."

_____ D. "Engage in low-impact, low-energy exercise three or four times a week."

_____ E. "Eat a healthy diet that is rich in fruits and vegetables."

_____ F. "Avoid high altitudes, such as mountainous areas."

_____ G. "Avoid smoking and tobacco use, including vaping."

_____ H. "Dress appropriately for the temperature that you are in."

4 Clotting
Deep Vein Thrombosis

Exemplar 4. Deep Vein Thrombosis (Medical-Surgical Nursing: Middle-Age Adult)

Thinking Exercise 4-1

A 38-year-old female client was admitted 3 days ago with severe abdominal pain, fever, and nausea. She was diagnosed with a small bowel obstruction and received general anesthesia yesterday during an exploratory laparotomy to remove adhesions. According to admission documents, the client has a 29 pack-year smoking history as well as chronic obstructive pulmonary disease, for which she takes fluticasone and albuterol; endometriosis, for which she takes ibuprofen and oral contraceptives; and a BMI of 36. The client lives alone and works at a telecommunication call center. The shift report indicates that the patient had a difficult recovery after surgery and has been on bedrest since admission. Initial nursing shift assessment findings include:

- Abdominal incision approximated and healing
- Hypoactive bowel sounds × 4
- Reports pain in right calf
- Nasogastric tube to low continuous suction
- Dependent edema in back and hips
- Reports incisional tenderness
- Left leg is cooler than right leg
- Dry unproductive cough
- Right lower extremity edema
- Reports passing flatus

Highlight or place a check mark next to the assessment findings that require follow-up by the nurse.

Thinking Exercise 4-2

A 38-year-old female client was admitted 3 days ago with severe abdominal pain, fever, and nausea. She was diagnosed with a small bowel obstruction, received general anesthesia yesterday during an exploratory laparotomy, experienced a difficult recovery after surgery, and has been on bedrest since admission. Venous duplex ultrasonography of her lower extremities and laboratory studies are completed. Results from these diagnostic tests include the following data:

Hemoglobin	17 g/dL (170 g/L)
Hematocrit	43% (0.43)
WBC count	5500 mm³ (5.5 × 10⁹/L)
Platelets	165,000/mm³ (165 × 10⁹/L)
aPTT	32 sec
PT	11.5 sec
INR	0.9
BUN	15 mg/dL (4.4 mmol/L)
Creatinine	0.6 mg/dL (53 mcmol/L)
Venous duplex ultrasonography	Conclusion: Right lower extremity deep vein thrombosis

The primary health care provider prescribes:
- Heparin 80 units/kg IV bolus followed by heparin 18 units/kg/hr IV infusion
- Fecal occult test
- Morning labs: CBC, PT/INR, aPTT, BUN, and creatinine

For each action below, use an X to specify whether the action would be <u>Indicated</u> (appropriate or necessary), <u>Contraindicated</u> (could be harmful), or <u>Non-Essential</u> (makes no difference or not necessary) for the client's care at this time.

Nursing Action	Indicated	Contraindicated	Non-Essential
Apply sequential compression devices to bilateral lower extremities.			
Teach the client to avoid foods high in vitamin K.			
Plan to check the client's platelet count in the morning.			
Use ice packs and massage techniques to decrease leg swelling and pain.			
Assess for hematuria and blood in the client's stool.			
Place client's legs in a dependent position when sitting in a chair.			
Monitor the client's intake and urinary output.			

Thinking Exercise 4-3

A 38-year-old female client, while recovering from a small bowel obstruction and an exploratory laparotomy, is diagnosed with a right lower extremity deep vein thrombosis. The client has several questions about her diagnosis and care. **Indicate which nursing response listed in the far-left column is appropriate for each client question. Note that not all responses will be used.**

Nurse's Responses	Client Questions	Appropriate Nurse's Response for Each Client Question
1 "There is an oral version of heparin called warfarin. I will ask your provider about your request."	"My doctor said I needed to stop smoking. How does smoking have anything to do with my swollen leg?"	
2 Heparin cannot be absorbed by your gastrointestinal tract. It has to be given via IV or injection to be effective."	"What can I do to help decrease the swelling in my leg?"	
3 "The fecal occult test makes sure that you are not hemorrhaging."	"I read on the Internet that I should not move my leg because the clot will dislodge and go to my lungs. Is that true?"	
4 "You have many risk factors for a DVT including smoking, oral contraceptive use, recent surgery with general anesthesia, and ongoing bedrest."	"Why are you testing my stool?"	

Continued

Nurse's Responses	Client Questions	Appropriate Nurse's Response for Each Client Question
5 "Nicotine causes your blood vessels to constrict or narrow, which makes it easier for blood clots to become stuck in the vein."	"Why can't this blood thinning medication be given orally?"	
6 "Elevating your legs when in bed and the chair will help."		
7 "When a clot dislodges and moves to your lung it is called a pulmonary embolism. This is a serious complication of a deep vein thrombosis."		
8 "Increasing your activity slowly may decease your fear. Let's start with getting out of bed and then a short walk later today."		
9 "Swelling will decrease when the clot is gone, and the medication you are on will dissolve the clot."		
10 "If you have pain when I flex your foot then you should stay in bed until the swelling decreases."		
11 "Heparin is a blood thinner and can cause internal bleeding. This test helps us monitor for microscopic blood in your stool."		

Thinking Exercise 4-4

A 38-year-old female client was diagnosed with a right lower extremity deep vein thrombosis after surgery 2 days ago. This morning the nurse reviews the client's electronic health record to complete a shift assessment. Data from the health record include a prescription from the primary health care provider for warfarin 5 mg orally every day, and the following laboratory results:

Hemoglobin	17 g/dL (170 g/L)
Hematocrit	44% (0.44)
WBC count	5550 mm³ (5.5 × 10⁹/L)
Platelets	160,000 mm³ (160 × 10⁹/L)
aPTT	40 sec
PT	12 sec
INR	0.9
BUN	16 mg/dL (4.5 mmol/L)
Creatinine	0.6 mg/dL (53 mcmol/L)

Choose the most likely options for the information missing from the statement below by selecting from the lists of options provided.

When assessing a client for complications of a deep vein thrombosis, the nurse recognizes _____1_____ and _____2_____ as signs of _____ __3_____ , and _____4_____ and _____5_____ as signs of _____6_____ , which can occur as a result of heparin therapy.

Options for 1 and 2	Options for 3
Bradycardia	Aortic aneurysm
Chest pain	Stroke
Confusion	Mitral valve prolapse
Hypotension	Pneumonia
Occult blood	Pulmonary embolism
aPTT >70 sec	
Unilateral edema	
Shortness of breath	

Options for 4 and 5	Options for 6
Calf pain	Coronary artery disease
Dilated superficial veins	Dehydration
Ecchymosis	Gastroesophageal reflux disease
Groin discomfort	Heparin-induced thrombocytopenia
Hematuria	Hemorrhage
Nausea	
Phlebitis	

Thinking Exercise 4-5

A 38-year-old female client was diagnosed with a right lower extremity deep vein thrombosis (DVT) after surgery. Five days later the heparin infusion is discontinued and the nurse prepares to discharge the client on warfarin. Which health teaching will the nurse include as part of discharge planning related to the client's DVT management and prevention of a new DVT? **Select all that apply.**

_____ A. "Elevate your legs on a couple of pillows when in bed."

_____ B. "Wear knee-high graduated compression stockings."

_____ C. "Apply prolonged pressure over cuts and nosebleeds."

_____ D. "Weigh yourself each morning on the same scale."

_____ E. "Avoid eating foods that are high in fat and cholesterol."

_____ F. "Increase your activity slowly and rest when needed."

_____ G. "Take over-the-counter pain medications for mild pain."

_____ H. "Keep your scheduled appointment at the Coumadin (Warfarin) clinic."

_____ I. "Contact your primary health care provider if your stool is black and tarry."

_____ J. "If you miss a dose of warfarin, take a double dose the following day."

_____ K. "Monitor your heart rate and blood pressure daily."

Exemplar 5A. Asthma (Pediatric Nursing: School-Age Child)

Thinking Exercise 5A-1

The nurse is assessing a 6-year-old male client with a history of asthma who was brought to the emergency department (ED) and reports shortness of breath during a soccer game. The nurse completes a triage assessment with the following data.

Vital Signs	
Temperature	99.2°F (37.1°C)
Heart rate	96 beats/min
Respirations	32 breaths/min
Blood pressure	97/66 mm Hg
Oxygen saturation	89% (on room air)
Health History	• Born at 30 weeks' gestation • History of asthma • Multiple environmental allergens • Allergic to penicillin • Immunizations are current

Physical/Psychosocial Assessment Findings

- Child reports no pain
- Child is restless and refuses to lie down in bed
- Wheezing in both lungs
- Minimal air movement noted in lower lobes bilaterally
- Child only nods head "yes" or "no" to questions
- Parents are at the bedside and providing comfort
- Parents deny that the child was exposed to any triggers
- Peak flow meter results are <50% of child's baseline
- Moderate intercostal retractions

Highlight or place a check mark next to the assessment findings that require follow-up by the nurse.

Thinking Exercise 5A-2

A 6-year-old asthmatic male client who was presented to the emergency department (ED) and reported shortness of breath during a soccer game is admitted to the pediatric unit. On arrival to the unit, the nurse begins the process for admission. In addition to the information obtained from the ED, the nurse notes that the client appears to be anxious and breathes predominantly through his mouth. The nurse notes wheezing throughout all lung fields and slightly diminished breath sounds in the lower lobes. **Use an X to indicate whether the nursing actions listed below are <u>Emergent</u> (appropriate or immediately necessary) or <u>Not Emergent</u> (not appropriate or not immediately necessary) for the client's care at this time.**

Nursing Action	Emergent	Not Emergent
Place nasal cannula to provide humidified oxygen in response to rescue treatment.		
Administer methylprednisolone per the primary health care provider's prescription.		
Titrate oxygen to keep oxygen saturation >90%.		
Teach the child to use a pursed-lip breathing technique.		
Administer albuterol per hospital protocol.		
Allow the child to assume the most comfortable upright position.		
Insert a peripheral intravenous line.		
Enter the primary health care provider's NPO order into the electronic health record.		
Encourage the family to change the child's clothing to promote comfort.		

Thinking Exercise 5A-3

The nurse is assessing a 6-year-old male client who had an asthma attack. Initial actions were performed on admission to stabilize the child's respiratory status. **For each assessment finding, use an X to indicate whether the intervention was <u>Effective</u> (helped to meet expected outcomes), <u>Ineffective</u> (did not help to meet expected outcomes), or <u>Unrelated</u> (not related to the expected outcomes).**

Assessment Finding	Effective	Ineffective	Unrelated
Oxygen saturation = 94%			
Child playing quietly on electronic device			
Heart rate = 121 beats/min			
Respirations = 26 breaths/min			
Blood pressure = 118/66 mm Hg			
Temperature = 100.4°F (38.0°C)			
Intermittent wheezing in lower lobes bilaterally			

Thinking Exercise 5A-4

A 6-year-old male client's mother provides the nurse with a partial list of the medications he has been taking at home for asthma, but she is unable to remember some of the information. The nurse provides health teaching to both parents regarding the child's medication while in the hospital and for home use. **Choose the *most likely* option for the information missing from the table below by selecting from the lists of choices provided.**

Medication	Dose, Route, Frequency	Drug Action	Health Teaching
methylprednisolone	0.5–1 mg/kg/dose IV every 6 hr	Reverses airflow obstruction by decreasing inflammation	**1**
albuterol	0.025 mcg/kg/dose via nebulizer every 4 hr and every 2 hr PRN	**2**	Monitor your child for increased heart rate and jitteriness.
montelukast sodium	**3**	Reduces inflammation and bronchoconstriction	The drug is for long-term treatment, not for acute exacerbations; be aware that it can cause depression and suicidal thinking and behavior.
4	10 mg/kg/dose orally every 4–6 hr as needed for pain or temperature >101°F (38.2°C)	Decreases pain and fever	Do not exceed 75 mg/kg/day to prevent liver damage.

Options for 1	Options for 2
Monitor your child's breathing.	Prevents pulmonary infection
Do not schedule vaccines when your child is taking corticosteroids.	Reduces wheezing by dilating smooth muscles of the airways
Monitor for gastrointestinal bleeding.	Reduces swelling in alveoli
Administer dose via intramuscular injection.	Increases respiratory rate
Administer dose via subcutaneous injection.	Reduces effect of allergens as triggers

Options for 3	Options for 4
0.6–1.5 mg/kg/day IV	Ibuprofen
1–2 puffs via inhalation as needed	Aspirin (ASA)
5-mg chewable tablet once daily	Acetaminophen
2 mg/kg/dose IV twice daily	Amlodipine
10–15 mg/kg/dose IV once daily	Hydrocodone

Thinking Exercise 5A-5

The nurse begins to develop a plan of care and identify teaching needs to review with the parents of a 6-year-old male client with asthma. What would the nurse include in the teaching plan? **Select all that apply.**

_____ A. The need for allergy testing to identify asthmatic triggers

_____ B. The need for early identification of symptomatic cough

_____ C. Home medications, including dosing and precautions

_____ D. Promoting a calm environment and quiet daily activities for the child during hospitalization

_____ E. Reassuring the parents that the child will outgrow his asthma

_____ F. Need for follow-up with pulmonary function testing

_____ G. Encouraging deep-breathing exercises for the child

Exemplar 5B. Chronic Obstructive Pulmonary Disease (Medical-Surgical Nursing: Middle-Age Adult)

Thinking Exercise 5B-1

A 47-year-old Caucasian female presents to the ED with an abrasion requiring stitches on her head. The client provides an overview of her health history, which includes 22 pack-years of cigarette smoking, dyspepsia, chronic obstructive pulmonary disease (COPD), cholecystectomy last year, and amputation of the two lateral fingers on her right hand due to an accident approximately 4 years ago. She provides an incomplete list of home medications to the nurse. **Choose the *most likely* options for the information missing from the table by selecting from the lists of options provided.**

Medication	Dose, Route, Frequency	Drug Class	Drug Action
Guaifenesin	200 mg orally every 4 hr	Mucolytic agent	**1**
Tiotropium	18 mcg as a dry powder inhalation once daily	Anticholinergic drug	**2**
Montelukast sodium	10-mg tablet orally once daily	**3**	Reduces bronchoconstriction and inflammation
Fluticasone Propionate	100 mcg via inhalation twice daily	**4**	Decreases inflammation
Albuterol	**5**	Beta₂-adrenergic agonist	Reduces bronchoconstriction
6	40 mg orally once daily	Proton pump inhibitor	Reduces acid reflux

Options for 1	Options for 2	Options for 3
Reduces chest congestion	Prevents asthma attacks	Beta₂-adrenergic agonist
Manages hay fever	Maintains relief of bronchospasm	Leukotriene modifier
Reduces neurologic pain	Replaces pancreatic enzymes	Methylxanthine
Decreases sinus pressure	Prevents pulmonary hypertension	Mineralocorticoid
Reduces wheezing	Manages urinary retention	Tricyclic antidepressant

Options for 4	Options for 5	Options for 6
Angiotensin-converting enzyme inhibitor	0.86 mg as a nebulizer inhalation every 6 hr	Omeprazole
Adrenergic blocker	1 puff as a dry powder inhalant PRN every 6–8 hr	Cimetidine
Glucocorticoid	20 mg orally every 8 hr	Famotidine
Histamine blocker	2 puffs as an inhalation PRN every 4–6 hr	Magnesium phosphate
Nonsteroidal anti-inflammatory drug (NSAID)	40 mg orally 30 min before exercising	Bismuth

Thinking Exercise 5B-2

A 47-year-old Caucasian female presents to the ED with an abrasion requiring stitches on her head. The client provides an overview of her health history, which includes 22 pack-years of cigarette smoking, dyspepsia, chronic obstructive pulmonary disease (COPD), cholecystectomy last year, and amputation of the two lateral fingers on her right hand due to an accident approximately 4 years ago. The nurse's initial assessment findings include:

- Labored breathing
- Denies headache
- Oxygen saturation = 88% (on room air)
- Unable to read the admission paperwork without her glasses
- Pupils equal, round, and reactive to light
- Arterial blood gas = pH = 7.37, $Paco_2$ = 48 mm Hg, Pao_2 = 81.2 mm Hg, HCO_3 = 20.6 mEq/L (20.6 mmol/L)
- Leaning forward with hands on upper thighs
- Chest symmetrically rises with each breath
- Respirations = 26 breaths/min
- Denies fever and chills
- Blood pressure = 142/57 mm Hg
- Heart rate = 95 beats/min

Highlight or place a check mark next to the assessment findings that require follow-up by the nurse.

Thinking Exercise 5B-3

A 47-year-old Caucasian female presents to the emergency department (ED) with an abrasion requiring stitches on her head. The client is a forklift operator for a local manufacturing company and was involved in a work-related accident. She is alert and oriented. Her speech is clear, but she becomes breathless when answering questions. The client provides an overview of her health history, which includes 22 pack-years of cigarette smoking, dyspepsia, chronic obstructive pulmonary disease (COPD), cholecystectomy last year, and amputation of the two lateral fingers on her right hand due to an accident approximately 4 years ago. She lives with a roommate and three dogs, enjoys grilling on the weekends, and drinks four to six beers a week. She is 5 feet 10 inches tall and weighs 123 lb. Which focused questions about the client's COPD will the nurse ask during the client's initial intake assessment? **Select all that apply.**

_____ A. "Do you have trouble doing things you enjoy due to shortness of breath?"

_____ B. "Does your employer follow OSHA protocols?"

_____ C. "What daily activities do you have difficulty performing?"

_____ D. "Do you have trouble digesting cholesterol and other fatty foods?"

_____ E. "Where do you sleep at night?"

_____ F. "Have you lost weight unexpectedly?"

_____ G. "Have you ever felt you should cut down on your drinking?"

_____ H. "Do you enjoy working as a forklift operator?"

_____ I. "What do you eat and drink on a typical day?"

Thinking Exercise 5B-4

A 47-year-old Caucasian female presents to the ED with an abrasion requiring stitches on her head and an exacerbation of chronic obstructive pulmonary disease (COPD). Her health history includes 22 pack-years of cigarette smoking, dyspepsia, cholecystectomy last year, and amputation of the two lateral fingers on her right hand 4 years ago. **Indicate which nursing action listed in the far-left column is appropriate for each potential complication. Note that not all actions will be used.**

Nursing Action	Potential Complication	Appropriate Nursing Action for Each Complication
1 Teach pursed-lip breathing technique.	Respiratory infection	
2 Administer oxygen therapy.	Dysrhythmias	
3 Assist the client with ADLs.	Activity intolerance	
4 Provide five small meals each day.	Oral candidiasis	
5 Evaluate laboratory results for acid-base and electrolyte imbalances.	Hypoxemia	
6 Teach the client to swish and spit mouthwash three times a day.	Malnutrition	
7 Encourage paced self-care with periods of rest.	Anxiety	
8 Implement continued electrocardiographic monitoring.		
9 Ask the client to rinse her mouth after administering corticosteroid inhalants.		
10 Turn off the lights and ask the client to take slow, deep breaths.		
11 Provide protein shake after each meal.		
12 Teach the client to drink at least 2 L of fluid daily.		
13 Weigh the client each morning on the same scale.		
14 Help the client develop a plan for what she should do when symptoms occur.		

Thinking Exercise 5B-5

A 5-foot 8-inch, 265-pound male client is admitted to a telemetry unit with a diagnosis of pneumonia. He is 44 years old, lives with his wife and three children, quit smoking 8 years ago after smoking a pack of cigarettes a day for 18 years, and drives a semitruck long distances for a living. His past medical history includes gastrointestinal esophageal reflux disease, hyperlipidemia, metabolic syndrome, chronic obstructive pulmonary disease, and sleep apnea. He is alert and oriented, and reports feeling fatigue and discomfort in the right side of his chest. He is sitting up in a chair, refuses to lie in the bed, and asks for a BiPAP machine, which he uses at home, so that he can take a nap. **Choose the *most likely* options for the information missing from the text below by selecting from the two lists of options provided.**

Chronic obstructive pulmonary disease interferes with airflow and gas exchange, leading to increased _____1_____, _____2_____, and _____3_____. These physiologic changes increase the client's risk for _____4_____, _____5_____, and _____6_____.

Options for 1, 2, and 3	Options for 4, 5, and 6
Bicarbonate levels	Coronary artery disease
Blood pressure	Hypertension
Bronchodilation	Hypoxemia
Carbon dioxide levels	Left-sided heart failure
Oxygen levels	Metabolic acidosis
Pulmonary pressure	Pulmonary infection
Respiratory rate	Respiratory alkalosis
Sputum production	Right-sided heart failure

Thinking Exercise 5B-6

A 44-year-old client is admitted with pneumonia and an exacerbation of chronic obstructive pulmonary disease. His past medical history includes gastrointestinal esophageal reflux disease (GERD), hyperlipidemia, metabolic syndrome, chronic obstructive pulmonary disorder, and sleep apnea. He quit smoking 8 years ago after having smoked a pack of cigarettes a day for 18 years and drives a semitruck long distances for a living. Current assessment findings include:

Vital Signs	
Temperature	101.2°F (38.4°C)
Heart rate	106 beats/min
Blood pressure	144/79 mm Hg
Respirations	32 breaths/min
Oxygen saturation	84% (on room air)
PEF	52%
Physical Assessment Findings	
Respiratory assessment findings	Bilateral wheezing Reports dyspnea, denies pain Thick, tenacious secretions Chest diameter ratio 1:1
Other assessment findings	Bilateral lower extremity pitting edema
Laboratory Test Results	
Hemoglobin	18 g/dL (180 g/dL)
Hematocrit	42% (0.42 volume fraction)
Potassium	4.2 mEq/L (4.2 mmol/L)
pH	7.32
Pa_{O_2}	67 mm Hg
Pa_{CO_2}	60 mm Hg
HCO_3	22 mEq/L (22 mmol/L)

For each action below, use an X to specify whether the action would be <u>Indicated</u> (appropriate or necessary), <u>Contraindicated</u> (could be harmful), or <u>Non-Essential</u> (makes no difference or is not necessary) for the client's care at this time.

Nursing Action	Indicated	Contraindicated	Non-Essential
Obtain sputum samples for culture and sensitivity.			
Administer humidified oxygen via Venturi mask.			
Provide the client with smoking cessation education.			
Type and cross for blood products.			
Perform pulmonary function tests after administrating bronchodilator.			
Administer 20 mEq oral potassium chloride.			
Administer albuterol nebulizer 15 minutes before each meal.			
Implement vibratory positive expiratory pressure therapy.			
Place the client on a 1200-mL fluid restriction.			

Thinking Exercise 5B-7

A 5-foot 8-inch, 265-lb male client was admitted to a telemetry unit with a diagnosis of pneumonia. He is 44 years old, lives with his wife and three children, quit smoking 8 years ago after having smoked a pack of cigarettes a day for 18 years, and drives a semitruck long distances for a living. His past medical history includes gastrointestinal esophageal reflux disease (GERD), hyperlipidemia, metabolic syndrome, chronic obstructive pulmonary disorder, and sleep apnea. He is alert and oriented, refuses to lie in the bed, and states that he uses a BiPAP machine when he sleeps. Which statements will the nurse include in this client's health teaching? **Select all that apply.**

_____ A. "Lie on your back with a pillow against your stomach when performing coughing exercises."

_____ B. "Walk 20 minutes each day with periods of rest when you become too short of breath to continue."

_____ C. "It is okay to sleep in a recliner or with several pillows tucked behind your back."

_____ D. "Make sure your oxygen flow meter is never higher than 4 liters per minute."

_____ E. "There are many programs and products that can help you stop smoking."

_____ F. "Gargle and rinse your mouth with water after using your fluticasone propionate inhaler."

_____ G. "Use of a spacer with a dry powder inhaler improves administration into the lungs."

_____ H. "Wait 1 minute before taking a second dose of your albuterol inhaler."

Elimination
Benign Prostatic Hyperplasia

Thinking Exercise 6-1

A 77-year-old male client with a history of chronic obstructive pulmonary disease is evaluated in an ambulatory care clinic after having experienced urinary hesitancy and postvoid leaking. The client's home medications are ipratropium MDI 2 inhalations four times a day and cetirizine 10 mg daily. The client's International Prostate Symptom Score (I-PSS) is 15.

International Prostate Symptom Score (I-PSS)

In the Past Month		Score
Incomplete emptying	How often have you had the sensation of not emptying your bladder?	1—Less than 1 in 5 times
Frequency	How often have you had to urinate less than every 2 hours?	2—Less than half the time
Intermittency	How often have you found you stopped and started again several times when you urinated?	4—More than half the time
Urgency	How often have you found it difficult to postpone urination?	3—About half the time
Weak stream	How often have you had a weak urinary stream?	2—Less than half the time
Straining	How often have you had to strain to start urination?	1—Less than 1 in 5 times
Nocturia	How many times do you typically get up at night to urinate?	2—2 times
	Total I-PSS Score	**15**

I-PSS contact information and permission to use: MAPI Research Trust, Lyon, France. E-mail: gro.tsurt-ipam@tcatnoc Website: www.mapi-trust.org I-PSS 1_Standard_UK English_Mapi Institute_ID2831

The primary health care provider prescribes a urinalysis, urine culture, complete blood count, blood urea nitrogen and serum creatinine levels, postvoid bladder ultrasound, and transrectal ultrasound. **Use an X to indicate whether the nursing actions listed below are <u>Indicated</u> (appropriate or necessary), <u>Contraindicated</u> (could be harmful), or <u>Non-Essential</u> (make no difference or are not necessary) for the client's care at this time.**

Nursing Action	Indicated	Contraindicated	Non-Essential
Confirm that the client has a signed informed consent for the bladder sonography.			
Refrigerate the urinalysis sample if it cannot be sent to the laboratory immediately.			
Ensure the client understands that a transducer will be inserted into his rectum to view the prostate and surrounding structures.			
Insert an indwelling urinary catheter to obtain a urine culture specimen.			
Ask the client to urinate prior to performing the bladder ultrasound.			
Collect the client's urine for a 24-hour period.			

Thinking Exercise 6-2

A 77-year-old male client with a history of chronic obstructive pulmonary disease is evaluated in an ambulatory care clinic after having experienced urinary hesitancy and postvoid leaking. The client's home medications are ipratropium MDI 2 inhalations four times a day and cetirizine 10 mg daily. As a result of a transrectal ultrasound and laboratory testing, the client is diagnosed with benign prostatic hyperplasia and prescribed terazosin, an alpha$_1$ blocker. Which statements will the nurse include in this client's teaching related to his diagnosis and treatment plan? **Select all that apply.**

_____ A. "Terazosin can decrease your libido. Limit sexual intercourse to once a month."

_____ B. "Rise slowly when getting up from a chair or out of bed, and sit if you feel light-headed."

_____ C. "Urinate as soon as you feel the urge. Do not hold in your urine."

_____ D. Terazosin may cause high blood pressure. Keep all follow-up appointments."

_____ E. "Avoid drinking beverages that contain caffeine and alcohol."

_____ F. "Your allergy medications may cause urinary retention. Talk to your primary health care provider."

_____ G. Terazosin must build up in your system before you will see a benefit. It usually takes a couple of months.

Thinking Exercise 6-3

A 77-year-old male client with a history of chronic obstructive pulmonary disease was evaluated in an ambulatory clinic 6 months ago after having experienced urinary hesitancy and postvoid leaking. The client was diagnosed with benign prostatic hyperplasia and prescribed terazosin. Today he presents to the emergency department with acute mental confusion and dysuria. The client's initial assessment findings include:
- Oriented to self and his wife at the bedside
- Disoriented to place, time, and situation
- Moves all extremities with equal strength and to command
- Temperature = 101.4°F (38.5°C)

- Heart rate = 92 beats/min
- Blood pressure = 122/48 mm Hg
- Respirations = 18 breaths/min
- Oxygenation saturation = 92% (on room air)
- Reports lower back pain
- Lung fields clear
- Light yellow nasal drainage
- Reports needing to urinate multiple times each hour
- Urine output is less than 20 mL/hr
- Bladder ultrasound indicates 800 mL fluid in bladder

Highlight or place a check mark next to the assessment findings that require follow-up by the nurse.

Thinking Exercise 6-4

A 77-year-old male client with a history of chronic obstructive pulmonary disease was diagnosed with benign prostatic hyperplasia and prescribed terazosin. He presented to the emergency department 2 days ago with acute mental confusion and was diagnosed with acute urinary retention, urinary tract infection, hematuria, and hydronephrosis. The client underwent a transurethral resection of the prostate (TURP) procedure and has been transferred to the medical-surgical unit. **Indicate which nursing action listed in the far-left column is appropriate for the potential postoperative TURP complication. Note that not all actions will be used.**

Nursing Action	Potential Postoperative Complication	Appropriate Nursing Action for Each Postoperative Complication
1 Maintain the rate of continuous bladder irrigation to keep the urine clear.	Urinary catheter obstruction	
2 Subtract the amount of irrigating solution that was instilled to determine actual urinary output.	Bladder spasm	
3 Discontinue the urinary catheter within 24 hours of the procedure.	Immobility	
4 Ask the client to contract his bladder muscle and attempt to void.	Urine blood clots	
5 Assess the three-way urinary catheter for kinks and blood clots.	Pain	
6 Help the client to get out of bed, ambulate, and sit in a chair as soon as permitted after surgery.		
7 Assess for pain every 2 hours and administer pain medication as needed.		
8 Keep the three-way urinary catheter attached to the client's thigh and encourage the client to relax his bladder muscles.		
9 Perform passive range-of-motion activities while client is in bed.		
10 Teach the client's wife to use the patient-controlled analgesia pump.		

Thinking Exercise 6-5

A 77-year-old male client with a history of chronic obstructive pulmonary disease was evaluated in an ambulatory clinic 6 months ago after having experienced urinary hesitancy and postvoid leaking. The client underwent a transurethral resection of the prostate (TURP) procedure yesterday. During shift change, the nurse notices that the output from the client's three-way urinary catheter is bright red and thick with multiple clots. Which **priority** actions will the nurse take? **Select all that apply.**

_____ A. Manually irrigate the urinary catheter with normal saline solution.

_____ B. Remove the urinary catheter that has clots and place a new one.

_____ C. Increase the inflow of the bladder irrigating solution.

_____ D. Ask the client to contract his bladder muscles and attempt to void.

_____ E. Dispose of the bloody output in a biohazard bag.

_____ F. Report the finding to the surgeon immediately

_____ G. Monitor the client's hemoglobin and hematocrit levels.

Thinking Exercise 6-6

A 77-year-old male client with a history of chronic obstructive pulmonary disease was evaluated in an ambulatory clinic 6 months ago after having experienced urinary hesitancy and postvoid leaking. The client was diagnosed with benign prostatic hyperplasia and prescribed terazosin. He presented to the emergency department several days ago and was diagnosed with acute urinary retention, urinary tract infection, hematuria, and hydronephrosis. The client underwent a transurethral resection of the prostate (TURP) procedure and is scheduled for discharge today. After providing discharge instructions to the client and his wife, the nurse assesses their understanding. **For each client statement, use an X to indicate whether the nurse's discharge instructions were <u>Effective</u> (helped the client understand the discharge instructions), <u>Ineffective</u> (did not help the client understand the discharge instructions), or <u>Unrelated</u> (not related to the discharge teaching).**

Client's Statement	Effective	Ineffective	Unrelated
"I may still experience overflow incontinence due to ongoing urinary retention."			
"I will follow up with my primary health care provider if I experience erectile dysfunction."			
"I will drink at least 2000 mL of water daily to keep hydrated and my urine color clear."			
"Kegel exercises can only be performed by women and will not help me strengthen my sphincter muscle."			
"I may have temporary dribbling of urine and will wear an incontinence pad until I am confident that this has resolved."			
"I plan to walk for 30 minutes each day and rest if I experience pain or shortness of breath."			

Thinking Exercise 7A-1

A 42-year-old female client is evaluated in the emergency department. She reports nausea, dyspepsia, and upper abdominal discomfort for the past 2 weeks. Her current medication list includes a liquid antacid, metformin, orlistat, and simvastatin. Initial assessment findings include the following:

Vital Signs	
Temperature	98.6°F (37°C)
Heart rate	89 beats/min
Respirations	14 breaths/min
Blood pressure	135/45 mm Hg
Oxygen saturation	96% (on room air)
Physical Assessment Findings	
Abdominal assessment	Abdomen is soft and round Abdominal pain 7/10 Reports abdominal pain is worse after meals
Respiratory assessment	Lung fields clear throughout
Laboratory Test Results	
White blood cell count	15,000 mm³ (15 × 10⁹/L)
Finger stick blood glucose (FSBG)	190 mg/dL (10.5 mmol/L)

Ultrasonography of the upper right abdominal quadrant indicates acute cholecystitis. The client is scheduled for a hepatobiliary iminodiacetic acid (HIDA) scan. The nurse initiates client care while awaiting this procedure. **Use an X to indicate whether the nursing actions listed below are Indicated (appropriate or necessary), Contraindicated (could be harmful), or Non-Essential (make no difference or are not necessary) for the client's care at this time.**

Nursing Action	Indicated	Contraindicated	Non-Essential
Request a high-fiber, low-fat lunch tray from dietary services.			
Insert an intravenous catheter and initiate a normal saline infusion.			
Administer morphine 2 mg intravenously as needed to manage pain.			
Obtain blood and urine cultures for bacterial and viral testing.			
Administer metformin 500 mg orally.			

Thinking Exercise 7A-2

A 42-year-old female client is evaluated in the emergency department. She reports nausea, dyspepsia, and upper abdominal discomfort for the past 2 weeks. The client is diagnosed with cholecystitis secondary to cholelithiasis and cystic duct obstruction. A laparoscopic cholecystectomy is scheduled. The client has several questions about her diagnosis and the scheduled procedure. **Indicate which nursing response listed in the far-left column is appropriate for the client's question. Note that not all actions will be used.**

Nurse's Responses	Client Questions	Appropriate Nurse's Response for Each Client Question
1 "During surgery you will not be able to move. This device stimulates muscle contraction so that your legs do not become sore."	"The surgeon said that he's removing my gallbladder. Will this surgery leave a large scar on my belly?"	
2 "A small midline incision at your umbilicus will be the one incision. This incision should not scar."	"The nursing assistant provided this machine that massages my legs. What is it for?"	
3 "You have several other risk factors. You are taking simvastatin for your high cholesterol and orlistat to lose weight. Have you lost a lot of weight recently?"	"Will I need to be on a special diet after my gallbladder is removed?"	
4 "You will want to avoid or decrease fatty and fried foods."	"I have non–insulin-depended diabetes. Why are you giving me insulin?"	
5 "The surgeon will attempt to remove your gallbladder through your belly button. If there are complications, then the surgeon will have to open your entire abdomen."	"I looked up cholecystitis on the Internet and it said I'm at risk because I'm female, 40, and fat. That sounds like every woman I know. Why me?"	
6 "The metformin you used to take was not controlling your blood sugar levels. Therefore the primary health care provider prescribed insulin."		
7 "That is an external pneumatic compression device that keeps blood from pooling in your legs during and after surgery."		
8 "A diet high in protein will help you heal after surgery."		
9 "We can control your blood sugar levels more closely with insulin while you are taking nothing by mouth."		
10 "Diabetes mellitus also puts you at risk. Your blood sugar levels need to be controlled appropriately."		
11 "It is a minimally invasive procedure requiring a couple of small incisions. I will ask the surgeon to speak with you again."		
12 "When clients with diabetes mellitus type 2 are sick, they become insulin dependent."		
13 "You should follow a diabetic diet. I will consult the registered dietitian nutritionist to explain what that is."		
14 "I can understand why you are questioning this. Would you like to speak with a chaplain?"		

Thinking Exercise 7A-3

A 42-year-old female client was evaluated in the emergency department yesterday with reports of nausea, dyspepsia, and upper abdominal discomfort for the past 2 weeks. She was diagnosed with cholecystitis secondary to cholelithiasis and cystic duct obstruction and is currently recovering from a laparoscopic cholecystectomy in the post-anesthesia care unit (PACU). **For each assessment finding, use an X to indicate whether the implemented intervention by the nurse was Effective (helped to meet expected outcomes), Ineffective (did not help to meet expected outcomes), or Unrelated (not related to the expected outcomes).**

Assessment Findings	Effective	Ineffective	Unrelated
Alert, oriented, and moving all extremities			
Stridor present on auscultation			
Urine output of 100 mL/hr			
Incisional pain reported 6/10			
Asks to use incentive spirometer			
Denies nausea or vomiting			

Thinking Exercise 7A-4

A 42-year-old female client was diagnosed with cholecystitis secondary to cholelithiasis and cystic duct obstruction, and underwent a laparoscopic cholecystectomy yesterday. The nurse completes a shift assessment and notes the following findings:
- Alert, oriented, speech clear and appropriate
- Temperature = 101.4°F (38.5°C)
- Heart rate = 86 beats/min
- Respirations = 12 breaths/min
- Blood pressure = 129/47 mm Hg
- Oxygen saturation = 96% (on room air)
- Abdominal pain = 8/10 (on a 0 to 10 pain scale)
- Vomiting bile-colored emesis
- Incision clean and intact with wound closure strips
- Urine output 75 mL/hr
- Urine dark yellow-orange
- Finger stick blood glucose (FSBG) = 120 mg/dL (6.7 mmol/L)

Highlight or place a check mark next to the assessment findings that require follow-up by the nurse.

Thinking Exercise 7A-5

A 42-year-old female client was diagnosed with cholecystitis secondary to cholelithiasis and cystic duct obstruction, and underwent a laparoscopic cholecystectomy 2 days ago. The client experiences symptoms of postcholecystectomy syndrome and is diagnosed with a common bile duct leak. The nurse prepares the client for endoscopic retrograde cholangiopancreatography (ERCP). Which actions will the nurse take to prepare the client for this procedure? **Select all that apply.**

_____ A. Do not allow the client anything by mouth for 6 to 8 hours before the procedure.

_____ B. Evaluate the client's intravenous site for patency.

_____ C. Administer ibuprofen and alprazolam to minimize pain and anxiety during the procedure.

_____ D. Ask the client if she is allergic to iodine, shellfish, or contrast media.

_____ E. Remind the client not to drive for at least 12 hours after the procedure.

_____ F. Explain how a cannula will be inserted into the common bile duct and contrast will be injected.

_____ G. Teach the client that she can eat and drink after the procedure once her gag reflex returns.

_____ H. Verify that an informed consent form has been signed by the client.

Exemplar 7B. Peptic Ulcer Disease (Medical-Surgical Nursing: Middle-Age Adult)

Thinking Exercise 7B-1

A 48-year-old female client is admitted to a telemetry unit after a syncopal episode during church service. She is married, has two elementary school children, and works for the public defender's office. Her past medical history includes atrial fibrillation, dyspepsia, chronic back pain, and a recent urinary tract infection. The client denies alcohol or cigarette use and jokes that she is addicted to caffeine. She drinks approximately eight 12-ounce carbonated beverages daily. She provides a list of her current medications, but the list is not complete. **Choose the _most likely_ options for the information missing from the table below by selecting from the lists of options provided.**

Medication	Dose, Route, Frequency	Drug Class	Indication
Warfarin	2.5 mg orally every day	Anticoagulant	1
2	400 mg orally every 6–8 hr as needed for pain	Nonsteroidal anti-inflammatory drug	Chronic back pain
Famotidine	20 mg orally twice a day	3	Gastric acid reflux
Trimethoprim/ sulfamethoxazole	4	Anti-infective agent	Urinary tract infection
Verapamil	40-mg oral extended-release tablet once daily	Calcium channel blocker	5

Options for 1	Options for 2	Options for 3
Atrial fibrillation	Acetaminophen	Antacid
Stroke	Aspirin	$Beta_2$-adrenergic agonist
Coronary artery disease	Ibuprofen	H_2 antagonist
Peripheral vascular disease	Oxycodone	Mucosal protectant
Pulmonary embolism	Prednisone	Proton pump inhibitor

Options for 4	Options for 5
40/200 mg orally three times daily	Angina pectoris
100 mg as a vaginal suppository once daily	Peptic ulcer disease
160/800 mg orally twice daily	Pulmonary edema
350-mg extended release tablet orally once daily	Cirrhosis
400/80 mg as an oral suspension every 6 hr	Urinary retention

Thinking Exercise 7B-2

A 48-year-old female client is admitted to a telemetry unit after a syncopal episode. She is married, has two elementary school children, and works for the public defender's office. Her past medical history includes atrial fibrillation, dyspepsia, chronic back pain, and a recent urinary tract infection. She denies alcohol or cigarette use and jokes that she is addicted to caffeine. She drinks approximately eight 12-ounce carbonated beverages daily. Her home medication list includes warfarin. The client is diagnosed as having probable peptic ulcer disease. The report from the emergency department includes the following assessment data:

- Alert and oriented $\times$ 3
- Speech clear and appropriate
- Heart rate = 104 beats/min
- Atrial fibrillation
- Blood pressure = 99/46 mm Hg
- Oxygen saturation = 94% (on room air)
- Denies dizziness or lightheadedness
- Reports abdominal discomfort
- Stool positive for occult blood and *H. pylori* bacteria
- Hemoglobin = 15 g/dL (150 g/L)
- Hematocrit = 38% (0.38)
- INR = 2.5

Based on the above assessment data, which **priority** questions will the nurse include in an initial assessment? **Select all that apply.**

_____ A. "Are you experiencing burning from your urinary infection?"

_____ B. "How long have you been taking warfarin?"

_____ C. "Does your indigestion keep you from sleeping at night?"

_____ D. "What is the cause of your chronic back pain?"

_____ E. "Have you ever been told that you need to lose weight?"

_____ F. "When did your abdominal discomfort start?"

_____ G. "Did you experience cardiac palpitations or chest pain before you passed out?"

_____ H. "How many meals do you eat every day?"

Thinking Exercise 7B-3

A 48-year-old female client is admitted to a telemetry unit after a syncopal episode. Based on her history and the presence of *H. pylori* bacteria, the client is diagnosed as having probable peptic ulcer disease. Shortly after the nurse completes an initial assessment, the client vomits 300 mL coffee-ground emesis. **Choose the *most likely* options for the information missing from the statement below by selecting from the lists of options provided.**

Massive bleeding from gastric or duodenal ulcers presents as _____1_____, and minimal bleeding from these ulcers can present as _____2_____. If massive upper GI bleeding occurs, the client may experience _____3_____ as a result of _____4_____ and _____5_____. The nurse would administer _____6_____ and _____7_____ as needed, start two large-bore intravenous lines for _____8_____ fluids and _____9_____ replacement, and monitor _____10_____, _____11_____, and _____12_____.

Options for 1 and 2	Options for 3, 4, and 5	Options for 6, 7, 8, and 9	Options for 10, 11, and 12
Anorexia	Angina	Antacid	Creatinine clearance
Chest pain	Coronary artery disease	Blood	Hematocrit
Dyspepsia	Dizziness	Calcium	Intake of fluids
Hematemesis	Dumping syndrome	Chest compressions	Number of visitors
Melena	Hypotension	Hypertonic	Oxygen saturation
Steatorrhea	Indigestion	Hypotonic	Pulmonary congestion
	Nausea	Isotonic	Respiratory rate
	Respiratory distress	Nitroglycerine	Vital signs
	Tachycardia	Oxygen	Vomiting
		Potassium	
		Proton pump inhibitor	
		Respiratory support	

Thinking Exercise 7B-4

A 48-year-old female client is admitted to a telemetry unit after a syncopal episode and is suspected of having peptic ulcer disease. A nasogastric tube connected to low continuous wall suction is placed and drains 100 to 150 mL/hr of coffee-ground secretions from the client's stomach. The primary health care provider schedules an esophagogastroduodenoscopy (EGD). After teaching the client about the procedure, the nurse assesses the client's understanding. **For each client response, use an X to indicate whether the nurse's teaching was Effective (helped the client understand the procedure), Ineffective (did not help the client understand the procedure), or Unrelated (not related to the health teaching about the procedure).**

Client's Response	Effective	Ineffective	Unrelated
"The primary health care provider will explain the procedure to me and answer my questions before I sign the consent form."			
"I will not eat or drink anything for 6 to 8 hours before the procedure, but I will be able to drink water right after it is done."			
"During the procedure a small flexible tube will be inserted into my colon."			
"The procedure is short so I don't have to worry about caffeine withdrawal."			
"My vital signs and breathing will be monitored by a specialized endoscopy nurse during the procedure."			
"This test will allow the primary health care provider to see any ulcers inside my esophagus, my stomach, and the upper part of my intestines."			

Thinking Exercise 7B-5

A 48-year-old female client was admitted to a telemetry unit yesterday after a syncopal episode and is suspected of having peptic ulcer disease. She returns to the telemetry unit after an esophagogastro-duodenoscopy (EGD). **For each nursing action below, use an X to specify whether the action would be** <u>Indicated</u> **(appropriate or necessary),** <u>Contraindicated</u> **(could be harmful), or** <u>Non-Essential</u> **(makes no difference or is not necessary) for the client's care at this time.**

Nursing Action	Indicated	Contraindicated	Non-Essential
Administer throat lozenges as needed for throat discomfort.			
Keep the client NPO until the client's gag reflex returns.			
Discontinue intravenous fluids if the client becomes nauseated and vomits.			
Encourage the spouse to be at the bedside when the sedation is wearing off.			
Monitor vital signs every 30 minutes until the client is fully wake and stable.			
Keep the client in a supine position with the head of the bed lower than 30 degrees.			

Thinking Exercise 7B-6

A 48-year-old female client was admitted to a telemetry unit 4 days ago after a syncopal episode during church services. She is married, has two elementary school children, and works for the public defender's office. Her past medical history includes atrial fibrillation, dyspepsia, chronic back pain, and a recent urinary tract infection. She denies alcohol or cigarette use and jokes that she is addicted to caffeine. She drinks approximately eight 12-ounce carbonated beverages daily. The client had an esophagogas-troduodenoscopy (EGD) 2 days ago and the nasogastric tube was discontinued yesterday. The client's discharge prescriptions include low-dose warfarin, verapamil, and omeprazole. Which of the following instructions will the nurse include in this client's discharge teaching instructions? **Select all that apply.**

_____ A. "Contact your primary health care provider if you experience sharp, sudden, or severe abdominal pain."

_____ B. "Fluids that contain caffeine, such as carbonated beverages, increase stomach acid; you need to decrease your intake of caffeinated beverages."

_____ C. "Keep a journal of stool color, consistency, and frequency, and share this information with your primary health care provider at your follow-up visit."

_____ D. "Certain foods such as tomatoes and onions can help decrease dyspepsia and your risk for future peptic ulcers."

_____ E. "Contact your primary health care provider if you experience muscle cramps or tremors."

_____ F. "Take the prescribed dose of omeprazole 2 hours after each meal for the greatest therapeutic effect."

_____ G. "Stop taking your warfarin until you follow up with your cardiologist to evaluate therapeutic versus adverse effects of continued use."

_____ H. "Talk to your primary health care provider about therapies for your chronic back pain that do not increase your risk for peptic ulcers."

Mobility
Common Health Problems

Exemplar 8A. Fractured Hip/Open Reduction Internal Fixation (Medical-Surgical Nursing: Older Adult)

Thinking Exercise 8A-1

An 80-year-old woman was admitted to the local community hospital following a motor vehicle crash. Her injuries include a left fractured hip, left compound fractured wrist, and multiple contusions and lacerations. The nurse notes that preoperative Buck traction has been applied to the client's left leg with two weights of 5 lb (2.3 kg) each. Her left lower arm has an external fixator to manage the open wound while the fracture heals. **For each nursing action below, use an X to specify whether the action would be <u>Indicated</u> (appropriate or necessary), <u>Contraindicated</u> (could be harmful), or <u>Non-Essential</u> (makes no difference or not necessary) for the client's care at this time.**

Nursing Action	Indicated	Contraindicated	Non-Essential
Remove traction weights when turning the client.			
Assess pin sites of external fixator for signs and symptoms of infection.			
Take the client's temperature every hour.			
Check the cast to ensure that it is not too tight.			
Manage the client's pain with analgesia.			
Assist the client when she is ambulating with her walker.			
Check all traction ropes and knots every shift for intactness.			

Thinking Exercise 8A-2

An 80-year-old woman was admitted to the local community hospital following a motor vehicle crash. Her injuries include a left fractured hip, left compound fractured wrist, and multiple contusions and lacerations. As part of the history and client assessment, the nurse asked her daughter about current medications that her mother is taking. The daughter provides incomplete information. **Choose the *most likely* options for the information missing from the table below by selecting from the lists of options provided.**

Medication	Dose, Route, Frequency	Drug Class	Indication
1	100 mg orally once at bedtime	Nonopioid centrally acting analgesic	Moderate-to-severe back pain and osteoarthritis
Sofosbuvir/velpatasvir	400 mg/100 mg orally once daily	NS5A inhibitor	**2**
Risedronate	5 mg orally once daily	**3**	Osteopenia/osteoporosis
Metoprolol	**4**	Beta blocker	Hypertension
5	20 mg orally twice daily	Sulfonylurea	Diabetes mellitus type 2

Options for 1	Options for 2	Options for 3
gabapentin	GERD	Calcium supplement
morphine	Pancreatitis	Bisphosphonate
tramadol	Stroke	Hyperparathyroidism
naproxen	Gonorrhea	Biguanide
oxycodone	Hepatitis C	Potassium supplement
ibuprofen	Ulcerative colitis	Biologic immune modifier

Options for 4	Options for 5
500 mg orally 3 times daily	Glipizide
5 mg sublingually twice daily	Lovastatin
100 mg orally once daily	Insulin
2 g orally once daily	Metformin
4 mg transdermal patch	Gemfibrozil
twice daily	Prednisone
0.25 mg orally 4 times daily	

Thinking Exercise 8A-3

An 80-year-old woman was admitted to the local community hospital following a motor vehicle crash. Her injuries included a left fractured hip and left compound fractured wrist, which were both surgically repaired 2 days ago. The client is alert and oriented × 3; she gets out of bed to a chair with assistance at least two times a day. The nurse's note from the previous shift includes these comments regarding the client's skin assessment.

> **Nurses' Notes**
>
> 3/16/20   0600
> Client has 1 in (2.2 cm) reddened area on coccyx that does not blanch. Both heels have bluish coloration and feel soft and "mushy." Superficial lacerations on her upper arms and chest are beginning to heal.
>   — L.B. Adams, RN

Which of the following nursing actions are indicated for the client at this time? **Select all that apply.**

_____ A. Teach the assistive personnel to avoid positioning the client in a supine position.

_____ B. Limit the client's time sitting in a chair to no more than 1 hour at a time.

_____ C. While the client is in bed, position her heels to be off of the bed at all times.

_____ D. Teach the client and family to increase her nutritional intake of carbohydrates.

_____ E. Consult with the registered dietitian nutritionist for possible oral nutritional supplement.

_____ F. Obtain a foot board or other device to prevent plantar flexion of her feet.

_____ G. Apply a pressure-reducing mattress overlay for the client's bed.

Thinking Exercise 8A-4

An 80-year-old woman was admitted to the local community hospital following a motor vehicle crash. Her injuries included a left fractured hip and left compound fractured wrist, which were both surgically repaired 3 days ago. The client has been alert and oriented × 3; she gets out of bed to a chair with assistance at least two times a day. The nurse documents these findings as part of the shift assessment:

- Temperature = 100°F (37.8°C)
- Heart rate = 82 beats/min and regular
- Respirations = 22 breaths/min
- Blood pressure = 96/52 mm Hg
- Left hip wound dry and staples intact

- Redness around proximal end of left wrist incision
- Reports feeling unusually tired today
- Drowsy but easily awakened
- States that her pain is currently a 2 (on a 0 to 10 pain intensity scale)

Highlight or place a check mark next to the assessment findings that require follow-up by the nurse.

Thinking Exercise 8A-5

An 84-year-old man who sustained a right fractured hip and right fractured tibia had an open reduction, internal fixation (ORIF) for both fractures. For which of the following **acute** postoperative complications would the nurse monitor while the client is hospitalized? **Select all that apply.**

_____ A. Wound infection

_____ B. Venous thromboembolism

_____ C. Chronic osteomyelitis

_____ D. Acute compartment syndrome

_____ E. Ischemic bone necrosis

_____ F. Fat embolism syndrome

_____ G. Complex regional pain syndrome

_____ H. Skeletal muscle atrophy

Thinking Exercise 8A-6

An 84-year-old man who sustained a right fractured hip and right fractured tibia had an open reduction, internal fixation (ORIF) for both fractures. **Indicate which nursing action listed in the far-left column is appropriate for each potential postoperative complication. Note that not all actions will be used.**

Nursing Action	Potential Postoperative Complication	Appropriate Nursing Action for Postoperative Complication
1 Administer long-term antibiotic therapy.	Acute compartment syndrome	
2 Consult with a specialist to manage pain.	Deep vein thrombosis	
3 Administer IV sodium heparin.	Fat embolism syndrome	
4 Initiate IV fluids and oxygen therapy.	Complex regional pain syndrome	
5 Prepare the client for a fasciotomy.	Chronic osteomyelitis	
6 Remove the cause of the increased pressure, if possible.		
7 Prepare to administer a blood transfusion.		

Exemplar 8B. Fractured Radius and Medial Epicondyle (Pediatric Nursing: Preschool Child)

Thinking Exercise 8B-1

A 3-year-old female client presents to a secondary community-based clinic after reportedly having been involved in a sledding accident with her father. The father provides the child's medical history, which includes a diagnosis of type I osteogenesis imperfecta. The child is visibly upset, crying, guarding her right arm, and repeatedly saying that she wants to go see her mommy. What additional information would the nurse collect regarding the accident? **Select all that apply.**

_____ A. "Where did the accident happen?"

_____ B. "What time did the accident occur?"

_____ C. "Is the child covered under an insurance plan?"

_____ D. "How did the accident happen?"

_____ E. "Has the child had other fractures?"

_____ F. "Were other siblings involved in the accident?"

Thinking Exercise 8B-2

Radiographic results from a 3-year-old child's sledding accident reveal a complete and moderately displaced fracture of the right radius and a fracture of the right medial epicondyle, as well as old fractures that support the child's history of osteogenesis imperfecta. The nursing admission assessment reveals the following results:

- Temperature = 99.1°F (37°C)
- Respirations = 24 breaths/min
- Heart rate = 112 beats/min
- Blood pressure = 99/45 mm Hg
- Child is crying inconsolably with parents at the bedside
- Child points to her right elbow to signify where she hurts the most
- Right forearm is dirty, reddened, and swollen
- Capillary refill of right fingers is <5 sec and left fingers is <3 sec
- Right hand is slightly warm, left hand is very warm to touch
- Radial pulse is noted to be 2+ bilaterally
- Child reports that her right fingers feel like they are being "poked with stickers"
- Abrasions noted to right lower extremity

Highlight or place a check mark next to the assessment findings that require follow-up by the nurse.

Thinking Exercise 8B-3

The nurse is caring for a 3-year-old girl awaiting a procedure to reduce her fractures and cast placement after a sledding accident that resulted in fractures of the right radius and right medial epicondyle. **Choose the *most likely* options for the information missing from the statements below by selecting from the lists of options provided.**

Before the procedure, the nurse will protect the child from further injury by _____1_____ and _____2_____ to promote cooperation from the child. Parental presence throughout the preprocedure and postprocedure periods is an important aspect of providing client-centered care, and the nurse must _____3_____ at every stage. The nurse will use _____4_____ and _____5_____ of the operating suite or procedure unit to provide age-appropriate education to the child. Baseline assessment provides a comparison for postprocedure assessment and should include _____6_____ and _____7_____. The nurse would use the _____8_____ to assess the child's pain level.

Options for 1, 2, and 3	Options for 4, 5, 6, 7, and 8
Instruct the parents on what to expect	Vital signs
Show a video to the child	FLACC scale
Obtain informed consent	Puppets
Providing pain medication	Presence of nausea of vomiting
Applying traction to the right arm	Wong-Baker FACES Scale
Sedating the child	Pictures
Keeping both arms immobilized	Level of consciousness
Provide an iPad to the child	Children's books

Thinking Exercise 8B-4

The nurse is caring for a 3-year-old female client who had fracture reduction and long arm cast placement under deep sedation. The nurse is alert to the various complications associated with fractures, sedation, and cast placement for a preschool child. **Indicate which nursing action listed in the far-left column is appropriate for each potential postprocedure complication. Note that not all actions will be used.**

Nursing Action	Potential Complication	Appropriate Nursing Action for Each Potential Complication
1 Assess for signs of infection.	Circulatory impairment	
2 Encourage diet high in fat and protein.	Nerve impairment	
3 Place protective barrier around the sharp edges on the cast.	Decreased muscle strength	
4 Assess for equality of pulses, color of extremities, difficulty moving fingers, inconsolable crying.	Fracture nonunion	
5 Elevate the head of the bed and provide oxygen as needed.	Skin breakdown	
6 Elevate the right arm for the first 24 hours.		
7 Remove cast and obtain an arteriogram.		
8 Reassure parents that with normal activity the child will regain all mobility.		

Thinking Exercise 8B-5

The nurse is providing client education to the parents of a 3-year-old child following the placement of a synthetic long arm cast to the right arm. Which statement(s) by the parents indicate(s) a **need for additional teaching? Select all that apply.**

_____ A. "I need to call the doctor immediately for any severe pain that is unrelieved by analgesics."

_____ B. "I will encourage safer activities for my child to participate in."

_____ C. "I will give my child ibuprofen with a snack to prevent upset stomach."

_____ D. "I will apply heat to the outside of the cast to relieve pain, itching, and swelling."

_____ E. "I will put moleskin on the cast around the edges to protect her skin."

_____ F. "I will keep my child in bed for the next few days until she feels better."

_____ G. "I will be sure to elevate the right arm for the next 72 hours."

_____ H. "I will notify my primary health care provider if my child runs a fever or a foul odor is present from the cast."

_____ I. "I won't have to worry about keeping the cast dry because it is waterproof."

Thinking Exercise 8B-6

A mother brings her 3-year-old daughter to the pediatric orthopedics office for a 4-week follow-up visit for repeat radiographs of her right arm and to evaluate whether to remove the cast or reapply it for another 2 weeks. **For each assessment finding, use an X to indicate whether the intervention was Effective (helped to meet expected outcomes), Ineffective (did not help to meet expected outcomes), or Unrelated (not related to the expected outcomes).**

Assessment Finding	Effective	Ineffective	Unrelated
Radiograph of right radius displays extensive callus formation.			
Easily consoled by mother, but still hesitant with health care workers.			
Denies difficulty with urination.			
Radial pulses are 3+ and equal bilaterally.			
Difficulty bending right arm at the wrist and elbow.			
Small reddened, blistered area on the inner aspect of the right upper arm.			
Capillary refill is <3 sec in lower extremities.			
Mother reports that pain is well controlled with hydrocodone/acetaminophen elixir.			

Exemplar 8C. Osteoarthritis/Total Knee Arthroplasty (Medical-Surgical Nursing: Middle-Age Adult)

Thinking Exercise 8C-1

A 55-year-old woman has a long history of osteoarthritis (OA) in both knees, ankles, and feet owing to obesity and her job, which requires long periods of standing. She has been taking acetaminophen and ibuprofen for many years and states that her pain has continued to worsen. Both of her knees are very swollen, and the left knee is red and warm. Her primary health care provider plans to prescribe laboratory testing to determine if she also has rheumatoid arthritis. Which of the following nursing actions are appropriate for the client at this time? **Select all that apply.**

_____ A. Teach the client to use ice on her knees to decrease inflammation.

_____ B. Refer the client to an occupational therapist.

_____ C. Refer the client to a physical therapist.

_____ D. Tell the client to request an opioid analgesic from her primary health care provider.

_____ E. Remind the client to elevate her legs as often as possible to decrease swelling.

_____ F. Suggest that the client consider changing her job to one that allows her to sit more often.

_____ G. Refer the client to a registered dietitian nutritionist for a weight reduction plan.

Thinking Exercise 8C-2

A 55-year-old woman has a long history of osteoarthritis (OA) in both knees, ankles, and feet due to obesity and her job, which requires long periods of standing. She is scheduled for a left total knee arthroplasty next month. What preoperative health teaching by the nurse is appropriate for the client in preparation for this surgery? **Select all that apply.**

_____ A. "You will need to shower with a special solution the night prior to your surgery."

_____ B. "The physical therapist will teach you about postoperative leg exercises and how to ambulate with a walker."

_____ C. "You will need an elevated toilet to prevent you from bending your knees."

_____ D. "You will be on a blood thinner to prevent blood clots in your legs and lungs."

_____ E. "After surgery you will be placed on pain medication and a cold application for your surgical knee."

_____ F. "You should only be in the hospital after surgery for a few days."

_____ G. "Although not as common today, you may have a surgical drain near your incision that will be removed before hospital discharge."

_____ H. "When you progress to walking with a cane, use it on the affected surgical side."

Thinking Exercise 8C-3

A 55-year-old woman returns from the PACU after a left total knee arthroplasty. During surgery she had epidural anesthesia and is currently receiving patient-controlled analgesia (PCA) morphine for surgical pain, gabapentin, and acetaminophen. The client has a long history of osteoarthritis (OA) in both knees, ankles, and feet due to obesity and her job, which requires long periods of standing. The nurse notes the following assessment findings:

- Has no history of chronic health problems except OA
- Small amount of serosanguineous drainage present on surgical dressing
- Reports left knee pain of 6/10 on a 0 to 10 pain intensity scale
- Drowsy but arouses easily
- Reports that her legs and feet feel "heavy and numb"
- Reports "frequent waves of nausea"

Highlight or place a check mark next to the assessment findings that require follow-up by the nurse.

Thinking Exercise 8C-4

A 55-year-old woman returns from the PACU after a left total knee arthroplasty. During surgery she had epidural anesthesia and is currently receiving patient-controlled analgesia (PCA) morphine for surgical pain and acetaminophen for chronic joint pain. **Choose the _most likely_ options for the information missing from the table below by selecting from the lists of options provided.**

The nurse should monitor postoperative clients who have a total knee arthroplasty under epidural anesthesia for common complications that can occur during their hospital stay, including _____1_____ and _____2_____. Nursing interventions that can help prevent these complications are to _____3_____, _____4_____, and _____5_____.

Options for 1 and 2	Options for 3, 4, and 5
Respiratory infection	Encourage fluids
Venous thromboembolism	Administer a stool softener
Intestinal obstruction	Maintain an abduction pillow or device
Surgical knee dislocation	Ambulate the client early
Urinary retention	Administer an anticoagulant
Anemia	Refer to respiratory therapy

Thinking Exercise 8C-5

A 55-year-old woman had a left total knee arthroplasty 2 days ago. The nurse is planning to provide health teaching for the client in preparation for her discharge. **Use an X to indicate whether the health teachings below are Indicated (appropriate or necessary), Contraindicated (could be harmful), or Non-Essential (makes no difference or not necessary) before the client's discharge at this time.**

Health Teaching	Indicated	Contraindicated	Non-Essential
"Use the prescribed ambulatory aid such as a walker."			
"Use assistive/adaptive devices as needed (e.g., sock aids, shoehorns, dressing sticks, extenders)."			
"Do not put more weight on your affected leg than allowed and instructed."			
"Use heat as needed to the operative hip to decrease pain and promote healing."			
"Do not bend your hips more than 90 degrees."			
"Follow up with all physical therapy appointments as prescribed."			
"Inspect your surgical incision every day for increased redness, heat, or drainage; if any of these are present, call your surgeon immediately."			

Thinking Exercise 8C-6

A 55-year-old woman who had a left total knee arthroplasty has a follow-up appointment with the surgeon 6 weeks after surgery. The client has a long history of osteoarthritis (OA) in both knees, ankles, and feet due to obesity and her job, which requires long periods of standing. The office nurse interviews the client and performs a previsit assessment. **For each assessment finding, use an X to indicate whether the intervention was Effective (helped to meet expected outcomes), Ineffective (did not help to meet expected outcomes), or Unrelated (not related to the expected outcomes).**

Assessment Finding	Effective	Ineffective	Unrelated
Incision shows no sign of infection.			
Reports increased pain in her right (nonsurgical) knee.			
Surgical knee flexion is 110 degrees.			
Cannot straighten surgical leg.			
Reports having periods of insomnia.			
Surgical knee is less bruised and mildly swollen.			

Exemplar 8D. Parkinson Disease (Medical-Surgical Nursing/Mental Health Nursing: Older Adult)

Thinking Exercise 8D-1

A 71-year-old male client with moderate to late-stage Parkinson disease is admitted from home to the hospital with new-onset orthostatic hypotension and occasional dysphagia. On admission the nurse notes the following assessment findings:
- Lives at home with his wife who cares for him
- Needs assistance with ADLs on days when his rigidity is worse
- Walks short distances in the house using a walker
- Is alert and oriented × 3
- Has resting tremors in both arms and hands, but right hand is worse than the left (client is right-handed)
- Chokes at times when he eats
- Has fallen twice in the past week because of dizziness when he stands from a sitting or lying position

- Temperature = 98°F (36.7°C)
- Apical pulse = 76 beats/min and regular
- Blood pressure = 100/64 mm Hg (in supine position)
- States that he is not in pain

Highlight or place a check mark next to the assessment findings that require follow-up by the nurse.

Thinking Exercise 8D-2

A 71-year-old male client with moderate to late-stage Parkinson disease is admitted from home to the hospital with new-onset orthostatic hypotension and occasional dysphagia. His wife cares for him at home and provides an incomplete list of the client's medications. **Choose the *most likely* options for the information missing from the drug table by selecting from the lists of options provided.**

Medication	Dose, Route, Frequency	Drug Class	Indication
Levodopa/carbidopa	200 mg levodopa/50 mg carbidopa orally 1 tablet 4 times daily	Dopamine replacement	**1**
Baclofen	20 mg orally 3 times daily	Centrally acting muscle relaxant	**2**
Entacapone	200 mg orally 4 times daily	**3**	Parkinson disease
Venlafaxine XR	**4**	Serotonin-norepinephrine reuptake inhibitor (SNRI)	Depression
5	10 mg orally every evening at bedtime	Sedative-hypnotic	Insomnia/promotion of sleep

Options for 1	Options for 2	Options for 3
Muscle atrophy	Peripheral neuropathy	Antiviral agent
Parkinson disease	Pain	Antibacterial agent
Hypertension	Muscle spasticity	Loop diuretic
Bladder incontinence	Anorexia	Beta blocker
Dementia	Cardiac conduction	Anxiolytic agent
Delirium	Nausea and vomiting	COMT inhibitor

Options for 4	Options for 5
250 mg orally 3 times daily	Zolpidem
5 mg sublingually twice daily	Diazepam
100 mg via nasal spray 4 times a day	Nortriptyline
75 mg orally once daily	Oxybutynin
2-mg transdermal patch once daily	Naloxone
125 mg orally 4 times a day	Lorazepam

Thinking Exercise 8D-3

A 71-year-old male client with moderate to late-stage Parkinson disease is admitted from home to the hospital with new-onset orthostatic hypotension and occasional dysphagia. According to his wife, he needs assistance with ADLs on days when his rigidity is worse, and walks short distances in the house using a walker. **Choose the *most likely* options for the information missing from the statement below by selecting from the list of options provided. Note that not all options will be used.**

Because of the client's orthostatic hypotension and dysphagia, he is currently *most likely* at risk for _____ and _____. During his hospital stay, he is also *most likely* at risk for complications associated with impaired mobility, especially _____ and _____.

Options
Stroke
Pressure injury
Aspiration
Falling
Constipation
Urinary incontinence
Bleeding
Diabetes mellitus

Thinking Exercise 8D-4

A 71-year-old male client with moderate to late-stage Parkinson disease is admitted from home to the hospital with new-onset orthostatic hypotension and occasional dysphagia. According to his wife, he needs assistance with ADLs only on days when his rigidity is worse, and walks short distances in the house using a walker. Which of the following actions would the nurse take? **Select all that apply.**

_____ A. Consult with the speech-language pathologist for a swallowing evaluation.

_____ B. Remind the client and wife to call for nursing staff to help the client out of bed.

_____ C. Obtain a prescription for a different antihypertensive medication.

_____ D. Place the client on the hospital's fall precautions protocol.

_____ E. Refer the client for physical and occupational therapy evaluations.

_____ F. Place the client on a liquid diet to prevent choking.

_____ G. Remind the nursing staff to place the client in a sitting position during meals.

_____ H. Perform frequent orthostatic blood pressure checks.

Thinking Exercise 8D-5

A 71-year-old male client with moderate to late-stage Parkinson disease was admitted from home to the hospital yesterday with new-onset orthostatic hypotension and occasional dysphagia. This evening he says he has been "seeing things" in the room that he realized later that were not present. He states he has had the "visions" for over a month and they make him anxious and scared. **Use an X to indicate whether the nursing actions listed below are <u>Indicated</u> (appropriate or necessary), <u>Contraindicated</u> (could be harmful), or <u>Non-Essential</u> (make no difference or are not necessary) for the client's care at this time.**

Nursing Action	Indicated	Contraindicated	Non-Essential
Focus on reality and not the hallucination experience.			
Place the client in the least restrictive restraints.			
Request a prescription for pimavanserin.			
Refer the client to a mental health professional.			
Make eye contact if culturally appropriate.			
Document the client's report of hallucinations.			

Metabolism
Common Health Problems

Thinking Exercise 9A-1

A 46-year-old female client who was diagnosed with an upper respiratory infection yesterday and prescribed an antibiotic presents to the emergency department (ED) reporting, "I just don't feel right." The client has a history of diabetes mellitus type 2, hypertension, peripheral neuropathy, vascular disease, and retinopathy. She provides an incomplete list of home medications to the nurse. **Choose the most likely options for the information missing from the table by selecting from the lists of options provided.**

Medication	Dose, Route, Frequency	Drug Class	Drug Action
1	500-mg oral extended-release tablet once daily with evening meal	Biguanide	Decreases glucose production by the liver and increases tissue response to insulin
Aspirin	2	Salicylate	Minimizes platelet aggregation
Metoprolol	25-mg oral extended-release tablet once daily	Beta-adrenergic blocker	3
Exenatide	5-mcg subcutaneous injection twice daily before breakfast and dinner	4	Slows gastric emptying, stimulates insulin release, suppresses glucagon release, and reduces appetite
Glipizide	10 mg orally once daily with breakfast	Second-generation sulfonylurea	5
6	300 mg orally once daily before bed	Antiepileptic drug	Relieves neuropathic pain

Options for 1	Options for 2	Options for 3
Rosiglitazone	2.5 mg orally three times daily with meals	Blocks glucose synthesis
Glyburide	10 mg sublingually, may repeat in 15 minutes	Decreases atherosclerosis in peripheral blood vessels
Insulin regular	81 mg orally once daily	Treatment for angina
Sitagliptin	325 mg orally twice daily	Increases production of insulin from beta cells
Metformin	400-mg gel cap every 6–8 hr as needed	Reduces blood pressure
Empagliflozin	650 mg orally once daily at night	Decreases serum cholesterol
Insulin degludec		

Options for 4	Options for 5	Options for 6
Amylin mimetic	Delays emptying of gastric contents	Acetaminophen
Anticholinergic	Improves neurologic conductivity in the eye	Gabapentin
Dopamine agonist	Increases glucose production by the liver	Ibuprofen
Incretin mimetic	Promotes insulin secretion by the pancreas	Phenytoin
Thiazolidinedione	Treats hypoglycemia	Valproic acid
Calcium channel blocker	Prevents infection	Lisinopril

Thinking Exercise 9A-2

A 46-year-old woman who was diagnosed with an upper respiratory infection yesterday and prescribed an antibiotic presents to the ED reporting, "I just don't feel right." The client has a history of diabetes mellitus type 2, hypertension, peripheral neuropathy, vascular disease, and retinopathy. Initial nursing shift assessment and findings include:

- Alert and oriented
- Productive cough
- Serum blood glucose = 486 mg/dL (27.1 mmol/L)
- Hemoglobin A_{1c} = 6.8%
- Serum potassium = 3.5 mEq/L (3.5 mmol/L)
- Rhinitis with pale yellow, thick drainage
- Reports urinating multiple times every hour
- Burning pain from bilateral toes to mid-calves

Highlight or place a check mark next to the assessment findings that require follow-up by the nurse.

Thinking Exercise 9A-3

A 46-year-old woman who was diagnosed with an upper respiratory infection yesterday and prescribed an antibiotic presents to the ED, reporting "I just don't feel right." The client has a history of diabetes mellitus type 2, hypertension, peripheral neuropathy, vascular disease, and retinopathy. While in the ED the client becomes confused. Laboratory tests are prescribed with the following results:

- Serum glucose = 590 mg/dL (32.9 mmol/L)
- Serum osmolality = 340 mOsm/kg (340 mmol/kg)
- Serum ketones = Negative
- Serum pH = 7.43
- Blood urea nitrogen (BUN) = 50 mg/dL (18.1 mmol/L)
- Serum creatinine = 2 mg/dL (176 mcmol/L)

The primary health care provider prescribed 0.45% normal saline to be infused at 1 L/hr for 2 hours, then 200 mL/hr. **Choose the *most likely* options for the information missing from the text below by selecting from the lists of options provided.**

Priority treatment for a hyperglycemic-hyperosmolar state is fluid replacement. When administering large volumes of fluids, the nurse assesses for complications. _____1_____ can result from a large fluid volume shift from extracellular to intracellular spaces faster than brain cells can adapt. This complication presents as changes in _____2_____, changes in _____2_____, and _____2_____. Clients with heart failure are at risk for _____1_____, which manifests as _____2_____.

Options for 1	Options for 2
Cerebral edema	Angina
Coronary artery occlusion	Facial symmetry
Fluid overload	Hypotension
Stroke	Level of consciousness
Traumatic brain injury	Lower extremity mobility
GI bleeding	Pulmonary congestion
Chronic kidney disease	Pupil size, shape, or reaction
Diabetes insipidus	Seizure activity
	Urinary incontinence

Thinking Exercise 9A-4

A 46-year-old woman who was diagnosed with an upper respiratory infection yesterday and prescribed an antibiotic presents to the ED reporting, "I just don't feel right." The client has a history of diabetes mellitus type 2, hypertension, peripheral neuropathy, vascular disease, and retinopathy. On admission to a medical-surgical unit, the nurse implements a plan of care to prevent complications and maintain client safety while in the hospital. **Indicate which nursing action listed in the far-left column is appropriate to prevent each complication of diabetes mellitus and maintain client safety while in the hospital. Note that not all actions will be used.**

Nursing Action	Potential Complication	Appropriate Nursing Action for Each Complication
1 Teach the client to rise slowly from the bed.	Injury secondary to visual disturbances	
2 Coordinate meal-time insulin with food delivery and consumption.	Orthostatic hypotension	
3 Administer intravenous 5%D/NS at 200 mL/hr.	Renal insufficiency	
4 Ensure the path to the bathroom is well lit.	Hypoglycemia	
5 Assist the client in putting on nonslip socks.		
6 Administer 1 mg glucagon IM PRN for blood glucose 70–90 mg/dL (3.9–5.0 mmol/L).		
7 Administer angiotensin-converting enzyme (ACE) inhibitor as prescribed.		
8 Encourage the client to drink 240 mL of sugar-free liquids every hour.		

Thinking Exercise 9A-5

A 46-year-old female client admitted to the medical-surgical nursing unit for hyperglycemic-hyperosmolar state (HHS) has a history of diabetes mellitus type 2, hypertension, peripheral neuropathy, vascular disease, and retinopathy. The primary health care provider prescribed regular subcutaneous insulin with a sliding scale dose to be administered with meals and prior to bedtime. This morning the client's finger stick blood glucose level was 205 mg/dL (11.4 mmol/L) and the nurse administered insulin per the sliding scale below at 7:15 a.m. (0715).

Finger Stick Blood Glucose (mg/dL [mmol/L])	Regular Subcutaneous Insulin (units)
<150 (<8.3)	0
151–200 (8.4–11.1)	3
201–250 (11.2–13.9)	5
251–300 14.0–16/6)	8
301–350 (16.7–19.6)	10
351–400 (19.7–22.2)	12
>400	15

A dietary aide delivers the client's breakfast tray at 8:00 a.m. (0800) and immediately requests the nurse to the client's bedside. The nurse completes a focused assessment with the following results:

- Confused but follows simple commands
- Skin cool and clammy
- Tachycardia
- Reports vision is blurry

Use an X to indicate whether the nursing actions listed below are <u>Indicated</u> (appropriate or necessary), <u>Contraindicated</u> (could be harmful), or <u>Non-Essential</u> (make no difference or are not necessary) for the client's care at this time.

Nursing Action	Indicated	Contraindicated	Non-Essential
Help the client to drink 120 mL of fruit juice.			
Obtain the client's blood glucose level.			
Administer subcutaneous insulin per the sliding scale.			
Notify the primary health care provider.			
Initiate oxygen therapy per nasal cannula.			
Administer 1 mg intramuscular glucagon.			
Reassess glucose level 15 minutes after treatment.			

Thinking Exercise 9A-6

A 46-year-old woman presented to the emergency department several days ago with a respiratory infection that caused a hyperglycemic-hyperosmolar event. The client has a history of diabetes mellitus type 2, hypertension, peripheral neuropathy, vascular disease, and retinopathy. The nurse prepares to discharge the client today. After providing discharge instructions, the nurse assesses the client's understanding. **For each client statement, use an X to indicate whether the nurse's discharge instructions were <u>Effective</u> (helped the client understand the discharge instructions), <u>Ineffective</u> (did not help the client understand the discharge instructions), or <u>Unrelated</u> (not related to the discharge teachings).**

Client's Statements	Effective	Ineffective	Unrelated
"I will wash my feet, dry them thoroughly, and wear clean socks every day."			
"My antidiabetic medications allow me to eat whatever I desire."			
"I will take my glyburide dose with my first bite of breakfast."			
"It is okay for me to walk barefooted while inside my home."			
"I will weigh myself at the same time and on the same scale each day."			
"I will make sure that I take my antidiabetic medications even when I am sick."			

Exemplar 9B. Hyperthyroidism/Thyroidectomy (Medical-Surgical Nursing: Middle-Age Adult)

Thinking Exercise 9B-1

A 40-year-old female client has a family history of "thyroid problems" and is being seen by the primary health care provider for unintentional weight loss, irritability, and chest discomfort. Her probable diagnosis is hyperthyroidism, which the primary health care provider plans to confirm by laboratory testing. What additional physical assessment findings would the nurse expect to be present in this client? **Select all that apply.**

_____ A. Bradycardia

_____ B. Heat intolerance

_____ C. Hypotension

_____ D. Diaphoresis

_____ E. Anorexia

_____ F. Constipation

_____ G. Insomnia

_____ H. Decreased deep tendon reflexes

Thinking Exercise 9B-2

A 40-year-old female client has a family history of "thyroid problems" and is being seen by the primary health care provider for unintentional weight loss, irritability, and chest discomfort. Her probable diagnosis is non-Graves hyperthyroidism. Which serum laboratory test results support this client's probable diagnosis? **Select all that apply.**

_____ A. Increased calcium

_____ B. Increased total thyroxine

_____ C. Increased parathyroid hormone

_____ D. Increased thyroid-stimulating hormone

_____ E. Decreased phosphorus

_____ F. Decreased vitamin D_3

_____ G. Increased potassium

Thinking Exercise 9B-3

A 40-year-old female client has a family history of "thyroid problems" and is being seen by the primary health care provider for unintentional weight loss, irritability, and chest discomfort. Her primary health care provider prescribes methimazole for laboratory-confirmed hyperthyroidism. **Choose the _most likely_ options for the information missing from the statements below by selecting from the list of options provided.**

The nurse teaches the client about the common side effects of methimazole, which include signs and symptoms of _____. This drug can also cause adverse drug effects such as _____ and therefore should not be prescribed for women who are _____ _____.

Options
Taking an oral contraceptive
Hyperparathyroidism
Birth defects
Pregnant
Hypothyroidism
Infection
Liver toxicity

Thinking Exercise 9B-4

A 40-year-old female client has laboratory-confirmed hyperthyroidism that has not responded to drug therapy. As a result, she had a total thyroidectomy this morning. In planning for the client's care, the nurse anticipates possible surgical complications. **Indicate which nursing action listed in the far-left column is appropriate for each potential postoperative thyroidectomy complication. Note that not all actions will be used.**

Nursing Action	Potential Postoperative Complication	Appropriate Nursing Action for Each Postoperative Complication
1 Increase IV fluids and call the Rapid Response Team.	Acute respiratory distress	
2 Monitor the client every 2 hours and reassure the client that the problem is temporary.	Bleeding	
3 Start oxygen therapy immediately, suction if needed, and notify the Rapid Response Team.	Parathyroid gland injury	
4 Assess for signs of calcium deficiency and give IV calcium gluconate if needed.	Laryngeal nerve damage	
5 Prepare the client for additional surgery.	Thyroid storm	
6 Administer propranolol and corticosteroids and apply a cooling blanket.		
7 Prepare to administer an albumin transfusion.		

Thinking Exercise 9B-5

A 40-year-old woman had a total thyroidectomy for hyperthyroidism after medical management was not successful. The nurse is preparing to teach the client about her thyroid hormone replacement (levothyroxine). Which health teaching will the nurse include about this drug? **Select all that apply.**

_____ A. "You will only need to take the drug for about 3 to 6 months."

_____ B. "You will need to get frequent laboratory tests to monitor your thyroid hormone levels."

_____ C. "There are very few side effects of levothyroxine."

_____ D. "Don't take more of the drug than prescribed to prevent hyperthyroidism symptoms."

_____ E. "Check with your primary health care provider if you take any other medication or herb."

_____ F. "Some drugs may increase or decrease the absorption of levothyroxine."

_____ G. "Let your primary health care provider know if you have increased energy."

Cellular Regulation
Breast Cancer

Exemplar 10. Breast Cancer (Medical-Surgical Nursing: Middle-Age Adult)

Thinking Exercise 10-1

A 52-year-old postmenopausal woman is concerned about her risk for breast cancer. Her mother and sister had the disease and were found to be *BRCA2* positive. What additional factors may place the client at risk for breast cancer and should be part of the nurse's health teaching? **Select all that apply.**

_____ A. Advanced age

_____ B. Malnutrition

_____ C. Alcohol consumption

_____ D. Female gender

_____ E. Nulliparity (no pregnancies)

_____ F. Ashkenazi Jewish heritage

_____ G. Late menopause

_____ H. Recent hormone replacement therapy

Thinking Exercise 10-2

A 52-year-old postmenopausal woman is at high risk for developing breast cancer. The nurse teaches the client about the evidence-based guidelines for breast cancer screening and management. **Choose the *most likely* options for the information missing from the statements below by selecting from the lists of options provided.**

The client should practice _____1_____ and have annual _____1_____. A _____1_____ should be performed by the primary health care provider as part of regular annual health examinations. Options for reducing the client's risk for breast cancer include _____2_____, _____2_____, and _____2_____.

Options for 1	Options for 2
Genetic testing	Vaginal hysterectomy
Breast self-awareness	Prophylactic mastectomy
Mammography	Prophylactic oophorectomy
Breast MRI screening	Antiestrogen drug therapy
Bone density scan	Breast reduction
Clinical breast examination	Testosterone replacement

Thinking Exercise 10-3

A 55-year-old postmenopausal woman discovers a lump in her left breast. A breast biopsy reveals a tumor that is classified as *HER2* positive. As a result, the client chose to have a left mastectomy with breast reconstruction. She returns from the PACU with a Jackson-Pratt (JP) drain and large intact surgical dressing. **Use an X to indicate whether the nursing actions below are __Indicated__ (appropriate or necessary), __Contraindicated__ (could be harmful), or __Non-Essential__ (make no difference or are not necessary) for the client's care at this time.**

Nursing Action	Indicated	Contraindicated	Non-Essential
Apply oxygen therapy at 2 L/min.			
Monitor the amount and color of the JP drainage.			
Teach the staff to avoid taking blood pressures or drawing blood in the affected arm.			
Keep the client's head of the bed flat at all times.			
Elevate the affected arm on a pillow.			
Assess the surgical dressing for bleeding.			
Keep the client in bed for at least 48 hours.			
Begin teaching the client about how to perform postmastectomy exercises.			

Thinking Exercise 10-4

A 55-year-old postmenopausal female client who had a left mastectomy with breast reconstruction returns to the surgeon's office for a 6-week follow-up appointment. **For each assessment finding, use an X to indicate whether the interventions were __Effective__ (helped to meet expected outcomes), __Ineffective__ (did not help to meet expected outcomes), or __Unrelated__ (not related to the expected outcomes).**

Assessment Finding	Effective	Ineffective	Unrelated
Mastectomy and reconstruction incisions show no sign of infection			
Reports an inability to straighten her left elbow			
States that she occasionally feels sad			
Mastectomy and reconstruction incisions are healed without redness or drainage			
Left arm is very swollen and much larger than the right arm			
Reports frequent heart palpitations when she drinks caffeinated beverages			

Thinking Exercise 10-5

A 48-year-old female client chose breast-conserving surgery and whole-breast external beam radiation therapy for her early-stage breast cancer. What health teaching would the nurse include when preparing the client for this therapy? **Select all that apply.**

_____ A. "Keep away from children while receiving therapy because you will be radioactive."

_____ B. "Avoid exposing the irradiated skin to sun to prevent burning for at least a year."

_____ C. "Do not wash off the temporary ink markings until radiation therapy is completed."

_____ D. "Use mild soap and water to clean the irradiated area during therapy."

_____ E. "Be aware that radiation may cause fatigue and changes in appetite or taste."

_____ F. "You might want to purchase a wig because of the permanent hair loss that is expected."

_____ G. "Report esophageal burning or feeling like food is 'sticking' after it is swallowed."

Thinking Exercise 10-6

A 58-year-old postmenopausal female client who had breast surgery for invasive cancer is preparing to begin chemotherapy that includes doxorubicin, cyclophosphamide, and paclitaxel (AC-T therapy). **Choose the *most likely* options for the information missing from the statements below by selecting from the lists of options provided.**

The nurse would teach the client that doxorubicin, cyclophosphamide, and paclitaxel can cause _____1_____ toxicity. Therefore the client should report _____2_____ and _____3_____ to the primary health care provider immediately. In addition, all three chemotherapeutic drugs can cause _____4_____, which places the client at risk for _____5_____ and _____5_____.

Options for 1	Options for 2 and 3
Liver	Jaundice
Skin	Pruritus
Cardiac	Shortness of breath
Neurologic	Memory loss
Muscle	Edema
Vascular	Fever
	Paresis

Options for 4	Options for 5
Infection	Fever
Diabetes mellitus	Infection
Peptic ulcer disease	Clotting
Bone marrow suppression	Bleeding
Gangrene	Dyspnea
Stroke	Dysrhythmias
	Perforation

Thinking Exercise 11A-1

A 25-year-old female client experienced remission of her Crohn's disease for the past 2 years. She is a single mother of two small children and finds that she needs to go to bed at night when her children do because of increasing fatigue. Today she presents to the emergency department (ED) with reports of frequent diarrhea, severe abdominal pain, and low-grade fever. She is admitted to the hospital to rule out potentially life-threatening complications and to manage her chronic disease. **Indicate which nursing action listed in the far-left column is appropriate for each potential complication. Note that not all actions will be used.**

Nursing Action	Potential Complication	Appropriate Nursing Action for Each Complication
1 Administer blood or blood products via a large-bore IV catheter.	Enteroenteric fistula	
2 Observe stool for undigested food or undissolved medication.	Small bowel obstruction	
3 Administer IV sodium heparin.	Lower GI bleeding	
4 Monitor client for hematemesis.	Malabsorption	
5 Monitor for signs and symptoms of irritable bowel syndrome.		
6 Insert a nasogastric tube and connect to suction.		
7 Administer antibiotic therapy.		

Thinking Exercise 11A-2

A 25-year-old female client with Crohn's disease was admitted to the hospital yesterday to rule out potentially life-threatening complications and to manage her chronic disease. Selected client assessment findings on admission and this morning are listed below.

Assessment	Assessment Findings on Admission 24 Hours Ago	Current Assessment Findings
Temperature	100°F (37.8°C)	101.8°F (38.8°C)
Heart rate	78 beats/min	82 beats/min
Blood pressure	128/76 mm Hg	124/72 mm Hg
White blood cell count	9200/mm³ (9.2 × 10⁹/L)	13,500/mm³ (13.5 × 10⁹/L)
Sodium	138 mEq/L (138 mmol/L)	133 mEq/L (133 mmol/L)
Potassium	3.6 mEq/L (3.6 mmol/L)	3.2 mEq/L (3.2 mmol/L)

Highlight or place a check mark next to the assessment findings that require follow-up by the nurse.

Thinking Exercise 11A-3

A 25-year-old female client with Crohn's disease was admitted to the hospital 2 days ago to rule out potentially life-threatening complications and to manage her chronic disease. She was diagnosed as having lower GI bleeding this morning. **Use an X to indicate whether the nursing actions below are Indicated (appropriate or necessary), Contraindicated (could be harmful), or Non-Essential (make no difference or are not necessary) for the client's care at this time.**

Nursing Action	Indicated	Contraindicated	Non-Essential
Monitor the client's hemoglobin and hematocrit levels.			
Prepare to administer a blood or blood product transfusion.			
Decrease the rate of the IV infusion.			
Prepare the client for a GI bleeding scan.			
Monitor pulse and blood pressure frequently.			
Document the number of the client's daily stools.			

Thinking Exercise 11A-4

A 25-year-old female client with Crohn's disease was admitted to the hospital to rule out potentially life-threatening complications and to manage her chronic disease. Today the assistive personnel (AP) reported that the client has foul drainage from an open area on her lower abdomen. On closer inspection, the nurse finds that the client developed an enterocutaneous fistula from her small bowel to her skin. Which nursing actions are indicated for her care at this time? **Select all that apply.**

_____ A. Apply a skin barrier and pouch to collect drainage and protect the surrounding skin.

_____ B. Consult with the registered dietitian nutritionist to increase the client's caloric intake.

_____ C. Monitor the client for signs and symptoms of sepsis to prevent septic shock.

_____ D. Ensure that the staff takes daily weights in the morning using the same scale.

_____ E. Monitor fluid and electrolyte balance to identify dehydration or electrolyte imbalances.

_____ F. For copious fistula drainage, apply negative-pressure wound therapy.

_____ G. Provide oral enteral supplements to increase protein intake.

_____ H. Administer IV antibiotic therapy as prescribed.

Thinking Exercise 11A-5

A 25-year-old female client with Crohn's disease was admitted to the hospital to rule out potentially life-threatening complications and to manage her chronic disease. Her drug therapy regimen is being re-evaluated and changed to better control her disease. **Choose the *most likely* options for the information missing from the table by selecting from the lists of options provided.**

Medication	Dose, Route, Frequency	Drug Class	Indication
Sulfasalazine	2 g orally each day	5-ASA drug	**1**
Infliximab	5 mg/kg IV at 0, 2, and 6 weeks followed by maintenance infusions of 5 mg/kg every 8 weeks	**2**	Decreases inflammatory and immune response
Ciprofloxacin XR	500 mg orally each day	**3**	Manages infection
Methotrexate	**4**	Immunosuppressant	Decreases disease activity
5	750 mg orally 3 times a day	Antibiotic	Manages infection

Options for 1	Options for 2	Options for 3
Manages infection	Nonsteroidal anti-inflammatory drug (NSAID)	Calcium channel blocker
Decreases inflammatory response	Corticosteroid	Macrolide
Reduces fever	Biologic response modifier	Antihistamine
Decreases diarrheal stools	Antidiarrheal agent	Biguanide
Manages refractory disease	Antipyretic drug	Fluoroquinolone
Decreases pain	Anticholinergic drug	Aminoglycoside

Options for 4	Options for 5
200 mg/mL subcutaneously once daily	Doxycycline
200 mg orally once daily	Metronidazole
150 mg topically twice daily	Azithromycin
25 mg orally once weekly	Linezolid
10 mg orally once daily	Gentamicin
1 g by infusion once daily	Trimethoprim

Thinking Exercise 11A-6

A 46-year-old male client who has had a long history of Crohn's disease was recently diagnosed with colon cancer. Yesterday afternoon he had a colectomy and creation of a permanent colostomy and is receiving patient-controlled analgesia (PCA) to manage pain. Which nursing assessment findings will the nurse report **immediately** to the primary health care provider? **Select all that apply.**

_____ A. Colostomy has no effluent (drainage).

_____ B. Colostomy stoma is dark red-purplish.

_____ C. The nasogastric tube is draining a small amount of yellowish-green effluent.

_____ D. The client reports pain of 8/10 on a 0 to 10 pain intensity scale.

_____ E. The client states he is anxious about caring for the new ostomy.

_____ F. The colostomy stoma is slightly swollen with a small amount of bleeding.

_____ G. The colostomy stoma protrudes about ¾ in (2 cm) from the abdominal wall.

Exemplar 11B. Appendicitis/Appendectomy (Pediatric Nursing: Late School-Age Child)

Thinking Exercise 11B-1

The nurse is caring for a 10-year-old male client who was admitted to the hospital with report of acute pain in the lower right abdomen. His parents are Spanish speaking only. The interpreter reports that the child complained of pain "a few days" ago, but the pain subsided until today. His parents also report that the child is up-to-date on his immunizations and had a tonsillectomy and ear tubes at 2 years of age. The nurse reviews these admission assessment findings:

- Temperature = 102°F (40.2°C)
- Heart rate = 123 beats/min
- Respirations = 34 breaths/min
- Oxygen saturation = 93% (on room air)
- Weight = 58 lb (26.3 kg)
- Acute pain = 10/10 on a 0 to 10 pain scale
- CT scan with contrast = inflammation of the appendix with fecalith present; free fluid and a 3 mm × 5 mm area of localized fluid formation present
- WBCs = 18,800/mm³ (18.8 × 10⁹/L)
- Hemoglobin = 14.8 g/dL (148 g/L)
- Platelets = 202,000/mm³ (202 × 10⁹/L)
- Potassium = 3.9 mEq/L (3.9 mmol/L)
- CO_2 = 18 mEq/L (18 mmol/L)
- Creatinine = 0.7 mg/dL (88 mcmol/L)
- BUN = 17 mg/dL (6.2 mmol/L)

Highlight or place a check mark next to the assessment findings that require follow-up by the nurse.

Thinking Exercise 11B-2

The nurse is caring for a 10-year-old male client who was admitted to the hospital with report of acute pain in the lower right abdomen. His admission assessment data include:

- Temperature = 102°F (40.2°C)
- Heart rate = 123 beats/min
- Respirations = 34 breaths/min
- Oxygen saturation = 93% (on room air)
- Weight = 58 lb (26.3 kg)
- Acute pain = 10/10 on a 0 to10 pain scale
- CT scan with contrast = inflammation of the appendix with fecalith present; free fluid and a 3 mm × 5 mm area of localized fluid formation present
- WBCs = 18,800/mm³ (18.8 × 10⁹/L)
- Hemoglobin = 14.8 g/dL (148 g/L)
- Platelets = 202,000/mm³ (202 × 10⁹/L)
- Potassium = 3.9 mEq/L (3.9 mmol/L)
- CO_2 = 18 mEq/L (18 mmol/L)
- Creatinine = 0.7 mg/dL (88 mcmol/L)
- BUN = 17 mg/dL (6.2 mmol/L)

Choose the *most likely* options for the information missing from the statements below by selecting from the list of options provided.

The nurse recognizes that an _____ temperature and an elevated _____ are factors that complicate the treatment of appendicitis and need to be closely monitored. Failure to treat this health problem can lead to _____, peritonitis, and sepsis.

Options
Elevated
Subnormal
Pancreatitis
Peptic ulcer disease
Cholecystitis
Bowel obstruction
Hemoglobin
White blood cell count
Bilirubin

Thinking Exercise 11B-3

The nurse is caring for a 10-year-old male client who was admitted to the hospital with report of acute pain in the lower right abdomen. His admission diagnosis is probable appendicitis. Which of the following complications will the nurse anticipate when caring for this client? **Select all that apply.**

_____ A. Respiratory acidosis

_____ B. Infection

_____ C. Internal hemorrhage

_____ D. Chronic kidney disease

_____ E. Ruptured appendix

_____ F. Gastroenteritis

_____ G. Ulcerative colitis

_____ H. Dehydration

Thinking Exercise 11B-4

While caring for a 10-year-old male client 2 days after open appendectomy for a ruptured appendix, the nurse notes the following assessment findings:
- Temperature = 99.1°F (37.3°C)
- Heart rate = 92 beats/min
- Respirations = 16 breaths/min
- Oxygen saturation = 98% (on room air)
- Pain = 5/10 on a 0 to 10 pain intensity scale
- Weight = 51 lb (23.1 kg)

In addition, the child has been unable to tolerate clear liquids and reports vomiting, nausea, and abdominal pain. The nurse encourages the child to walk three times a day, but the child refuses. The nurse notes that the client is guarding his abdomen, has refused pain medication for the past 12 hours, and grimaces with any type of movement. On further questioning, the client tearfully shares that he is not taking pain medications because he doesn't want his parents to spend extra money on his care. **Use an X to indicate which of the potential nursing actions are essential and appropriate for the nurse to perform at this time for the client.**

Potential Nursing Action	Appropriate Nursing Action
Administer piperacillin and tazobactam intravenously.	
Monitor oxygen saturation and CO_2 levels.	
Encourage oral clear liquids.	
Give the child intravenous morphine IV push.	
Encourage the child to share his concerns with his parents.	
Maintain 5%D/0.45% NS with 20 mEq/L (20 mmol/L) of KCl at 66 mL/hr.	
Administer ondansetron immediately.	
Maintain accurate intake and output.	

Potential Nursing Action	Appropriate Nursing Action
Encourage visitors to help manage pain.	
Monitor daily weight using the same scale at the same time.	
Monitor stool count for the next 3 days.	
Explain to the child about how pain control and healing are interrelated.	
Encourage the use of incentive spirometer every 2 hours.	

Thinking Exercise 11B-5

The nurse is evaluating the progress of a 10-year-old male client following open appendectomy. He is currently being treated for an abdominal abscess, nausea and vomiting, and abdominal pain. The nurse reviews the following assessment data:

	Current	24 Hours Ago	48 Hours Ago
Serum Lab Results			
Hemoglobin	9.8 g/dL (98 g/L)	10.9 g/dL (109 g/L)	11.7 g/dL (117 g/L)
Hematocrit	35.1% (0.35)	41.8% (0.42)	44.6% (0.45)
Platelet count	148,000/mm^3 (148 × 10^9/L)	200,000/mm^3 (200 × 10^9/L)	211,000/mm^3 (211 × 10^9/L)
White blood cell count	12,700/ mm^3 (12.7 × 10^9/L)	12,200/ mm^3 (12.2 × 10^9/L)	11,700/ mm^3 (11.7 × 10^9/L)
Bands	11%	3%	0
Potassium	3.2 mEq/L (3.2 mmol/L)	3.4 mEq/L (3.4 mmol/L)	3.6 mEq/L (3.6 mmol/L)
Sodium	132 mEq/L (132 mmol/L)	129 mEq/L (129 mmol/L)	134 mEq/L (134 mmol/L)
Glucose	111 mg/dL	102 mg/dL	99 mg/dL
CO$_2$	20 mEq/L (20 mmol/L)	19 mEq/L (19 mmol/L)	16 mEq/L (16 mmol/L)
Prealbumin	18 mg/dL (180 mg/L)	22 mg/dL (220 mg/L)	24 mg/dL (240 mg/L)
Blood urea nitrogen	18 mg/dL (6.5 mmol/L)	12 mg/dL (4.4 mmol/L)	11 mg/dL (4.0 mmol/L)
Creatinine	1.02 mg/dL (89 mcmol/L)	0.6 mg/dL (53 mcmol/L)	0.45 mg/dL (40 mcmol/L)
Vital Signs			
Temperature	101.6°F (38.6°C)	100.1°F (37.8°C)	99.1°F (37.3°C)
Heart rate (beats/min)	98	90	92
Respirations (breaths/min)	16	18	16
Pain score	7	4	5
Daily weight (lb [kg])	53 (24.1)	50 (22.7)	51

Highlight or place a check mark next to the assessment findings that require follow-up by the nurse.

Thinking Exercise 11B-6

The nurse is evaluating the progress of a 10-year-old male client with an abdominal abscess, nausea and vomiting, and abdominal pain. **For each assessment finding, use an X to indicate whether the interventions were <u>Effective</u> (helped to meet expected outcomes), <u>Ineffective</u> (did not help to meet expected outcomes), or <u>Unrelated</u> (not related to the expected outcomes).**

Assessment Finding	Effective	Ineffective	Unrelated
Hemoglobin = 9.8 g/dL (98 g/L)			
Platelet count = 128,000/mm³ (128 × 10⁹/L)			
Bands = 11%			
Potassium = 3.2 mEq/L (3.2 mmol/L)			
Glucose = 111 mg/dL (6.2 mmol/L)			
CO_2 = 20 mEq/L (20 mmol/L)			
Creatinine = 1.02 mg/dL (89 mcmol/L)			
Prealbumin = 18 mg/dL (480 mg/L)			
Tolerating clear liquid diet			
Temperature = 101.6°F (38.6°C)			
Heart rate = 98 beats/min			
Respirations = 16 breaths/min			
Pain = 7 on a 0 to 10 pain intensity scale			
Incision site intact, red, and edematous with serous drainage under transparent dressing			
Child Life Specialist reports that school tutor for home has been arranged			
Client playing video game with sibling			

Infection

Common Health Problems

12

Infection

Common Health Problems

Exemplar 12A. Cellulitis (Medical-Surgical Nursing: Middle-Age Adult)

Thinking Exercise 12A-1

A 57-year-old female client had a large mole removed from her left upper arm by a dermatologist in the office 2 days ago. She has a history of atrial fibrillation, chronic heart failure, diabetes mellitus type 2, and multiple lower back surgeries for persistent back pain. This morning the client asked her daughter to drive her to the emergency department (ED) for severe radiating 8/10 pain in her entire left arm. When the nurse removes the bandage from the area, the nurse notes that the skin and tissue around the wound are reddened, very swollen, and warm. The wound drainage is foul smelling and greenish-yellow. The client's current temperature is 100.6°F (38.2°C), and she is admitted to the hospital with left upper arm cellulitis. **Choose the *most likely* options for the information missing from the statements below by selecting from the lists of options provided.**

Based on the nurse's assessment findings, the client is at risk for complications as a result of her cellulitis and wound, especially _____1_____ and _____1_____. Assessment findings for which the nurse would monitor include _____2_____, _____2_____, _____2_____, and _____2_____.

Options for 1	Options for 2
Neurovascular compromise	Increased temperature
Myocardial infarction	Chest pain
Diabetic ketoacidosis	Dyspnea
Sepsis	Left arm tingling and numbness
Hyperkalemia	Leukocytosis
Anemia	Diminished left radial pulse

Thinking Exercise 12A-2

A 57-year-old female client is admitted to the hospital with a left upper arm open wound infection (methicillin-resistant *Staphylococcus aureus* [MRSA]) and cellulitis. **Use an X to indicate whether the nursing actions listed below are <u>Indicated</u> (appropriate or necessary), <u>Contraindicated</u> (could be harmful), or <u>Non-Essential</u> (make no difference or are not necessary) for the client's care at this time.**

Nursing Action	Indicated	Contraindicated	Non-Essential
Place the client on Contact Precautions.			
Apply cold compresses on her left upper arm.			
Elevate the client's left arm on a pillow.			
Take a wound culture every shift to determine if the infection is improving.			

Continued

Nursing Action	Indicated	Contraindicated	Non-Essential
Initiate IV access for the client to receive fluids and antibiotic therapy.			
Administer subcutaneous sodium heparin every 12 hours.			

Thinking Exercise 12A-3

A 57-year-old female client is admitted to the hospital with a left upper arm open wound infection (methicillin-resistant *staphylococcus aureus* [MRSA] and several gram-negative bacteria) and cellulitis. The primary health care provider prescribes IV daptomycin and tobramycin to treat the infection. What health teaching will the nurse include for the client prior to administration of these drugs? **Select all that apply.**

_____ A. "We will be monitoring you for any nausea or diarrhea that may occur when taking these drugs."

_____ B. "Please let a nurse know if you have any ringing in your ears or have problems hearing while you are taking these drugs."

_____ C. "We will be carefully monitoring your kidney function while you are on this drug therapy."

_____ D. "Although very rare, let us know if your muscles feel weak or you feel them tightening."

_____ E. "We will be drawing blood frequently to measure drug levels to make sure they are effective."

_____ F. "We will be changing the IV site often to prevent your veins from getting irritated."

_____ G. "We will discontinue your maintenance IV after we make sure you don't have nausea and your fever comes down."

Thinking Exercise 12A-4

A 57-year-old female client admitted to the hospital with a left upper arm open wound infection (methicillin-resistant *Staphylococcus aureus* [MRSA] and several gram-negative bacteria) and cellulitis has been on IV daptomycin and tobramycin for less than 2 days. This morning she reports having frequent foul-smelling diarrhea and severe abdominal discomfort. **Choose the *most likely* options for the information missing from the statements below by selecting from the lists of options provided.**

Based on the nurse's assessment, the client most likely has _____1_____ as a result of antibiotic therapy. The most common drugs used to treat this problem are _____2_____ and _____2_____. The nurse would remind the nursing staff to _____3_____ and _____3_____ to prevent transmission to other clients on the hospital unit.

Options for 1	Options for 2	Options for 3
Pseudomembranous colitis	Clindamycin	Wear a mask when in the client's room
Crohn disease	Cefoxitin	Use strict hand hygiene measures.
Clostridium difficile infection	Vancomycin	Record the number of stools the client has each day
Viral gastroenteritis	Trimethoprim	Use strict Contact Precautions
Diverticulitis	Metronidazole	Teach the client to increase dietary fiber
Secondary bowel cancer	Tetracycline	Restrict oral fluids for the client to decrease stools

Thinking Exercise 12A-5

The nurse is reassessing a 57-year-old female client who was admitted to the hospital with a left upper arm open wound infection (methicillin-resistant *Staphylococcus aureus* [MRSA] and several gram-negative bacteria) and cellulitis 5 days ago. Tomorrow she is scheduled for discharge to home with her daughter to continue oral antibiotic therapy for another 10 days. **For each assessment finding, use an X to indicate whether the interventions were <u>Effective</u> (helped to meet expected outcomes), <u>Ineffective</u> (did not help to meet expected outcomes), or <u>Unrelated</u> (not related to the expected outcomes).**

Assessment Finding	Effective	Ineffective	Unrelated
Client's oral temperature this morning is 98°F (36.7°C).			
Client reports mild pain in upper left arm at 2/10 on a scale of 0 to 10.			
Client reports that she has had less diarrhea today than the past 2 days.			
Client's early morning finger stick blood glucose (FSBG) was 97 mg/dL (5.4 mmol/L).			
Client's left upper arm slightly reddened when compared with right upper arm.			
Client reports that her back is more achy since she came to the hospital.			

Thinking Exercise 12A-6

A 57-year-old female client was admitted to the hospital with a left upper arm open wound infection (methicillin-resistant *Staphylococcus aureus* [MRSA] and several gram-negative bacteria) and cellulitis 5 days ago. Her wound is packed and requires a dressing change twice a day. Tomorrow she is scheduled for discharge to home with her daughter to continue antibiotic therapy for another week. What health teaching will the nurse include as part of the discharge instructions for the client and her daughter? **Select all that apply.**

_____ A. "Use strict sterile technique when packing the wound and changing the dressing twice a day."

_____ B. "Stop taking the antibiotics when your arm feels better and is not reddened."

_____ C. "Notify your primary health care provider if your wound drainage is foul smelling or changes color."

_____ D. "Notify your primary health care provider if your diarrhea gets worse."

_____ E. "Avoid strenuous activity and take frequent reset periods."

_____ F. "Do not return to work until after your follow-up appointment."

_____ G. "Notify your primary health care provider if your arm feels numb or becomes more painful."

Exemplar 12B. Respiratory Syncytial Virus (RSV) (Pediatric Nursing: Infant)

Thinking Exercise 12B-1

A 2-month-old male infant is brought into the pediatrician's office for a routine well-child appointment and because of additional concerns that his mother has about the baby. The nurse notes the following data on completing a comprehensive history and assessment:

- Born at 32 weeks' gestation via spontaneous vaginal delivery
- Birth weight = 2054 g (4 lb 8.3 oz)
- Uncomplicated NICU stay for 5 weeks
- Mother reports that 7-year-old sibling has a "cold"
- Mother reports that the infant has not eaten well today
- Temporal temperature = 99.0°F (37.2°C)
- Heart rate = 156 beats/min
- Respirations = 66 breaths/min
- Weight = 3.45 kg (7 lb 9.6 oz)
- Nasal flaring
- Makes soft sounds with each exhalation
- Substernal retractions
- Pale pink mucous membranes
- Fontanels are soft and flat
- Quiet and arouses slightly during assessment

Highlight or place a check mark next to the assessment findings that require follow-up by the nurse.

Thinking Exercise 12B-2

The nurse is caring for a 2-month-old infant who has been admitted to the pediatric unit with respiratory distress. **Use an X to indicate whether the nursing actions below are <u>Indicated</u> (appropriate or necessary), <u>Contraindicated</u> (could be harmful), or <u>Non-Essential</u> (make no difference or are not necessary) for the client's care at this time.**

Nursing Action	Indicated	Contraindicated	Non-Essential
Provide parents with consent forms for immunizations.			
Obtain oxygen saturation level.			
Complete the growth chart.			
Assess for presence or history of rhinorrhea.			
Obtain manual blood pressure.			
Administer *Haemophilus influenzae* type b (Hib) vaccine.			
Administer varicella vaccine.			
Provide anticipatory guidance education for car seat safety.			
Provide parents with injury prevention education for infants.			
Suction infant to clear nasal passages.			
Provide oxygen for O_2 saturation less than 90%.			
Obtain a nasopharyngeal swab for culture.			

Thinking Exercise 12B-3

The primary health care provider prescribes acetaminophen for fussiness or fevers greater than 100.5°F (38°C). What are the essential elements of safe medication administration for an infant weighing 3.45 kg? **Choose the most likely options for the information missing from the statements below by selecting from the lists of options provided.**

To ensure _____1_____ dosages of medications, the nurse will practice _____2_____ medication administration principles. Per the primary health care provider's prescription, the nurse will give _____3_____ for fevers higher than 100.5°F (38°C) as needed. To provide an accurate dose, the nurse will calculate that to give ___4___ of acetaminophen with a 90 mg/0.9 mL solution, the nurse will administer ___5___ using a ___6___ oral syringe, or ___7___ of the medication.

Options for 1, 2, and 3	Options for 4, 5, 6, and 7
Ibuprofen	10 mg/kg per dose
Medication	7 doses each day
Aspirin	5–10 mg/kg every 3 hr
Pyretic	1.0 mL
Acetaminophen	0.35 mL
Safe	5 mg/kg per dose
Documentation	0.345 mL
Accurate	35 mg
Administration	3 mL
Assessment	20 mg/kg every 4 hr

Thinking Exercise 12B-4

A 2-month-old infant is admitted to the pediatric unit for respiratory distress. The nurse caring for the infant reviews the infant's lab test results and documents the following admission assessment findings:

Lab Test Results
- White blood cell count = 17,800 mm³ (17.8 × 10⁹/L)
- Hemoglobin = 11.6 g/dL (116 g/L)
- Hematocrit = 33.9% (0.34 volume fraction)
- Platelet count = 400,000 mm³ (400 × 10⁹/L)
- Viral PCR panel results = (−) adenovirus, (−) influenza A & B, (−) human metapneumovirus, (+) respiratory syncytial virus, (−) rhinovirus, (−) parainfluenza types 1 to 3
- Anteroposterior chest x-ray = interstitial perihilar markings

Assessment Findings
- Lung sounds are coarse; crackles and diminished breath sounds in lower lobes
- Respirations = 76 breaths/min
- Intercostal retracting
- Regular heart rate and rhythm
- Brachial and femoral pulses are 3+ and equal
- Pale mucous membranes
- Central capillary refill = 4–5 seconds

Based on these results, identify the appropriate nursing actions. **Use an X to indicate whether the nursing actions below are <u>Indicated</u> (appropriate or necessary), <u>Contraindicated</u> (could be harmful), or <u>Non-Essential</u> (make no difference or are not necessary) for the client's care at this time.**

Nursing Action	Indicated	Contraindicated	Non-Essential
Administer antibiotics.			
Monitor oxygen saturation and CO_2 levels.			
Encourage oral clear liquids.			
Maintain Contact and Droplet Precautions.			
Provide frequent oral suctioning.			
Perform deep suctioning two times daily.			
Administer albuterol.			
Maintain accurate intake and output.			
Encourage visitors.			
Administer opioid pain medication.			
Instruct the infant's mother to pump and store breast milk.			
Maintain 5%D/0.45% NS with 20 mEq of KCl per liter at 14 mL/hr.			

Thinking Exercise 12B-5

The nurse is evaluating the clinical outcomes for a 2-month-old infant who was admitted with respiratory syncytial virus (RSV) bronchiolitis. **For each assessment finding, use an X to indicate whether the interventions were <u>Effective</u> (helped to meet expected outcomes), <u>Ineffective</u> (did not help to meet expected outcomes), or <u>Unrelated</u> (not related to the expected outcomes).**

Assessment Finding	Effective	Ineffective	Unrelated
Oxygen saturation 94% on ¼ L/min via nasal cannula			
<2nd percentile for weight			
Temperature 99.0°F (37.2°C)			
Heart rate = 116 beats/min			
Respirations = 46 breaths/min			
Baby is awake and fussy			
17¾ inches or 45.4 cm in length			
Baby breast-feeds every 2–3 hr			
Weight is 3.41 kg (7 lb 8 oz)			

Thinking Exercise 12B-6

The nurse is providing discharge information to the family of a 2-month-old infant admitted with respiratory syncytial virus (RSV) bronchiolitis. What will the nurse include in discharge teaching for the family? **Select all that apply.**

_____ A. "Resume breast-feeding on demand."

_____ B. "Weigh your infant every day using the same scale at the same time."

_____ C. "Suction the infant's nose as needed to clear passages."

_____ D. "Contact the primary health care provider if rapid or difficulty breathing, excessive sleepiness, and/or poor feeding occur."

_____ E. "Return to the clinic for monthly infusions of palivizumab."

_____ F. "Keep the baby away from secondhand and thirdhand smoke."

_____ G. "Isolate your infant from all extended family members during flu and cold season."

_____ H. "Return to the clinic for deep nasopharyngeal suctioning in the morning and evening for the next 3 to 5 days."

_____ I. "Encourage good hand hygiene at all times."

Sensory Perception
Cataracts

Thinking Exercise 13-1

A 68-year-old male client presents at the ophthalmologist's office for his annual eye examination. He has worn glasses since the third grade and has severe astigmatism and photophobia. He currently wears progressive bifocal glasses to enable him to see both near and far away. He tells the office nurse that he is having increasing problems with seeing at night, especially when driving. During the night when he gets up to go to the bathroom, he sometimes "runs into walls or doors" because it is so dark in his bedroom. He has stubbed several toes and had "bumps" on his forehead as a result. What health teaching would the nurse include when helping the client **maintain safety at night**? **Select all that apply.**

_____ A. "Ask a family member or friend to drive you at night if you have to go out."

_____ B. "Use plug-in night lights in your bedroom and bathroom to help you see at night."

_____ C. "Buy or rent a bedside commode and place it near your bed for nighttime use."

_____ D. "Be sure that your bathroom floor has a nonskid surface and avoid using throw rugs."

_____ E. "Check that furniture or other obstacles are not in the path between your bed and the bathroom."

_____ F. "Use a large-print digital clock on your bed stand so that you'll know when you go to the bathroom."

_____ G. "Be sure that electric cords or electronic device charging cords are not present between your bed and the bathroom."

Thinking Exercise 13-2

A 68-year-old male client presents at the ophthalmologist's office for his annual eye examination. He has worn glasses since the third grade and has severe astigmatism and photophobia. He currently wears progressive bifocal glasses to enable him to see both close up and at a distance for a correction to 20/10 visual acuity. After the client's examination, the ophthalmologist reports that there is no evidence of disease and his optic nerves are intact and healthy. However, the client has a beginning cataract in his left eye which requires surgery to prevent his vision from worsening. As part of preoperative assessment, the nurse asks the client what medications he takes. He recalls most of his medication regimen, but the information is incomplete. **Choose the *most likely* options for the information missing from the table by selecting from the lists of options provided.**

Medication	Dose, Route, Frequency	Drug Class	Indication
Apremilast	30 mg orally twice daily	Phosphodiesterase type 4 (PDE-4) inhibitor	**1**
2	5–10 mg orally every 24 hr	Second-generation H$_1$ antagonist	Seasonal allergic rhinitis
Pantoprazole	**3**	Proton pump inhibitor	GERD
Sildenafil	50 mg orally PRN	Phosphodiesterase type 5 (PDE-5) inhibitor	**4**
Rivaroxaban	20 mg orally once daily with the evening meal	**5**	Nonvalvular atrial fibrillation

Options for 1	Options for 2	Options for 3
Contact dermatitis	Filgrastim	40 mg orally once daily
Hypertension	Amlodipine	150 mg orally twice daily
Psoriasis	Spironolactone	25 mg subcutaneously once weekly
Depression	Rifampin	300 mg orally once daily
Lupus erythematosus	Cetirizine	500 mg orally every 4 hr
Multiple sclerosis	Amphotericin B	250 mg orally every 6 hr

Options for 4	Options for 5
Benign prostatic hyperplasia	Benzodiazepine
Erectile dysfunction	5-Alpha-reductase inhibitor
Migraine headache	Xanthine oxidase inhibitor
Fever	Tricyclic antidepressant
Chest pain	Aminoglycoside
Nausea and vomiting	Direct factor Xa inhibitor

Thinking Exercise 13-3

A 68-year-old male client presents at the ophthalmologist's office for his annual eye examination. After the client's examination, the ophthalmologist reports that there is no evidence of disease and his optic nerves are intact and healthy. However, the client has a beginning cataract in his left eye and he is scheduled for surgery to prevent his vision from worsening. He is scheduled for cataract removal and insertion of an intraocular lens. What preoperative health teaching will the nurse include for this client? **Select all that apply.**

_____ A. "Check with the doctor about when you need to stop taking rivaroxaban a few days prior to surgery."

_____ B. "You will need to use eyedrops to dilate your pupils and paralyze your eye muscles the morning of surgery."

_____ C. "Be sure that someone drives you to the doctor's office and takes you home to stay with you for the first night."

_____ D. "You will be on patient-controlled analgesia for the first 24 hours after surgery."

_____ E. "You will need to wear dark glasses or sunglasses outdoors and in brightly lit rooms for several weeks after surgery."

_____ F. "Your operative eye will have a "bloodshot" appearance that will fade over time."

_____ G. "You may still need to wear corrective glasses or contact lenses after surgery."

_____ H. "You will have to put several kinds of eyedrops and/or ointments in your eyes a number of times each day for several weeks after surgery."

Thinking Exercise 13-4

A 68-year-old male client just had a left cataract removal and insertion of an intraocular lens. The nurse is preparing to teach the client's wife about his postoperative care. **Indicate which health teaching listed in the far-left column is appropriate for the potential postoperative complication. Note that not all choices will be used.**

Health Teaching	Potential Postoperative Complication	Appropriate Health Teaching for Each Potential Postoperative Complication
1 "Report increased swelling or redness of the operative eyelid."	Increased intraocular pressure	
2 "Encourage the client to eat high-protein foods to promote healing."	Infection	
3 "Remind the client to avoid coughing, sneezing, lifting, and sexual intercourse until after his follow-up visit."	Hemorrhage	
4 "Have the client sleep in a sitting position at all times until after the follow-up visit."	Eyelid swelling	
5 "Observe the eye bandage for any signs of bleeding."	Detached retina	
6 "Contact the surgeon immediately if the client has severe pain or sees floating particles in the operative eye."		
7 "Be sure the client takes his oral antibiotic for 14 days."		
8 "Contact the surgeon immediately if there is yellow or green discharge on the eye dressing when you change it."		

Thinking Exercise 13-5

A 68-year-old male client had a cataract removal and insertion of an intraocular lens 4 weeks ago and is being seen in the ophthalmologist's office for a surgical follow-up visit. **For each assessment finding, use an X to indicate whether the interventions were Effective (helped to meet expected outcomes), Ineffective (did not help to meet expected outcomes), or Unrelated (not related to the expected outcomes).**

Assessment Finding	Effective	Ineffective	Unrelated
Has no bleeding or discharge from the operative eye			
Operative eyelid is swollen but not reddened			
Vision in operative eye is improved			
Reports new-onset constipation			
Reports no sharp or sudden episodes of pain			
Reports no flashes of light or floating shapes			
Tearing eyes and nose from allergic response to pollen			
Reports frontal sinus headache			

Cognition
Common Health Problems

Exemplar 14A. Delirium (Mental Health Nursing: Older Adult)

Thinking Exercise 14A-1

A 79-year-old female client had an emergent colon resection for lower GI bleeding related to diverticulitis this morning. Her assigned nurse performs a postoperative client assessment and recognizes that she is at risk for delirium. Which of the following factors place the client at high risk for delirium at this time? **Select all that apply.**

_____ A. Older age

_____ B. Female

_____ C. Infection

_____ D. Surgery

_____ E. Substance use disorder

_____ F. Relocation from home to hospital

_____ G. Possible anemia

_____ H. Fluid overload

Thinking Exercise 14A-2

A 79-year-old female client had an emergent colon resection for lower GI bleeding related to diverticulitis this morning. The nurse notes the following client history:
- Lives independently in a senior housing apartment
- Part-time employee as a bookkeeper
- Hypertension controlled by hydrochlorothiazide and diet
- Two falls at home without major injury in the past 6 months
- Diabetes mellitus type 2 controlled by diet and metformin
- Appendectomy at 23 years of age
- Benign thyroid nodule removed at 38 years of age
- Vaginal hysterectomy at 56 years of age

Highlight or place a check mark next to the history data that would be of concern to the nurse.

Thinking Exercise 14A-3

A 79-year-old female client had an emergent colon resection for lower GI bleeding related to diverticulitis this morning. The night nurse receives the report and reads the following note in the electronic health record entered by the nurse who was assigned to the client during the day:

Nurses' Notes

1830 Client receiving basal morphine via PCA. Unable to verbalize her pain level, but client yells out when touched and tried to hit several staff members while changing her bed. Vomited small amount (about 30 mL) of yellowish-green emesis. Remains NPO with Ringer's lactate infusing at 100 mL/hr. Abdominal surgical dressing dry and intact, but abdomen is slightly distended with no bowel sounds × 4. Amber yellow urine draining from catheter. Blood pressure decreased from 154/88 at 1400 to 122/74 at 1800. No major changes in temperature or apical pulse. Postoperative lab results show that serum sodium level dropped from 137 mg/dL (137 mmol/L) preoperatively to 130 mg/dL (130 mmol/L). Dr. Jones aware and will check on client on rounds later this evening. ———————————————————————————————— J. Donner, RN

1900 Client found trying to climb out of bed. Continues to scream and cry out periodically. Attempted to pull out IV line. Reoriented client × 2. Calmer when daughter came in to visit. ———————— J. Donner, RN

Based on the above information, use an X to indicate whether the nursing actions listed below are Indicated (appropriate or necessary), Contraindicated (could be harmful), or Non-Essential (make no difference or are not necessary) for the client's care at this time.

Nursing Action	Indicated	Contraindicated	Non-Essential
Request that the surgeon change the client's analgesic medication to a nonopioid drug.			
Be sure that environmental orientation cues are available, such as a large clock, in the client's room.			
Place the client on fall precautions.			
Continue to monitor serum sodium levels.			
Monitor pulse and blood pressure every 1 to 2 hours.			
Request a prescription for an antipsychotic medication.			
Reorient the client frequently.			
Request that a family member or friend stay with the client at night.			
Prepare to administer a blood or blood product transfusion.			
Ask family to bring in familiar or favorite items that may help reorient or distract client from pulling out IV.			

Thinking Exercise 14A-4

A 79-year-old female client had an emergent colon resection for lower GI bleeding related to diverticulitis 2 days ago. The night nurse reports that the client is oriented to person and place but not time. When her family visited last evening, they reported that the client was "making more sense" in her conversation with them, and they are excited that she will be going home soon. This morning the day nurse assesses the client and finds that she is only oriented to person. She states that she is not having abdominal pain at this time. Before the nurse leaves her room, the client tells the nurse that she sees a "little man" sitting on her windowsill and asks why the man is there. **Choose the *most likely* options for the information missing from the statements below by selecting from the lists of options provided.**

The client is experiencing a visual hallucination most likely due to delirium. Her acute confusion is most likely the result of _____1_____, _____1_____, or _____1_____. The nurse would request a _____2_____, _____2_____, and _____2_____, and carefully monitor the client's _____2_____ and _____2_____.

Options for 1	Options for 2
Deep vein thrombosis	Platelet count
Urinary tract infection	CT scan
Thrombocytopenia	Urine culture
Opioid withdrawal	Sequential compression stockings
Anemia	Vital signs
Hypertension	Complete blood cell count
Electrolyte imbalance	Chest x-ray
Dementia	Basic metabolic panel (BMP)
Bowel perforation	Voiding pattern
Constipation	Stool count

Thinking Exercise 14A-5

The nurse is preparing a 79-year-old female client who had an emergent colon resection 5 days ago for discharge to her daughter's house. **For each assessment finding, use an X to indicate whether the interventions for the client's delirium were <u>Effective</u> (helped to meet expected outcomes), <u>Ineffective</u> (did not help to meet expected outcomes), or <u>Unrelated</u> (not related to the expected outcomes).**

Assessment Finding	Effective	Ineffective	Unrelated
Alert and oriented × 3			
Has not had additional hallucinations			
Had a small stool this morning			
Understands discharge instructions			
Has minimal surgical pain			
No episodes of screaming or crying out for the past 3 days			
Has short-term memory loss at times			

Exemplar 14B. Alzheimer's Disease (Mental Health Nursing: Middle-Age Adult)

Thinking Exercise 14B-1

A 54-year-old male client comes to the primary health care provider's office with report of having difficulty with math calculation and short-term memory loss for the past 5 to 6 months. He tells the office nurse that he has been very healthy throughout his life and successful in his construction business. When taking a history, the nurse notes the following data:

- Participated in football and ice hockey in high school and college
- Father died at 52 from lung cancer
- Mother resides in a nursing home due to chronic heart failure, chronic kidney disease, and late-stage Alzheimer's disease
- Married to the same woman for 30 years
- Has two children in college
- Fell off a ladder last year and suffered a mild concussion

- Is trying to lose weight following a "keto" diet due to new-onset hypertension
- Recently has had "problems with finding the right words at times"
- Had two benign polyps removed during a colonoscopy 3 years ago

Highlight or place a check mark next to the history data that would be of concern to the nurse.

Thinking Exercise 14B-2

A 54-year-old male client has had difficulty with math calculation, short-term memory loss, and word finding for the past 5 to 6 months. He was referred by his primary health care provider for a complete neurologic evaluation, which resulted in a diagnosis of probable Alzheimer's disease (AD). What health teaching about AD will the nurse include for the client? **Select all that apply.**

_____ A. "AD is a chronic disease that is not curable and gets worse over time."

_____ B. "With appropriate care and treatment, people with AD can live for many years."

_____ C. "You will need emotional support from family and friends as your disease progresses."

_____ D. "Drug therapy can stop the progression of the disease."

_____ E. "Diet therapy has been shown to slow the progression of the disease."

_____ F. "If you haven't already done so, you should plan advance directives."

_____ G. "You can expect to have incontinence in this mild or early stage of your disease."

_____ H. "The best approach now to manage your disease is to stay physically and mentally active."

Thinking Exercise 14B-3

A 58-year-old male client was diagnosed with Alzheimer's disease 4 years ago. He has continued working in his construction business but has reduced his time at the office to part-time. Recently his wife states that he has become lost several times while driving and makes judgment errors at work and at home. Today he presents to the primary health care provider with a new report of frequent headaches. As part of the history and client assessment, the nurse asks the client's wife about current medications that he is taking. The wife provides incomplete information. **Choose the *most likely* options for the information missing from the table by selecting from the lists of options provided.**

Medication	Dose, Route, Frequency	Drug Class	Indication
1	10 mg orally once at bedtime	Cholinesterase inhibitor	Alzheimer's disease
Enalapril	5 mg orally once each day	Angiotensin-converting enzyme inhibitor	**2**
Furosemide	20 mg orally once in the morning	**3**	Hypertension
Pantoprazole	**4**	Proton pump inhibitor	Gastroesophageal reflux disease (GERD)
5	200 mg orally 3–4 times each day	NSAID	Chronic low back pain and headaches

Options for 1	Options for 2	Options for 3
Gabapentin	Chronic heart failure	Thiazide-type diuretic
Selegiline	Hypertension	Cholinergic agent
Memantine	Peripheral vascular disease	Cardiac glycoside
Imipramine	Hypercholesterolemia	Beta blocker
Donepezil	Peripheral neuropathy	Potassium-sparing diuretic
Diazepam	Anemia	High-ceiling (loop) diuretic

Options for 4	Options for 5
250 mg IV every 6 hr	Acetaminophen
15 mg orally twice each day	Ibuprofen
150 mg orally twice each day	Tramadol
40 mg orally once each day	Morphine
100 mg orally before each meal	Codeine
50 mg via transdermal patch once each day	Cannabis

Thinking Exercise 14B-4

A 58-year-old male client was diagnosed with Alzheimer's disease 4 years ago. He has continued working in his construction business but has reduced his time at the office to part-time. Recently his wife states that he has become lost several times while driving and makes judgment errors at work and at home. The neurologist told her that the client is now in the middle stage of the disease. She also states that she is having more difficulty communicating with the client because he gets agitated at times and yells at her. Which of the following statements would help her more effectively communicate with the client? **Select all that apply.**

_____ A. "Use distraction when possible to prevent confrontation with the client."

_____ B. "Try to reorient the client to his surroundings as many times as needed each day."

_____ C. "Decrease stimulation at home to try to keep the client as calm as possible."

_____ D. "Limit the number of choices that the client has to prevent frustration."

_____ E. "Keep the television on at all times to help with client orientation."

_____ F. "Provide for rest periods to reduce the client's stress and prevent fatigue."

_____ G. "Provide structure and consistency in the client's daily routine."

_____ H. "Use simple, short sentences and one-step directions when communicating."

_____ I. "Validate the client's feelings as needed to prevent conflict."

Thinking Exercise 14B-5

A 59-year-old male client was diagnosed with Alzheimer's disease 5 years ago. His wife states that he became lost several times while driving and made judgment errors at work and at home. As a result he does not work anymore and she is his sole caregiver. The neurologist told her that the client is in the middle stage of the disease. The client's wife states that she is getting very tired and is afraid he will wander away from the house while she is sleeping. What health teaching would the nurse provide to help with caregiver stress? **Select all that apply.**

_____ A. "When possible, use humor to help get through each day."

_____ B. "Try to take one day at a time and not stress about the future."

_____ C. "Take a vacation with the client to distract him and provide a different environment."

_____ D. "Use relaxation strategies such as meditation, massage, and music therapy."

_____ E. "Ask a family member or close friend to stay with the client to provide respite time for you."

_____ F. "Contact the Alzheimer's Association to join a support group or obtain information."

_____ G. "Be realistic in your expectations of the client and look for positive aspects of each situation."

Mood and Affect
Depression

Exemplar 15. Depression (Mental Health Nursing: Adolescent)

Thinking Exercise 15-1

A 15-year-old female client and her mother come to the primary health care provider's office for the client's annual physical examination. The office nurse collects the client's history. Her mother reports that her artistic and talented daughter has become very moody, irritable, and often agitated over the past 6 months. She states that her daughter is failing the 10th grade and her artwork has become "very dark" by focusing only on death and pain. The client stays in her room with the door locked after school and spends numerous hours on various electronic devices. During a confidential nursing interview without her mother, the client states that her parents are very controlling and unreasonably strict because they "don't understand the needs of teenagers today." They do not let her have fun with her friends and she has sneaked out of the house to meet them on several occasions. The client states that she feels depressed most of the time. She plans to move out of her parents' house to live with her boyfriend next year. What questions would the nurse ask the client at this time to obtain additional assessment information? **Select all that apply.**

_____ A. "Have you ever taken drugs or alcohol? If so, how often and what did you use?"

_____ B. "Have you been feeling very tired or have you had little energy?"

_____ C. "Have you thought about harming yourself or others at any time?"

_____ D. "Do you feel sad or have periods of sadness?"

_____ E. "How is your appetite? Have you experienced loss of appetite?"

_____ F. "Why do you want to move out of your house and live with your boyfriend?"

_____ G. "Have you had sex with your boyfriend and/or another person?"

_____ H. "Do you have any problems sleeping? How many hours do you sleep each night?"

_____ I. "Does anything give you pleasure in your life? If so, what?"

_____ J. "Do you have any problems concentrating during school or when doing your school work?"

Thinking Exercise 15-2

A 15-year-old female client and her mother come to the primary health care provider's office for the client's annual physical examination. The office nurse collects the client's history. Her mother reports that her artistic and talented daughter has become very moody, irritable, and often agitated over the past 6 months. She states that her daughter is failing the 10th grade and her artwork has become "very dark" by focusing only on death and pain. The client stays in her room with the door locked after school and spends numerous hours on various electronic devices. The nurse's physical assessment findings include the following data:

- Client's mother has a history of anorexia nervosa and major depressive disorder
- Client's height = 5 ft, 8 in (172.7 cm)
- Client's weight = 102 lb (46.3 kg)
- Small parallel linear scars on both upper thighs
- Dry flaky skin on most of her body

- Last menstrual period = 2 weeks ago
- Hair dry and brittle
- Vital signs within normal limits

Highlight or place a check mark next to the assessment findings that require follow-up by the nurse and health care team.

Thinking Exercise 15-3

A 15-year-old female client was referred to a clinical psychologist for psychological evaluation for severe moodiness, irritability, isolation, and a focus on death and darkness in her artwork. The client is also underweight and has signs and symptoms of a possible eating disorder. As a result of a comprehensive psychological evaluation, she was diagnosed with major depressive disorder and mild bulimia nervosa. The primary health care provider prescribes fluoxetine 20 mg orally each day and psychological therapy for the client twice a week. **Choose the *most likely* options for the information missing from the statements below by selecting from the lists of options provided.**

Fluoxetine is a _____1_____ that can be effective for treating both depression and eating disorders. The nurse teaches the client and her parents that this drug can cause common side effects including _____2_____, _____2_____, and _____2_____. In addition, the nurse teaches them that this class of drugs makes clients at increased risk for _____3_____ and the client must be monitored closely. A rare and life-threatening adverse effect of fluoxetine is _____3_____, which can cause increased vital sign values, GI distress, seizures, and possibly apnea (death). Teach the client and family to call 911 if these signs and symptoms occur.

Options for 1	Options for 2	Options for 3
Monoamine oxidase inhibitor	Urinary retention	Myocardial infarction
Benzodiazepine	Weight gain	Thrombocytosis
Selective serotonin reuptake inhibitor	Sedation	Sepsis
Antipsychotic	Constipation	Pulmonary edema
Melatonin receptor agonist	Orthostatic hypotension	Serotonin syndrome
Barbiturate	Sexual dysfunction	Liver dysfunction
Tricyclic antidepressant	Dermatitis	Suicide
Antiepileptic drug	Nervousness	Sickle cell anemia

Thinking Exercise 15-4

A 15-year-old female client was referred to a clinical psychologist for psychological evaluation for severe moodiness, irritability, isolation, and a focus on death and darkness in her artwork. She states that she feels depressed most of the time. The client is also underweight and has signs and symptoms of a possible eating disorder. As a result of a comprehensive psychological evaluation, she was diagnosed with major depressive disorder and mild bulimia nervosa. The primary health care provider prescribed fluoxetine 20 mg orally each day and psychological therapy for the client twice a week. On her first visit, the therapist asked questions to determine the client's suicidal potential. Which of the following screening questions are appropriate for a client to determine the risk for suicide? **Select all that apply.**

_____ A. "What is it like for you when you feel depressed?"

_____ B. "When you are feeling sad, what thoughts are going through your mind?"

_____ C. "Have you ever thought of taking your own life?"

_____ D. "Do you have a way to carry out a plan for taking your own life?"

_____ E. "Have you ever attempted suicide?"

_____ F. "Have you been thinking about death recently?"

_____ G. "Why does your artwork look dark and focus on death?"

Thinking Exercise 15-5

A 15-year-old female client was referred to a clinical psychologist for psychological evaluation for severe moodiness, irritability, isolation, and a focus on death and darkness in her artwork. She states that she feels depressed most of the time. The client is also underweight and has signs and symptoms of a possible eating disorder. As a result of a comprehensive psychological evaluation, she was diagnosed with major depressive disorder and mild bulimia nervosa. The primary health care provider prescribes fluoxetine 20 mg orally each day and psychological therapy for the client twice a week. On her first visit, the therapist asked questions about her cutting behavior. Which of the following screening questions are appropriate for a client to determine the likelihood for continued cutting or other nonsuicidal self-injury? **Select all that apply.**

_____ A. "Have you recently engaged in cutting behaviors?"

_____ B. "How often do you cut yourself?"

_____ C. "Are you usually with friends when cutting or by yourself?"

_____ D. "Why do you feel that you need to cut yourself?"

_____ E. "What do you use to make the cuts on your legs?"

_____ F. "Have you ever cut yourself deeper than you expected?"

Thinking Exercise 15-6

A 15-year-old female client was diagnosed with major depressive disorders and anorexia nervosa. The primary health care provider prescribed fluoxetine 20 mg orally each day and psychological therapy for the client twice a week. **For each assessment finding, use an X to indicate whether the interventions were _Effective_ (helped to meet expected outcomes), _Ineffective_ (did not help to meet expected outcomes), or _Unrelated_ (not related to the expected outcomes).**

Assessment Finding	Effective	Ineffective	Unrelated
Continues to engage in cutting behaviors at times			
Adheres to the treatment plan each week			
Gained 10 lb (2.3 kg) in 2 months			
Has dinner with the family most nights			
Grades in school improving			
Acne worsened during the past month			
Joined the tennis team at school			

Stress and Coping
Generalized Anxiety Disorder

Exemplar 16. Generalized Anxiety Disorder (Mental Health Nursing: Young Adult)

Thinking Exercise 16-1

A 32-year-old female client visits her primary health care provider for her annual physical examination. On initial assessment by the nurse, the following data were recorded:

- VS within normal limits
- Height = 5 ft, 7 in (170.2 cm)
- Weight = 126 lb (57.2 kg)
- History of migraines that are controlled by drug therapy (one to two headaches a month)
- History of depression as a teenager but currently not being treated for this problem
- States that she has been extremely worried most days for the past 7 to 8 months about many day-to-day things and reports having difficulty controlling the worry
- Married for 1½ years and is starting out her practice as a clinical psychologist
- Husband lost his job 6 months ago due to his company's closure; remains unemployed
- Has student loans from graduate school and is having problems making payments
- Wants to get pregnant someday but feels too stressed to think about it now
- Is having problems sleeping—either getting to sleep or staying asleep
- Has been taking melatonin to help her sleep but is finding it only slightly effective
- Denies using illicit drugs or other substances; has an occasional glass of wine to help her relax
- Reports always feeling tired and having problems concentrating at work
- Has no problems with appetite and states that she eats healthily as much as she can

Highlight or place a check mark next to the assessment findings that require follow-up by the nurse and health care team.

Thinking Exercise 16-2

A 32-year-old female client visits her primary health care provider for her annual physical examination. At the end of her visit, the provider determined that the client has generalized anxiety disorder (GAD). **Choose the *most likely* options for the information missing from the statements below by selecting from the lists of options provided.**

The nurse teaches the client that nonpharmacologic interventions for managing GAD include _____1_____, _____1_____, and _____1_____. If the client needs drug therapy to treat her mental health problem, the first-line drug classes used are _____2_____ and _____2_____. _____2_____ is another preferred drug for GAD. Unlike other anxiolytics, this drug is not a central nervous system depressant, has no abuse potential, and can be used on a long-term basis.

Options for 1	Options for 2
Cognitive behavioral therapy	Benzodiazepines
Herbal supplements	Selective serotonin reuptake inhibitors
Copper bracelets	Butorphanol
Biofeedback	Stimulants
Vitamin supplements	Clorazepate
Relaxation techniques	Serotonin-norepinephrine reuptake inhibitors
Keto diet	Buspirone
High-protein diet	Alprazolam

Thinking Exercise 16-3

A 32-year-old female client visits her primary health care provider for her annual physical examination. At the end of her visit, the provider determines that the client has generalized anxiety disorder (GAD) and prescribes venlafaxine XR 37.5 mg orally once a day as an initial dose. **Indicate which health teaching about venlafaxine listed in the far-left column is *appropriate* for the nurse to provide for the client at this time.**

Potential Health Teaching	Appropriate Health Teaching
"Your drug dosage will likely be increased based on how well this dosage reduces your anxiety."	
"Take the drug in the morning on an empty stomach to decrease the risk of nausea."	
"If you begin thinking about harming yourself, let your primary health care provider know immediately."	
"This drug may decrease your appetite, so monitor your weight."	
"This drug can make you sleepy."	
"Follow up with your primary health care provider to check your blood pressure, which may increase."	

Thinking Exercise 16-4

A 32-year-old female client visits her primary health care provider for follow-up regarding the response to her daily dosing of venlafaxine XR 37.5 mg for generalized anxiety disorder. The provider increased the venlafaxine dosage because the client reports that her anxiety has not decreased. The nurse reviews the client's current list of drugs, which includes:
- Propranolol 40 mg orally twice a day for migraine headache prevention
- Naratriptan 2.5 mg orally PRN for abortive therapy for migraine headache
- Eszopiclone 1 mg orally at bedtime for insomnia
- Ibuprofen 600 mg orally once a day for chronic ankle pain
- Venlafaxine XR 75 mg orally for generalized anxiety disorder

Based on the nurse's review for potential drug-drug or drug-supplement interactions or potential adverse effects, what health teaching will the nurse need to provide? **Select all that apply.**

_____ A. "Report dizziness and lightheadedness to your primary health care provider."

_____ B. "Expect your heart rate to increase with the increase in your medication for anxiety."

_____ C. "Avoid taking any over-the-counter drugs for cough and colds, especially those containing dextromethorphan."

_____ D. "Do not take St. John's wort or ginseng while taking your prescribed medications."

_____ E. "Seek medical attention immediately if you experience increased temperature, tremors, diarrhea, profuse sweating, or dilated pupils."

_____ F. "Take acetaminophen instead of ibuprofen for your chronic ankle pain."

_____ G. "Avoid vitamin supplements while taking your prescribed medications."

_____ H. "Monitor your blood pressure at home because a higher dosage of venlafaxine can increase blood pressure."

Thinking Exercise 16-5

A 32-year-old female client visited her primary health care provider for her annual physical examination. At the end of her visit, the provider determined that the client has generalized anxiety disorder (GAD) and prescribed venlafaxine XR 37.5 mg orally once a day as an initial dose. The client returns today to the primary health care provider's office for follow-up 6 weeks after beginning drug therapy. **For each assessment finding, use an X to indicate whether the interventions were <u>Effective</u> (helped to meet expected outcomes), <u>Ineffective</u> (did not help to meet expected outcomes), or <u>Unrelated</u> (not related to the expected outcomes).**

Assessment Finding	Effective	Ineffective	Unrelated
Unintentional weight loss of 10 lb (4.5 kg) in the past 6 weeks			
Sleeping pattern improving			
Feels less worried most of the time			
Participates in yoga class 3 to 4 days a week			
No longer eating red meat in her diet			
Husband starting new job next week			
Has decided to try to get pregnant starting next month			
Was able to pay her student loan payment last month			

**Exemplar 17. Uterine Leiomyoma/Hysterectomy
(Medical-Surgical Nursing: Middle-Age Adult)**

Thinking Exercise 17-1

A 54-year-old postmenopausal female client visits her primary health care provider with a report of heavy vaginal bleeding for the past 3 weeks. The nurse takes the client's history and performs an abdominal assessment in preparation for a more thorough pelvic examination by the primary health care provider. The client states that she has a history of uterine fibroids. Which of the following additional assessment data would the nurse expect for this client? **Select all that apply.**

_____ A. Feeling of pelvic pressure

_____ B. Diarrhea

_____ C. Urinary incontinence

_____ D. Abdominal bloating

_____ E. Anemia

_____ F. Cramping pain

_____ G. Nausea

_____ H. Anorexia

_____ I. Urolithiasis

Thinking Exercise 17-2

A 54-year-old postmenopausal female client visits her primary health care provider with a report of heavy vaginal bleeding for the past 3 weeks. Last week she had a transvaginal ultrasound and MRI, which verified two large uterine leiomyomas (fibroids). The primary health care provider recommended that the client have a laparoscopic hysterectomy. The nurse takes a medication history from the client, who can recall only some of the information. **Choose the *most likely* options for the information missing from the table by selecting from the lists of options provided.**

Medication	Dose, Route, Frequency	Drug Class	Indication
1	50 mcg orally once daily 30–60 min before breakfast	Thyroid replacement drug	Hypothyroidism
Dabigatran	150 mg orally twice daily	Direct thrombin inhibitor	2
Citalopram	40 mg orally once daily	3	Depression
Lisinopril	4	Angiotensin-converting enzyme inhibitor	Hypertension
5	40 mg orally once daily	HMG-CoA reductase inhibitor	Hypercholesterolemia

Options for 1	Options for 2	Options for 3
Methimazole	GERD	Tricyclic antidepressant
Levothyroxine	Stroke	Bisphosphonate
Propylthiouracil	Heart failure	Selective serotonin reuptake inhibitor
Prolactin	Peripheral vascular disease	Biguanide
Vasopressin	Hepatitis C	Beta-adrenergic blocking agent
Tolvaptan	Arial fibrillation	Biologic immune modifier

Options for 4	Options for 5
500 mg orally 3 times daily	Glipizide
5 mg sublingually twice daily	Tramadol
10 mg orally once daily	Cisplatin
40 mg orally once daily	Rifampin
4 mg orally twice daily	Gemfibrozil
0.25 mg orally 3 times daily	Simvastatin

Thinking Exercise 17-3

A 54-year-old postmenopausal female client visited her primary health care provider with a report of heavy vaginal bleeding for the previous 3 weeks. At her surgeon's recommendation, she was scheduled for a laparoscopic hysterectomy this afternoon due to two large uterine leiomyomas (fibroids). During surgery, the surgeon found excessive abdominal adhesions and performed an open abdominal laparotomy and hysterectomy instead of using a laparoscopic approach. The client was admitted to the surgical unit, where the nurse performs a postoperative assessment and health teaching. Which health teaching will the nurse provide for the client to help prevent postoperative complications? **Select all that apply.**

_____ A. "You'll be here in the hospital for at least 3 days."

_____ B. "Be sure to use your incentive spirometer every 1 to 2 hours."

_____ C. "Your compression devices will help prevent blood clots."

_____ D. "We'll be giving you a laxative to help you go to the bathroom."

_____ E. "We'll be helping you get out of bed this evening."

_____ F. "Be sure to drink plenty of fluids to prevent dehydration."

_____ G. "We'll be checking your blood count to make sure you aren't anemic."

_____ H. "Be sure to do your deep breathing exercises every 1 to 2 hours."

_____ I. "We'll take your IV out once you can drink without nausea and urinate."

Thinking Exercise 17-4

A 54-year-old postmenopausal female client visited her primary health care provider with a report of heavy vaginal bleeding for the previous 3 weeks. At her surgeon's recommendation, she was scheduled for a laparoscopic hysterectomy yesterday afternoon due to two large uterine leiomyomas (fibroids). During surgery, the surgeon found excessive abdominal adhesions and performed an abdominal laparotomy and hysterectomy instead of using a laparoscopic approach. This morning the open nurse reads the night nurse's notes below:

Nurses' Notes

4/21/20 0545 Alert and oriented, sleeping intermittently throughout the night after receiving analgesic. Stated that her abdominal pain decreased from a 7 to a 2. Abdominal dressing clean, dry, and intact. Drinking fluids without nausea or vomiting. Voided × 3. Has not eaten much solid food yet but looking forward to breakfast. Will be discharged today if she tolerates food. Husband is coming to pick her up when ready.

————————————————————————————————— S.B. Jenkins, RN,C

The day nurse plans to provide health teaching in preparation for the client's discharge. **Choose the *most likely* options for the information missing from the statements below by selecting from the lists of options provided.**

The nurse teaches the client to monitor for potential postoperative complications such as _____1_____, _____1_____, and _____1_____. The client should contact the primary health care provider if any of these signs and symptoms occur: _____2_____, _____2_____, and _____2_____.

Options for 1	Options for 2
Intestinal obstruction	Elevated temperature
Acute kidney injury	Hiccups
Venous thromboembolism	Diaphoresis
Acute cholecystitis	Heart palpitations
Vaginitis	Reddened swollen calf
Infection	Severe abdominal pain and swelling
Menopause	Absence of menstrual periods
Internal abdominal bleeding	Increased blood pressure
Menarche	Vaginal itching

Thinking Exercise 17-5

A 54-year-old postmenopausal female client has a follow-up appointment with the surgeon 6 weeks after her open hysterectomy for uterine leiomyomas. The office nurse interviews the client and performs a previsit assessment. **For each assessment finding, use an X to indicate whether the interventions were <u>Effective</u> (helped to meet expected outcomes), <u>Ineffective</u> (did not help to meet expected outcomes), or <u>Unrelated</u> (not related to the expected outcomes).**

Assessment Finding	Effective	Ineffective	Unrelated
Incision healed without infection			
Urinary incontinence			
Normal body temperature			
No vaginal bleeding			
Reports having periods of flatus			
Reports occasional constipation			

Reproduction
Childbearing Family

Exemplar 18A. Uncomplicated Prenatal Woman

Thinking Exercise 18A-1

A 36-year-old female client arrives at her primary health care provider's office for her initial prenatal visit at 9 weeks' gestation. The nurse collects and records the following health and obstetric history:

Health History
- Allergies: None
- Current medications: Sertraline daily, acetaminophen, and naproxen sodium as needed for headache pain
- Past health history: Tonsillectomy as a child, asthma
- Family health history: Ovarian cancer—grandmother

Obstetric History
- LMP: 12/12/2019

Date of Delivery	Weeks of Gestation	Sex	Delivery Style and Any Complications	Fetal Demise (Yes [Y] or No [N])
2/21/2010	41	F	SVD and none	N
4/16/2012	21	F	SVD and none	Y
8/8/2014	36	M	C/S and dizygotic twin	N
8/8/2014	36	F	C/S and dizygotic twin	N

Based on the client's obstetric history from the table above, choose the *most likely* options for the information missing from the statements below by selecting from the lists of options provided.

The client's gravida is ____1____ and her parity is ____2____. The number of term deliveries is ____3____, the number of preterm deliveries is ____4____, the number of aborted deliveries is ____5____, and the number of living children is ____6____. The client's estimated date of delivery is _____7_____.

Options for 1, 2, and 3	Options for 4, 5, and 6	Options for 7
1	0	March 5, 2020
2	1	August 29, 2020
3	2	September 19, 2020
4	3	September 26, 2020

Thinking Exercise 18A-2

A 36-year-old female client has her initial prenatal primary health care provider visit at 9 weeks' gestation. Which prenatal care activities would the nurse likely include in today's visit? **Select all that apply.**

_____ A. Provide nutrition education.

_____ B. Obtain a midstream urinalysis.

_____ C. Send a blood sample for a complete blood count.

_____ D. Send a blood sample for alpha-fetoprotein (AFP) testing.

_____ E. Advise the client to have DNA testing.

_____ F. Assist the primary health care provider in collecting specimens for vaginal culture.

_____ G. Complete an obstetric ultrasound.

_____ H. Enter a prescription to obtain the client's blood typing.

Thinking Exercise 18A-3

A 36-year-old female client has her initial prenatal primary health care provider visit at 9 weeks' gestation. The nurse completes the initial assessment of the client and reviews the client's health and obstetric history.

Health History
- Allergies: None
- Current medications: Sertraline daily, acetaminophen, and naproxen sodium as needed for headache pain
- Past health history: Tonsillectomy as a child, asthma
- Family health history: Ovarian cancer—grandmother

Obstetric History
- LMP: 12/12/2019

Date of Delivery	Weeks of Gestation	Sex	Delivery Style and Any Complications	Fetal Demise (Yes [Y] or No [N])
2/21/2010	41	F	SVD and none	N
4/16/2012	21	F	SVD and none	Y
8/8/2014	36	M	C/S and dizygotic twin	N
8/8/2014	36	F	C/S and dizygotic twin	N

For each health assessment finding below, use an X to indicate whether it <u>Requires Nursing Follow-Up</u> (could be harmful to the client) or is <u>Expected</u> (no follow-up is required) for the client at this time.

Assessment Findings	Expected	Requires Nursing Follow-Up
Temperature = 98.6°F (37°C)		
Respiratory rate = 14 breaths/min		
Heart rate = 76 beats/min		
Blood pressure = 132/78 mm Hg		

Assessment Findings	Expected	Requires Nursing Follow-Up
Timing of initial visit (9 weeks)		
Previous term delivery(s)		
Previous preterm delivery(s)		
Estimated date of delivery (EDD)		
Height: 66 in (167.64 cm)		
Daily sertraline		
Acetaminophen as needed for pain		
Naproxen sodium as needed for pain		

Thinking Exercise 18A-4

The nurse provides health teaching for a 36-year-old female client during her initial prenatal primary health care provider visit at 9 weeks' gestation. **Choose the *most likely* options for the information missing from the statements below by selecting from the lists of options provided.**

During the client's first trimester, routine prenatal visits will be every _____1_____ week(s). The primary health care provider will prescribe an ultrasound to check for fetal _____2_____ that could indicate fetal anomalies. The client can expect to hear the heartbeat during the second trimester and feel fetal _____3_____ after 16 weeks. A noninvasive way to monitor the _____4_____ of the fetus is by measuring the _____5_____ height and is done at every visit after _____6_____ weeks' gestation but may have a _____7_____ -week margin of error.

Options for 1, 6, and 7	Options for 2, 3, 4, and 5
1	Growth
2	Respirations
4	Movements
6	Fundal
12	Circumference
16	Heart rate
20	Viability
	Anatomy
	Gender

Thinking Exercise 18A-5

The nurse is preparing a 41-year-old female client and her husband for various testing that will be done throughout the pregnancy to monitor for maternal and fetal well-being. The client is a gravida 3 para 2 (G3P2) with a history of cephalopelvic disproportion and previous cesarean section. She is currently at 15⁶⁄₇ weeks' gestation. **Choose the *most likely* options for the information missing from the table below by selecting from the lists of options provided.**

Diagnostic Test	Indication	Nursing Implications
1	Used to evaluate the viability of the fetus and the placenta's ability to perfuse the fetus.	Place client on external fetal monitor and instruct her to push the button every time the fetus moves.
Alpha-fetoprotein	**2**	Perform test after 10 weeks' gestation and include gestation with serum sample.
Fetal biophysical profile	Used to identify if a fetus is in distress and assesses fetal heart rate reactivity, breathing and body movements, muscle tone, and amniotic fluid volume.	**3**
5	Done at 8–12 wk for pregnancies associated with high risk for genetic defects.	Potential complications include spontaneous or accidental abortion.
Amniocentesis	**4**	Test is contraindicated in clients with abruptio placentae and may cause amniotic fluid emboli.
Glucose tolerance test	Can be used to evaluate clients with hypoglycemia.	**6**

Options for 1	Options for 2	Options for 3
Fetal contraction stress test Chorionic villus sampling Fetal nonstress test Chromosome karyotype	Screening marker used to identify increased risk for birth defects Used to measure fetal maturity, fetal distress, and risk for respiratory distress syndrome Serum screen used to monitor clients at high risk for failed pregnancy Reveals the chromosomal makeup of the fetus to determine chromosomal defects	Hypotension may cause false-positive results and may induce premature labor. Instruct client to eat 2 to 3 hours prior to examination. Specimens may be obtained from fluid, fetal tissue, or venipuncture. Instruct the client to fast for 12 hours prior to the test. The overall score will dictate if and when the test has to be repeated.

Options for 4	Options for 5	Options for 6
Used to measure fetal maturity, fetal distress, and risk for respiratory distress syndrome Reveals the chromosomal makeup of the fetus to determine chromosomal defects Multiple marker screen to identify increased risk for birth defects Serum screen used to monitor clients at high risk for failed pregnancy	Human chorionic gonadotropin (HCG) Fetal nonstress test Chromosome karyotype Chorionic villus sampling	Hypotension may cause false-positive results and may induce premature labor. Instruct the client to fast for 12 hours prior to the test. Perform test after 10 weeks' gestation and include gestation with serum sample.

Thinking Exercise 18A-6

A 36-year-old primigravida client has a 36-week obstetric appointment. The nurse assesses the woman's and fetal overall well-being. **For each assessment finding, use an X to indicate whether health teaching and screening tests were <u>Effective</u> (helped to meet expected outcomes), <u>Ineffective</u> (did not help to meet expected outcomes), or <u>Unrelated</u> (were not related to the expected outcomes).**

Assessment Findings	Effective	Ineffective	Unrelated
Temperature = 98.6°F (37°C)			
Blood pressure = 142/88 mm Hg			
Client reports six fetal kicks every hour			
Group B streptococci (+)			

Assessment Findings	Effective	Ineffective	Unrelated
1-hour glucose tolerance test results = 133 mg/dL (10 mmol/L)			
Client reports having car seat, clothes, diapers, and bassinet			
Client plans to breast-feed			
Urinalysis results = 3+ protein, negative for bacteria			
Client denies completing childbirth preparation class			

Exemplar 18B. Complicated Prenatal Woman

Thinking Exercise 18B-1

The nurse performs an assessment of a 21-year-old gravida 2 para 1 (G2P1) client at 28 weeks' gestation. The client tells the nurse that she is concerned about dizziness and a headache that persists even with acetaminophen administration. **For each health assessment finding below, use an X to indicate whether it <u>Requires Nursing Follow-Up</u> (could be harmful to client) or is <u>Expected</u> (no follow-up is required) for the client at this time.**

Assessment Findings	Expected	Requires Nursing Follow-Up
Temperature = 98°F (36.7°C)		
Heart rate = 100 beats/min		
Respiratory rate = 22 breaths/min		
Blood pressure = 168/98 mm Hg		
Headache rated at 8/10 on a 0 to 10 pain scale		
Constant epigastric pain		
Hemoglobin = 11 g/dL (110 g/L)		
Platelets = 128,000/mm³ (128 × 10⁹/L)		
Urine protein = 2+		
Urine ketones = 1+		
Clonus = negative		
DTRs = 2+ in lower and upper extremities		
Breath sounds = clear in all fields		
Visual disturbances		
Client reports that primary health care provider is "watching my blood pressure"		

Thinking Exercise 18B-2

The nurse performs an assessment of a 21-year-old gravida 2 para 1 (G2P1) client at 28 weeks' gestation. The client tells the nurse that she is concerned about dizziness and a headache that persists even with acetaminophen administration. The nurse documents the following client assessment findings:

Vital Signs	
Temperature	98°F (36.7°C)
Heart rate	100 beats/min
Respirations	22 breaths/min
Blood pressure	168/98 mm Hg
Oxygen saturation	100% (on room air)
Laboratory Test Results	
Hemoglobin	11.0 g/dL (110 g/L)
Platelets	128,000/mm³ (128 × 10⁹/L)
Urine protein	2+
Urine ketones	1+
Blood type	A negative

Physical Assessment Findings
- Reports headache as 8/10 on a 0 to 10 pain scale
- Reports epigastric pain that is constant
- Breath sounds clear in all lung fields
- No clonus, DTRs 2+ in lower and upper extremities
- States that her obstetric provider has been "watching her blood pressure"
- Reports seeing "stars" sometimes

Based on these assessment findings, which of the following actions would the nurse take? **Select all that apply.**

_____ A. Administer an antihypertensive medication per protocol.

_____ B. Check the client for muscle twitching and tingling.

_____ C. Request prescription for blood pressure parameters.

_____ D. Check the client's eyesight for blurriness.

_____ E. Compare the client's prenatal and current blood pressure values.

_____ F. Place the client in a flat position on her back to increase blood pressure.

_____ G. Teach the client that blood pressures usually increase significantly in the third trimester.

Thinking Exercise 18B-3

The nurse reviews the following assessment findings for a 21-year-old pregnant client at 28 weeks' gestation who is concerned about dizziness and a headache that persists even with acetaminophen administration.

Vital Signs

Temperature	98°F (36.7°C)
Heart rate	100 beats/min
Respirations	22 breaths/min
Blood pressure	168/98 mm Hg
Oxygen saturation	100% (on room air)

Laboratory Test Results

Hemoglobin	11.0 g/dL (110 g/L)
Platelets	128,000/mm³ (128 × 10⁹/L)
Urine protein	2+
Urine ketones	1+
Blood type	A negative

Physical Assessment Findings

- Reports headache as 8/10 on a 0 to 10 pain scale
- Reports epigastric pain that is constant
- Breath sounds clear in all lung fields
- No clonus, DTRs 2+ in lower and upper extremities
- States that her obstetric provider has been "watching her blood pressure"
- Reports seeing "stars" sometimes

The nurse wants to encourage optimal outcomes for both mother and baby. Based on the assessment findings above, what **priority** nursing actions are needed to prevent worsening of the client's symptoms? **Select all that apply.**

_____ A. Administer magnesium sulfate per protocol.

_____ B. Position the client in reverse Trendelenburg.

_____ C. Assess deep tendon reflexes to establish a baseline.

_____ D. Encourage increased oral fluid intake of water.

_____ E. Teach the client to avoid foods high in fat.

_____ F. Schedule a nonstress test weekly.

Thinking Exercise 18B-4

A client who is 29 weeks pregnant presents to the primary health care provider's office for her regularly scheduled visit. The nurse reviews the following documented assessment findings:

Assessment Findings

Temperature	98.4°F (36.9°C)
Blood type	A negative
Hep B status	Negative
Current blood pressure	152/92 mm Hg
Prepregnancy blood pressure	120/68 mm Hg
Previous deliveries	G4P3 (G4 T1 P2 A0 L2)
Rubella status	Nonimmune
Group B strep	Will test at a later date
Fetal movement	Yes
Fundal height	28 cm

Highlight or place a check mark next to the assessment findings that require follow-up by the nurse.

Thinking Exercise 18B-5

A 25-year-old primigravida had an incomplete abortion at 12 weeks' gestation. After initial stabilization on admission to the hospital, a vacuum extraction with curettage was performed to remove retained placental tissue. When the client has questions about the loss of her fetus and the procedure, how will the nurse therapeutically and truthfully respond? **Use an X to indicate whether the nurse's responses below are __Therapeutic__ or __Nontherapeutic__.**

Nurse's Response	Therapeutic	Nontherapeutic
"Spontaneous abortions are for the best and you are lucky it happened early."		
"You can always have other children."		
"We will be monitoring your bleeding for your safety."		
"Fluid replacement and nutrition are important for your physical healing."		
"Talking to someone you trust is vital for your mental healing."		
"Who can I call to be with you during this time?"		

Exemplar 18C. Uncomplicated Intrapartum Care

Thinking Exercise 18C-1

The nurse is caring for a 34-year-old laboring woman and provides health teaching about the stages of labor. **Complete the statements below by selecting from the lists of options provided.**

The first stage of labor lasts from the time _____1_____ begins to the time when the _____2_____ is fully dilated. The second stage of labor lasts from the time of full cervical _____1_____ to the birth of the _____3_____. The third stage of labor lasts from the _____3_____'s birth to the expulsion of the _____4_____. The fourth stage of labor begins with the delivery of the _____4_____ and includes at least the first ___5___ hours after birth.

Options for 1	Options for 2	Options for 3	Options for 4	Options for 5
Dilation	Vagina	Placenta	Infant	2
Change	Cervix	Umbilical cord	Placenta	3
Station	Fundus	Infant	Fundus	5
Contractions	Fetus	Uterus	Umbilical cord	8
Fetal movement	Uterus	Fundus	Uterus	24

Thinking Exercise 18C-2

A 19-year-old nulliparous client is being sent home from the hospital after being monitored for 2 hours with no cervical change. She is at 36 5/7 weeks' gestation and has had occasional prenatal care. She states that she is "terrified of going into labor in public." **Place a check mark to indicate what health teaching by the nurse is __Indicated__ or __Non-Essential__ before discharge that would alert the client about the need to return to the hospital.**

Health Teaching	Indicated	Non-Essential
Contractions every 5 minutes for at least an hour with a pattern of increasing regularity, frequency, duration, and intensity		
Awakening less than twice per night with the need to urinate		
Any gush or trickle of fluid from the vagina		
Vaginal bleeding		
"Nesting" or feeling the need to clean		
Feeling the baby move more than usual		
Decreased fetal movement		
Any feeling that something is wrong		

Thinking Exercise 18C-3

The nurse is caring for a client who is having her first child. The client asks about what the fetal monitor tracing is showing the health care team. An external monitor is being used for contractions and fetal heart rate. The monitor strip shows the following:

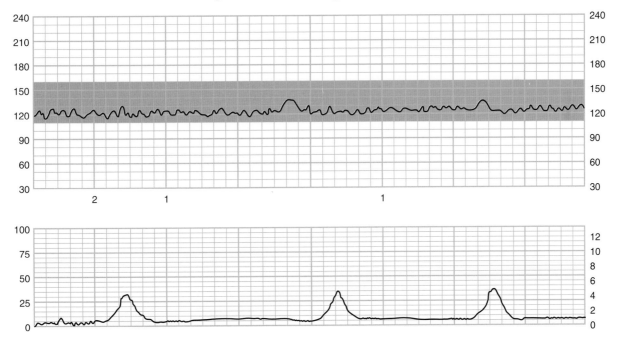

Which of the following statements are appropriate for the nurse when interpreting the fetal monitoring strip results? **Select all that apply.**

_____ A. "We are concerned about your fetus's oxygenation because of absent variability."

_____ B. "We can see that you are having contractions every minute."

_____ C. "Your contraction pattern is every 4 to 5 minutes."

_____ D. "The beat-to-beat difference in your baby's heartbeat shows that there is variability."

_____ E. "The decelerations have been reported to your primary health care provider."

_____ F. "The contractions are not strong enough to cause cervical change."

_____ G. "An average fetal heart rate is 110 to 160, and your baby has a baseline of 120."

Thinking Exercise 18C-4

The nurse evaluates the following external fetal monitor strip of the client at 40 weeks' gestation who is contracting and in active labor.

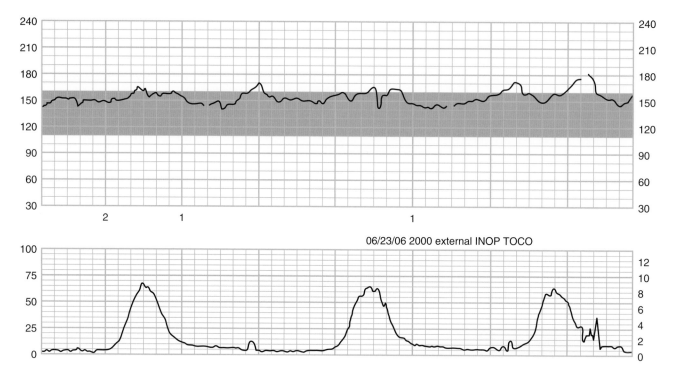

06/23/06 2000 external INOP TOCO

Which statements correctly describe the **fetal heart rate** in this strip and would be documented by the nurse? **Select all that apply.**

_____ A. "The fetal heart rate is tachycardic and needs to be evaluated."

_____ B. "The fetal heart rate shows accelerations."

_____ C. "The type of accelerations are a positive indicator of fetal well-being."

_____ D. "The decelerations are common with contractions."

_____ E. "The marked variability of this fetus is abnormal for this stage of labor."

_____ F. "No fetal decelerations in the heart rate are present."

_____ G. "The normal fetal heart rate is any rate above 120 beats per minute."

_____ H. "The baseline fetal heart rate is 145 beats per minute."

_____ I. "All decelerations indicate fetal compromise."

Thinking Exercise 18C-5

The nurse evaluates the following fetal monitoring strip for a laboring client at 40³⁄₇ weeks' gestation.

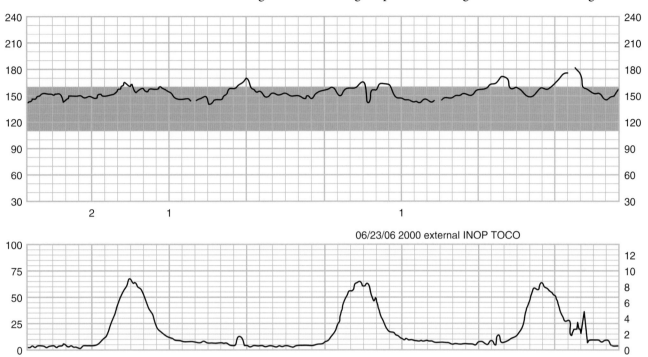

06/23/06 2000 external INOP TOCO

Which statements correctly describe the **contraction pattern** in this strip and would be provided by the nurse in a report to the primary health care provider? **Select all that apply.**

_____ A. "Contractions are strong in intensity."

_____ B. "Contraction frequency is every 2 to 3 minutes."

_____ C. "The duration of contractions is 3 to 4 minutes."

_____ D. "Cervical change is occurring with this contraction pattern."

_____ E. "There is adequate resting tone at this time."

_____ F. "The duration of contractions is 50 to 70 seconds."

_____ G. "This contraction pattern shows false labor."

_____ H. "Contraction frequency is every 60 seconds."

_____ I. "This marked contraction pattern shows pushing efforts."

Exemplar 18D. Complicated Intrapartum Care

Thinking Exercise 18D-1

The nurse assesses and documents the following findings for a client at 39 weeks' gestation during the active stage of labor:

Assessment Findings	
Temperature	98°F (36.7°C)
Heart rate	100 beats/min

Continued

Assessment Findings	
Respirations	22 breaths/min
Blood pressure	144/78 mm Hg
Oxygen saturation	100% (on room air)
Pain level	3/10 on 0 to 10 pain scale
Cervical dilation	5 cm
Cervical effacement	90%
Fetal station	−3

The client's membranes rupture and the umbilical cord is found to be protruding from the vaginal opening. **Use an X for the nursing actions below that are <u>Anticipated</u> (appropriate or necessary), <u>Contraindicated</u> (could be harmful), or <u>Non-Essential</u> (make no difference or are not necessary) for the client's care at this time.**

Nursing Action	Anticipated	Contraindicated	Non-Essential
Apply pressure to fetal presenting part and off of the cord.			
Apply oxygen to client at 10 L per mask.			
Encourage client's support person to remain calm.			
Attempt to replace cord back into the client's uterus.			
Remove pressure from the client's cervix after 60 seconds.			
Remain with client until delivery of the infant.			

Thinking Exercise 18D-2

The nurse is caring for a client with the diagnosis of polyhydramnios during the active stage of labor. **Indicate which nursing action(s) listed in the far-left column is (are) appropriate for managing each potential intrapartum complication. Note that not all actions will be used and <u>some actions will be used multiple times.</u>**

Nursing Action	Potential Intrapartum Complication	Appropriate Nursing Action(s) for Each Intrapartum Complication
1 Apply pressure to fetal presenting part and off of the cord.	Prolapsed cord	
2 Apply oxygen to client at 10 L per mask.	Abruptio placentae	
3 Encourage client's support person to leave the room.	Eclampsia seizure	

Nursing Action	Potential Intrapartum Complication	Appropriate Nursing Action(s) for Each Intrapartum Complication
4 Compare the client's prenatal and current blood pressure values.	Chorioamnionitis	
5 Monitor blood glucose levels hourly.		
6 Attempt to replace cord back into the client's uterus.		
7 Remove pressure off the client's cervix after 60 seconds.		
8 Remain with client until delivery of the infant.		
9 Titrate or administer magnesium sulfate.		
10 Administer ampicillin.		

Thinking Exercise 18D-3

The nurse is caring for a client who is having her fourth child during the active stage of labor. The client reports shortness of breath and chest pain. She states, "This feels different than any delivery before." Which of the following actions would the nurse take? **Select all that apply.**

_____ A. Assess the client's oxygen saturation.

_____ B. Apply oxygen to the client at 10 L per mask

_____ C. Encourage the client's support person to leave the room.

_____ D. Attempt to position the client with her head lower than her uterus.

_____ E. Compare the client's prenatal and current blood pressure values.

_____ F. Check membrane status.

_____ G. Remain with the client while contacting the primary health care provider immediately.

Thinking Exercise 18D-4

A 21-year-old G4P1 client at 24 weeks' gestation reports having lower back pain over the past 2 days and was referred to the labor and delivery assessment center for evaluation. The nurse reviews the prenatal record below to identify any possible maternal risk factors for preterm labor.

Height	63 in (160 cm)
Prepregnancy weight, current weight	103 lb (46.8 kg), 110 lb (50 kg)
Medical history	None significant
Obstetric history	12/2016 SAB 12 weeks 11/2017 Vaginal delivery 30 weeks 12/2018 SAB at 16 weeks Diagnosed 11/2018 with incompetent cervix No previous uterine surgery

Continued

Present pregnancy	Twin pregnancy
	Vaginal spotting after cerclage placement at 14 weeks
	Hgb 12–13 g/dL (120–130 g/L) throughout pregnancy
	Hct 35.8%–39% throughout pregnancy
	Blood pressures 110–120/60–70 mm Hg throughout pregnancy
	No rupture of membranes
	No fetal or placental abnormalities
	Prenatal care started at 8 weeks' gestation
	Hispanic descent
	Smokes approximately 1 pack per day (PPD)
	Employed as a Certified Nursing Assistant, working night shift, 12 hours, full-time in a long-term care facility
	Denies substance use

Highlight or place a check mark next to the assessment findings that require follow-up by the nurse.

Thinking Exercise 18D-5

The nurse is caring for a client at 32 weeks' gestation. The client reports regular contractions over the past 8 hours and has dilated from 1 cm to 2 cm. Betamethasone has been prescribed for the client. What health teaching will the nurse provide about this drug? **Select all that apply.**

_____ A. "This drug will help decrease contractions."

_____ B. "This drug will help to accelerate fetal lung maturity."

_____ C. "This drug will help reduce the incidence and severity of respiratory distress for the fetus."

_____ D. "You'll need to take this drug twice each day as a tablet."

_____ E. "I'll need to give the drug to you by injection two times and 24 hours apart."

_____ F. "This drug will lessen the severity of any complications of prematurity."

_____ G. "The benefits of this drug are greatest within 6 hours of administration."

Exemplar 18E. Uncomplicated Postpartum Care

Thinking Exercise 18E-1

The nurse performs a fundal assessment on a postpartum client. **Complete the statements below by selecting from the lists of options provided.**

First, the nurse asks the client to empty her _____1_____ to prevent _____2_____ displacement. Next, the nurse assists the client to a _____3_____ position with her knees flexed. Then, the nurse applies clean gloves and lower the perineal pads to observe lochia as the _____4_____ is palpated. To _____5_____ and anchor the lower uterine segment, the nurse's non-dominant hand is placed above the woman's symphysis pubis. Finally, palpation begins at the _____6_____ and the nurse gently palpates until the _____4_____ is located.

Options for 1	Options for 2	Options for 3	Options for 4	Options for 5	Options for 6
Uterus	Uterus	High Fowler	Fundus	Palpate	Bladder
Bladder	Bladder	Prone	Bladder	Displace	Umbilicus
Amniotic fluid	Amniotic fluid	Supine	Bowels	Support	Ribs
Bowels	Bowels	Semi-Fowler	Perineum	Invert	Gallbladder

Thinking Exercise 18E-2

A postpartum client delivered her sixth infant via cesarean section 5 hours ago. She delivered her last four children via cesarean section, including the current infant, and all infants weighed over 9 lb (4082 g). When assessing this client, which of the following factors place her at an increased risk for hemorrhage? **Select all that apply.**

_____ A. Grand multiparity

_____ B. Prolonged labor

_____ C. Overdistention of the uterus

_____ D. Retained placental fragments

_____ E. Operative cesarean delivery

_____ F. Preeclampsia

_____ G. History of postpartum hemorrhage

Thinking Exercise 18E-3

A client delivered her newborn 30 hours ago vaginally and experienced a second-degree laceration that was repaired. She has chosen to breast-feed her infant and is preparing for hospital discharge soon. The nurse assesses her discharge teaching and intervention follow-up needs. **For each health assessment finding below, use an X to indicate whether it <u>Requires Nursing Follow-Up</u> (could be harmful to client) or is <u>Expected</u> (no follow-up is required) for the client at this time.**

Assessment Findings	Expected	Requires Nursing Follow-Up
Temperature: 98.6°F (37°C)		
Blood type is A negative		
Hepatitis B status is negative		
Blood pressure = 132/78 mm Hg		
Had a total of four prenatal visits		
Had one previous term delivery		
Rubella status is nonimmune		
Uses ibuprofen and oxycodone regularly for pain		
No colostrum noted with hand expression		
No running water available at her home		

Thinking Exercise 18E-4

A client delivered her first baby 36 hours ago at 2:21 a.m. (0221) via cesarean delivery for failure to progress. Although she was able to dilate to 8 cm, she was not able to progress past the second stage of labor. Her birth plan included wanting a safe vaginal delivery. The nurse reviews the following assessment data to determine the client's adaptation to being a new mother:
- Continues to rate her pain at 5/10 (on a 0 to 10 pain scale) with medication administration
- Having trouble sleeping
- Has large support system

- Has first baby in family
- Has read "what to expect the first year"
- Babysat once for a neighbor's 6-year-old
- Has a positive attitude
- Father of the baby not involved
- Infant boy has many characteristics of father of the baby
- Cesarean birth
- Term infant with no issues

Highlight or place a check mark next to the assessment findings that require follow-up by the nurse.

Thinking Exercise 18E-5

The nurse is preparing to discharge the client and her newborn following a spontaneous vaginal delivery 26 hours ago and evaluates the effectiveness of the client's postpartum care. **For each assessment finding, use an X to indicate whether the interventions were Effective (helped to meet expected outcomes), Ineffective (did not help to meet expected outcomes), or Unrelated (not related to the expected outcomes).**

Assessment Finding	Effective	Ineffective	Unrelated
Temperature = 98.2°F (36.8°C)			
Pain = 2 (on a 0 to 10 pain scale)			
Lochia = serosa, moderate amount			
Nipples are tender with blisters			
No clots noted in past 24 hours			
Fundus is firm and 2 fingerbreadths below the umbilicus			
1+ pitting edema in lower extremities bilaterally			
Client denies difficulty urinating			
Family present at bedside			
Blood glucose = 96 mg/dL (5.3 mmol/L)			

Exemplar 18F. Complicated Postpartum Care

Thinking Exercise 18F-1

The nurse is caring for a client after a spontaneous vaginal delivery of a term fetus. The client's pregnancy blood pressure at that time was 150/85 mm Hg. The client has been on magnesium sulfate therapy for preeclampsia for the past 8 hours per protocol. Current assessment data are as follows:

Vital Signs	
Temperature	98°F (36.7°C)
Heart rate	100 beats/min
Respirations	22 breaths/min
Blood pressure	198/104 mm Hg
Oxygen saturation	100% (on room air)
Pain level	8/10 (on 0 to 10 pain scale) (headache)

Based on the client's current assessment findings, which of the following actions would the nurse take? **Select all that apply.**

_____ A. Notify the primary health care provider of change in vital signs.

_____ B. Administer antihypertensive medication per protocol.

_____ C. Administer acetaminophen.

_____ D. Encourage the client to empty her bladder.

_____ E. Draw a magnesium level as ordered.

_____ F. Position client in a high-Fowler position to decrease blood pressure.

_____ G. Remain with client until new prescriptions are received.

Thinking Exercise 18F-2

The nurse is taking care of a 30-year-old client who gave birth vaginally 8 hours ago. The nurse reviews her assessment findings as listed below:

- Gravida 6 para 5 (G6P5)
- 9-lb (4082-g) new baby
- Delivered vaginally via an intact perineum
- Precipitous birth within 30 minutes of arrival at hospital
- Breast-feeding successfully
- Postbirth hemoglobin 12.4 g/dL (124 g/L)
- Postdelivery hemoglobin 11.2 g/dL (112 g/L)
- Fundus firms with massage
- Large clots expelled with recent fundal check
- Feeling light-headed and dizzy when getting up to go to the bathroom
- Temperature 98.7°F (37°C)

Highlight or place a check mark next to the assessment findings that require follow-up by the nurse.

Thinking Exercise 18F-3

The nurse is caring for a 34-year-old gravida 8 para 6 postpartum client with a blood pressure of 170/94 mm Hg who gave birth vaginally 2 hours ago. The quantitative blood loss (QBL) during delivery was 350 mL, with a 2-hour recovery QBL of 250 mL. The client continues to have a slow trickle of bright red blood from her vagina. Which of the following actions will the nurse take? **Select all that apply.**

_____ A. Administer additional oxytocin per protocol.

_____ B. Perform a fundal assessment.

_____ C. Administer misoprostol rectally per protocol.

_____ D. Administer methylergonovine intramuscularly per protocol.

_____ E. Assess deep tendon reflexes.

_____ F. Administer dinoprostone intravenously per protocol.

_____ G. Notify the primary health care provider.

Thinking Exercise 18F-4

When discharging a 2-day postpartum client, the nurse would teach her to notify the primary health care provider if which signs and symptoms of postpartum affective mood disorder occur? **Select all that apply.**

_____ A. Feelings of sadness and crying

_____ B. Feelings of extra energy and cleaning the house

_____ C. Inability to sleep through the night

_____ D. Easily distracted, difficulty concentrating

_____ E. Dreams of harming self or infant

_____ F. Feelings of wanting to protect infant from outside disturbances

_____ G. Supplementing feedings at night to encourage maternal rest

_____ H. Nightmares about the pregnancy or delivery

Thinking Exercise 18F-5

The nurse is preparing to discharge the client and her newborn following an emergency cesarean section (postoperative day 4) that was complicated by postpartum hemorrhage without transfusion. Her hemoglobin level before delivery was 14 g/dL (140 g/L). The nurse evaluates the effectiveness of the client's postpartum care. **For each assessment finding, use an X to indicate whether the interventions were <u>Effective</u> (helped to meet expected outcomes), <u>Ineffective</u> (did not help to meet expected outcomes), or <u>Unrelated</u> (not related to the expected outcomes).**

Assessment Findings	Effective	Ineffective	Unrelated
Heart rate = 82 beats/min			
Blood pressure = 112/67 mm Hg			
Reports feeling light-headed and dizzy when getting up to go to the bathroom			
Hemoglobin = 9.7 g/dL (97 g/L)			
Incision is clean, dry, slightly pink with staples intact			
Pain = 4 (on a 0 to 10 pain scale) after ibuprofen for pain relief			
Reports breast-feeding is going well; newborn is gaining weight			
Verbalizes that she will take iron supplements with orange juice until next appointment with primary health care provider			

Exemplar 18G. Uncomplicated Newborn Care

Thinking Exercise 18G-1

The nurse is caring for a newborn born at 39 weeks' gestation 1 hour ago. What evidence-based care will the nurse provide to the newborn during the transitional period? **Select all that apply.**

_____ A. Administer hepatitis B vaccine per protocol.

_____ B. Assess for hypoxia.

_____ C. Administer oxygen therapy per protocol.

_____ D. Perform a gestational assessment.

_____ E. Administer intramuscular vitamin K per protocol.

_____ F. Complete an otoacoustic test.

_____ G. Encourage skin-to-skin contact with the baby's mother.

_____ H. Complete congenital cardiac heart defect screening.

_____ I. Place identification and security safety bands on the newborn.

Thinking Exercise 18G-2

The nurse completes a routine infant assessment approximately 12 hours after birth. **Use an X to indicate whether the assessment findings below are <u>Expected</u> (finding within usual limits or parameters), a <u>Common Variation</u> (finding that may or may not indicate an abnormality, usually transitory), or <u>Unexpected</u> (finding that is abnormal and could be harmful) for the infant at this time.**

Assessment Findings	Expected	Common Variation	Unexpected
Heart rate = 134 beats/min			
Pale mucous membranes			
Bluish tint of fingers and toes			
Jittery activity			
Fontanels are soft with edema of soft scalp tissue			
Cries without tears			
Positive red reflex			
Large dark bluish areas of pigmentation on lower back			
Small white bumps along the midline of the hard palate			

Thinking Exercise 18G-3

Nursing care for an infant during the first 24 to 48 hours after birth includes frequent assessments. **Complete the statements below by selecting from the lists of options provided.**

To accurately assess the newborn, the nurse will count heart rate and respirations for _____1_____ seconds, measure the weight of the baby _____2_____ clothes or diaper at the same time of day daily, and monitor the feeding patterns of the newborn daily. These feeding patterns are then compared with _____3_____ intake to identify _____4_____ growth difficulties.

Options for 1	Options for 2, 3, and 4
5	Potential
10	Without
15	Appropriate for gestational age
30	Expected
60	Calories per kilogram

Thinking Exercise 18G-4

The nurse is caring for a maternal/newborn couplet with the following birth delivery data:
- Mother's blood type: O positive
- Gestational age: 38 weeks
- Spontaneous, precipitous vaginal delivery
- Weight = 9 lb 13 oz (4.46 kg)

The nurse identifies screening tests that are needed for newborn infants. **Use an X to indicate whether the screening tests below are <u>Anticipated</u> (appropriate or necessary), <u>Contraindicated</u> (could be harmful), or <u>Non-Essential</u> (make no difference or are not necessary) for the newborn at this time.**

Screening Tests	Anticipated	Contraindicated	Non-Essential
Type and screen blood			
Metabolic panel			
Bilirubin			
Car seat screening			
Pulse oximetry			
Urinalysis			
Hearing			
Fingerprints			
Blood glucose			

Thinking Exercise 18G-5

The nurse is preparing to discharge the client and her newborn following a spontaneous vaginal delivery at 40 weeks' gestation and evaluates the effectiveness of the newborn's care. **For each assessment finding, use an X to indicate whether the interventions were <u>Effective</u> (helped to meet expected outcomes), <u>Ineffective</u> (did not help to meet expected outcomes), or <u>Unrelated</u> (were not related to the expected outcomes).**

Assessment Finding	Effective	Ineffective	Unrelated
Temperature = 99.1°F (37.2°C)			
Heart rate = 144 beats/min			
Respirations = 54 breaths/min			
Pulse oximetry = 99% (on room air)			
Bilirubin = 14 mg/dL (205 mcmol/L)			
Birth weight = 9 lb 13 oz (4.46 kg) Current weight = 9 lb 6 oz (4.29 kg)			
Baby has minimal periods of wakefulness			
Breast-feeding every 2.5–3 hr			
Urine output = 4 wet diapers in 12 hours			
Bowel movement = dark green, thick, and large amount			
Baby has had photographs taken			
Security safety bands are intact			

Clinical Judgment for Clients Across the Life Span Experiencing Complex Multisystem Health Problems

Perfusion
Complex Health Problems

Exemplar 19A. Myocardial Infarction (Medical-Surgical Nursing: Middle-Age Adult)

Thinking Exercise 19A-1

A 56-year-old obese female client reports chest pain, back pain, and shortness of breath. Her history reveals that the client was diagnosed with diabetes mellitus type 2 over 10 years ago. Current vital signs for the client are:

- Temperature = 98.9°F (37.2°C),
- Heart rate = 132 beats/min
- Blood pressure = 189/100 mm Hg
- Respirations = 26 breaths/min
- Oxygen saturation = 90% (on room air)

Use an X to indicate whether the nursing actions below are <u>Indicated</u> (appropriate or necessary), <u>Contraindicated</u> (could be harmful), or <u>Non-Essential</u> (make no difference or are not necessary) for the client's care at this time.

Nursing Action	Indicated	Contraindicated	Non-Essential
Apply supplemental oxygen.			
Assess pain intensity level.			
Conduct a head-to-toe assessment.			
Obtain an electrocardiogram (ECG).			
Obtain a comprehensive metabolic profile (CMP).			
Obtain a chest x-ray.			
Insert an indwelling urinary catheter.			

Thinking Exercise 19A-2

A 56-year-old obese female client reports chest pain, back pain, and shortness of breath. Her history reveals that the client was diagnosed with diabetes mellitus type 2 over 10 years ago. The nurse reviews the following laboratory results for the client over the past 24 hours.

Laboratory Test	Current	6 Hours Ago	24 Hours Ago
Hemoglobin	12.5 g/dL (7.5 mmol/L)	12.8 g/dL (7.6 mmol/L)	12.4 g/dL (7.5 mmol/L)
Platelet count	221,000/mm³ (221 × 10⁹/L)	223,000/mm³ (223 × 10⁹/L)	222,0000/mm³ (222 × 10⁹/L)
White blood cell (WBC) count	10,200/mm³ (10.2 × 10⁹/L)	10,300/mm³ (10.3 × 10⁹/L)	10,200/mm³ (10.2 × 10⁹/L)
Partial thromboplastin time (aPTT)	65 sec	70 sec	68 sec
Troponin T	8.0 ng/mL (8.0 mcg/L)	0.4 ng/mL (0.4 mcg/L)	0.1 ng/mL (0.1 mcg/L)
Creatine kinase MB (CKMB)	195 U/L (195 IU/L)	170 U/L (170 IU/L)	170 U/L (170 IU/L)
Serum magnesium	1.1 mEq/L (0.55 mmol/L)	1.5 mEq/L (0.75 mmol/L)	1.7 mEq/L (0.85 mmol/L)

Highlight or place a check mark next to the laboratory findings that require follow-up by the nurse.

Thinking Exercise 19A-3

Based on ECG and laboratory findings, a 56-year-old obese female diabetic client is diagnosed with myocardial infarction (MI) and taken to the cardiac catheterization laboratory for a successful percutaneous coronary intervention for her coronary artery blockage. The primary health care provider used the client's right wrist for catheter access. During the client's recovery, the nurse evaluates her progress and observes for potential postprocedure complications. **Indicate which nursing action listed in the far-left column is appropriate to help prevent or monitor for each potential postprocedure complication. Note that not all actions will be used.**

Nursing Action	Potential Postprocedure Complication	Appropriate Nursing Action for Prevention of Postprocedure Complication
1 Assess the neurovascular status of the right hand.	Acute kidney injury	
2 Maintain continuous cardiac telemetry monitoring.	Dysrhythmia	
3 Increase the intravenous fluid rate of infusion.	Hypotension	
4 Monitor level of consciousness and vital signs.	Stroke	
5 Maintain sequential or pneumatic compression devices.	Procedure site hematoma	
6 Monitor oxygen saturation.		
7 Monitor urine output.		

Thinking Exercise 19A-4

Based on ECG and laboratory findings, a 56-year-old obese female diabetic client is diagnosed with myocardial infarction (MI). She had a successful percutaneous coronary intervention for her coronary artery blockage. The nurse reviews the client's newly prescribed medication list and plans health teaching for the client. **For each drug listed in the table below, select the drug's _Purpose_ and _Common Side/Adverse Effect_. Note that options may be used more than once.**

Medication	Purpose	Common Side/Adverse Effect
Aspirin		
Atorvastatin		
Carvedilol		
Clopidogrel		
Lisinopril		

Options for Purpose	Options for Common Side/Adverse Effect
Prevent platelet aggregation	Black tarry stools or bleeding gums
Decrease the force of cardiac contraction	Increased shortness of breath
Reduce the risk of recurrent myocardial infarction	Swelling of the tongue and throat
Prevent the development of heart failure	Unexplained muscle pain, cramping, or tenderness
	Pulmonary embolus

Thinking Exercise 19A-5

The family members of a 56-year-old female client who had a myocardial infarction (MI) ask questions about what could have been done to avoid the client's MI. The nurse plans to include education about modifiable risk factors for coronary artery disease. Which of the following statements will the nurse include for this client? **Select all that apply.**

_____ A. "Decrease smoking and/or tobacco use, including vaping."

_____ B. "Lower sodium and fatty food consumption."

_____ C. "Eat foods that increase your low-density lipoprotein level."

_____ D. "Increase exercise periods to three to four times each week."

_____ E. "Work to control your hemoglobin A_{1c} level."

_____ F. "Regularly monitor your blood pressure."

_____ G. "Begin a high-protein, low-carbohydrate diet."

_____ H. "Implement a weight reduction program."

Exemplar 19B. Atrial Fibrillation/Stroke (Medical-Surgical Nursing: Older Adult)

Thinking Exercise 19 B-1

Complete the following sentences by choosing the *most likely* option for the missing information from the lists of options provided.

A 75-year-old male client is diagnosed with new-onset atrial fibrillation. The nurse would administer _____1_____ IV push to convert this dysrhythmia to normal sinus rhythm. However, this drug puts the client at risk for immediate _____2_____ and _____3_____, and therefore it should be injected over _____4_____.

Options for 1	Options for 2	Options for 3	Options for 4
Amlodipine	Bradycardia	Bronchospasm	0.5 to 1 minutes
Carvedilol	Dehydration	Hypertension	1 to 2 minutes
Clevidipine	Diarrhea	Hypotension	2 to 3 minutes
Diltiazem	Increased T-wave height	Nausea/vomiting	3 to 4 minutes
Sodium heparin	Seizure	Pulmonary embolism	4 to 5 minutes
Lidocaine	Tachycardia	Shortened QRS interval	5 to 10 minutes

Thinking Exercise 19B-2

Complete the following sentences by choosing the *most likely* option for the missing information from the lists of options provided.

A 75-year-old male client is diagnosed with new-onset atrial fibrillation. The nurse understands that atrial fibrillation puts the client at increased risk for _____1_____ and _____2_____. In addition to medication administration, vital sign checks, and focused cardiac assessments, the nurse implements _____3_____ and prepares for possible _____4_____.

Options for 1	Options for 2	Options for 3	Options for 4
Bradycardia	Bowel obstruction	A full liquid diet	Cardiac catheterization
Embolus formation	Heart failure	Isolation precautions	Cardioversion
Low serum potassium	Hypothermia	Limb precautions	Carotid sinus massage
Peripheral neuropathy	Increased urine output	One-to-one monitoring	Endotracheal intubation
Premature ventricular	Mental status changes	Strict intake and output	Urinary catheterization
contractions	Respiratory acidosis	Telemetry	Transcutaneous pacing
Vasospasm			

Thinking Exercise 19B-3

A 75-year-old male client is diagnosed with new-onset atrial fibrillation and directly admitted to the hospital for cardiac conversion. While the client is hospitalized for cardiac conversion, what health teaching will the nurse provide for the client and family? **Select all that apply.**

_____ A. Bleeding Precautions

_____ B. Need to reposition slowly

_____ C. Need for daily weights

_____ D. Need to take pulse and blood pressure daily

_____ E. Need to avoid leafy green vegetables in diet

_____ F. Signs and symptoms of stroke

_____ G. Procedure for using incentive spirometry

_____ H. Skin care and local burn treatment, if needed

Thinking Exercise 19B-4

A 75-year-old male client is diagnosed with new-onset atrial fibrillation. Despite drug therapy and cardioversion, the client remains in atrial fibrillation. The nurse understands that atrial fibrillation increases the client's risk for stroke and educates the client on modifiable risk factors for developing stroke. Which of the following modifiable risk factors does the nurse include in health teaching for this client? **Select all that apply.**

_____ A. Smoking

_____ B. Obesity

_____ C. Sedentary lifestyle

_____ D. Heavy alcohol use

_____ E. Antihistamine use

_____ F. Illegal substance use

_____ G. History of stroke

_____ H. History of hypertension

Thinking Exercise 19B-5

The nurse is conducting a home health visit with an 82-year-old male client who has a history of atrial fibrillation, hypertension, and chronic kidney disease stage 2 for medication management and blood pressure check. When the nurse arrives, the client is having difficulty walking upright, reports "the worst headache I've ever had," and states he has trouble seeing out of his left eye. He states the problems started just after he woke up at 7:00 a.m. (0700). The client took 2 acetaminophen tablets to ease the pain at 7:30 a.m. (0730), but they did not have any effect. The nurse performs a head-to-toe assessment and documents the findings. Selected client assessment findings are presented in the table below.

Vital Signs	
Temperature	97.9°F (36.6°C)
Heart rate	110 beats/min
Respirations	26 breaths/min
Blood pressure	195/100 mm Hg
Oxygen saturation	91% (on room air)
Pain	10/10 headache on right side of head that is constant and sharp and "nothing makes it better"
Physical Assessment Findings	
Glasgow Coma Scale score	14
Pupil size and response	Right eye = 3 mm and reactive to light Left eye = 6 mm and sluggish
Level of consciousness	Alert
Orientation	2/3 (alert to person and place)
Heart sounds	S_1/S_2
Lung sounds	Clear bilaterally
Pulses—radial	+2
Bowel sounds	Present and active × 4
Edema	Absent
Pulses—pedal	+2
Skin	Clean, dry, and intact
Hand grasp	Unequal: strong on right, weak on left
Foot strength	Unequal: strong on right, weak on left

Highlight or place a check mark next to the assessment findings that require follow-up by the nurse.

Thinking Exercise 19B-6

The nurse is conducting a home health visit with an 82-year-old male client who has a history of atrial fibrillation, hypertension, and chronic kidney disease stage 2 for medication management and a blood pressure check. When the nurse arrives, the client is having difficulty walking upright, reports "the worst headache I've ever had," and states he has trouble seeing out of his left eye. He states the problems started just after he woke up at 7:00 a.m. (0700). The client took 2 acetaminophen tablets to ease the pain at 7:30 a.m. (0730), but they did not have any effect. The home health nurse calls 911 and administers 325 mg of aspirin. The EMS arrives at the client's home at 9:45 a.m. (0945), obtains a report from the nurse, and transports the client to the nearest emergency department (ED). Before arrival, the paramedic gives the ED nurse the following report:

Vital Signs	
Temperature	97.9°F (36.6°C)
Heart rate	110 beats/min
Respirations	26 breaths/min
Blood pressure	195/100 mm Hg
Oxygen saturation	91% (on room air)
Pain	10/10 headache on right side of head that is constant, sharp, and "nothing makes it better"
Physical Assessment Findings	
Glasgow Coma Scale score	14
PERRLA	Right eye = 3 mm and reactive to light Left eye = 6 mm and sluggish
Level of consciousness	Alert
Orientation	2/3 (oriented to person and place)
Heart sounds	S_1/S_2
Lung sounds	Clear bilaterally
Pulses—radial	+2
Bowel sounds	Present and active × 4
Edema	Absent
Pulses—pedal	+2
Skin	Clean, dry, and intact
Hand grasp	Unequal: strong on right, weak on left
Foot strength	Unequal: strong on right, weak on left

Use an X to indicate whether the nursing actions below are <u>Indicated</u> (appropriate or necessary), <u>Contraindicated</u> (could be harmful), or <u>Non-Essential</u> (make no difference or are not necessary) for the client's care at this time.

Nursing Action	Indicated	Contraindicated	Non-Essential
Apply supplemental oxygen.			
Call Imaging for stat CT and MRI.			
Perform the National Institutes of Health (NIH) Stroke Scale Neurologic Exam.			
Obtain a comprehensive metabolic panel (CMP).			
Provide a low-stimulation room.			
Keep the head of the client's bed (HOB) at less than 20 degrees.			
Establish IV access.			

Exemplar 19C. Hypovolemic Shock (Medical-Surgical Nursing: Older Adult)

Thinking Exercise 19C-1

The nurse is assessing a 68-year-old female client who reports severe lower back and flank pain, excessive thirst, shortness of breath, anxiety, and weakness. The nurse reviews the following assessment findings:

Vital Signs	
Temperature	97.9°F (36.6°C)
Heart rate	110 beats/min
Respirations	26 breaths/min
Blood pressure	96/70 mm Hg
Oxygen saturation	92% (on room air)

Physical Assessment Findings

- Oral mucosa pale
- Breath sounds clear
- Capillary refill 4 seconds
- Radial pulses weak bilaterally
- Lower back pain 9/10
- Bowel sounds hypoactive × 4

Use an X to indicate whether the nursing actions below are <u>Indicated</u> (appropriate or necessary), <u>Contraindicated</u> (could be harmful), or <u>Non-Essential</u> (make no difference or are not necessary) for the client's care at this time.

Nursing Action	Indicated	Contraindicated	Non-Essential
Administer a normal saline 1000-mL bolus.			
Administer oxygen via nasal cannula (NC).			
Draw type and screen for possible blood transfusion.			
Ambulate the client to the toilet.			
Position the head of the bed at 45–60 degrees.			
Frequently check client mental status and level of consciousness (LOC).			
Educate the client about incentive spirometry.			

Thinking Exercise 19C-2

An 83-year-old female client was transferred to the medical ICU from a skilled nursing facility. Previously at the facility, the client reported weakness and shortness of breath. The assistive personnel (AP) reported that the client had several black tarry stools and increasing pallor. The client's primary health care provider prescribed a hemoglobin check; the results were 5.0 g/dL (3.0 mmol/L).

The client's vital signs on admission were:

Heart rate	125 beats/min
Blood pressure	85/50 mm Hg
Respirations	32 breaths/min
Oxygen saturation	88% (on 2 L NC)
Temperature	97.0°F (36.1°C)

On arrival at the hospital, a recheck of the client's hemoglobin level was 4.8 g/dL (2.9 mmol/L). The client was diagnosed with GI bleeding and hypovolemic shock. The nurse needs to complete the client's admission paperwork, but the medication administration record (MAR) from the skilled nursing facility was damaged in the transfer and some of the information is missing. **Choose the *most likely* options for the information missing from the table by selecting from the lists of options provided.**

Medication	Dose, Route, Frequency	Drug Class	Indication
Aspirin	**1**	Antiplatelet agent	Primary prevention of myocardial infarction and ischemic stroke
2	850 mg orally twice a day	Biguanide	Diabetes mellitus to lower blood glucose
Metoprolol/hydrochlorothiazide	100 mg/50 mg orally once daily	Beta-adrenergic blocker/diuretic	**3**
Naproxen sodium	250 mg orally PRN twice a day	**4**	Osteoarthritic pain
Rivaroxaban	10 mg orally once daily	Thrombin inhibitor	**5**

Options for 1	Options for 2	Options for 3
50 mg orally once daily	Glyburide	Angina pectoris
81 mg orally once daily	Glipizide	Coronary artery disease
100 mg orally twice a day	Regular insulin	Heart block
250 mg orally once daily	Metformin	Hyperlipidemia
500 mg orally 4 times a day	Sitagliptin	Hypertension

Options for 4	Options for 5
Antibiotic	Prevention of Alzheimer disease
Glucocorticoid	Prevention of bronchospasm
Immunosuppressant	Prevention of embolic events
NSAID	Prevention of Parkinson disease
Sulfonylurea	Prevention of vasospasm

Thinking Exercise 19C-3

An 83-year-old female client was admitted to the medical ICU with GI bleeding and hypovolemic shock. Which of the following medications will the nurse **avoid** giving to the client? **Select all that apply.**

_____ A. Atorvastatin 10 mg orally once daily

_____ B. Levothyroxine 75 mcg orally once daily

_____ C. Lisinopril 10 mg orally once daily

_____ D. Metformin 850 mg orally twice a day

_____ E. Metoprolol/hydrochlorothiazide 100 mg/50 mg orally once daily

_____ F. Naproxen sodium 250 mg, orally PRN twice a day

_____ G. Rivaroxaban 10 mg orally once daily

_____ H. Omeprazole 40 mg orally once daily

_____ I. Sertraline 50 mg orally once daily

Thinking Exercise 19C-4

An 83-year-old female client was transferred to the medical ICU from a skilled nursing facility. Previously at the facility, the client reported weakness and shortness of breath. The assistive personnel (AP) reported that the client had several black tarry stools and increasing pallor. The client's primary health care provider prescribed a hemoglobin check; the results were 5.0 g/dL (3.0 mmol/L).

On arrival at the hospital, a recheck of the client's hemoglobin level was 4.8 g/dL (2.9 mmol/L) and the client was diagnosed with GI bleeding and hypovolemic shock. In addition to hemoglobin, the following results were posted from the laboratory:

Laboratory Test Results	Current
Platelet count	221,000/mm³ (221 × 10⁹/L)
White blood cell count	10,200/mm³ (10.2 × 10⁹/L)
Prothrombin time	25 sec
International normalized ratio (INR)	7
Blood urea nitrogen	60 mg/dL (21.3 mmol/L)
Creatinine	3 mg/dL (265 mcmol/L)
Potassium	4.9 mEq/L (4.9 mmol/L)
Sodium	145 mEq/L (145 mmol/L)
Lactate	40 mg/dL (4.4 mmol/L)

Highlight or place a check mark next to the laboratory findings that require follow-up by the nurse.

Thinking Exercise 19C-5

An 83-year-old female client was transferred to the medical ICU from a skilled nursing facility with report of weakness, shortness of breath, black tarry stool, and pallor. On arrival at the hospital, her hemoglobin level was 4.8 g/dL (2.9 mmol/L). The client was diagnosed with GI bleeding and hypovolemic shock. The nurse infuses 4 units of packed red blood cells and 2 units of platelets and performs a head-to-toe assessment. Selected client assessment findings are presented in the table below:

Vital Signs	At Admission	1 Hour After Transfusion
Heart rate	125 beats/min	125 beats/min
Blood pressure	85/50 mm Hg	160/95 mm Hg
Respirations	32 breaths/min	28 breaths/min
Oxygen saturation	88% (on 2 L nasal cannula)	88% (on 4 L nasal cannula)
Temperature	97.0°F (36.1°C)	99.0°F (37.2°C)

Physical Assessment Findings	
Glasgow Coma Scale score	14
PERRLA	3 mm and reactive to light
Level of consciousness	Alert
Orientation	2/3 (oriented to person and place)
Heart sounds	S_1/S_2 present
Lung sounds	Crackles bilaterally in lower lobes
Pulses—Radial	+3
Bowel sounds	Present and active × 4
Edema	Absent
Pulses—Pedal	+3
Skin	Clean, dry, and intact
Hand grasp	Equal and strong
Foot strength	Equal and strong

Highlight or place a check mark next to the assessment findings that require follow-up by the nurse.

Thinking Exercise 19C-6

An 83-year-old female client has a history of GI bleeding and is at continued risk for additional bleeding episodes. The nursing team has provided client and family health teaching during the client's hospital stay about safety measures she will need to follow after discharge. Which statements by the client indicate a need for further teaching? **Select all that apply.**

_____ A. "I will be sure to floss every day."

_____ B. "I will take my aspirin for pain as needed."

_____ C. "I can volunteer in the gymnasium with activities again."

_____ D. "If I get bumped, I will apply ice for an hour."

_____ E. "I should use a rectal suppository to relieve constipation."

_____ F. "I will notify my primary health provider if I see blood in my urine."

_____ G. "I will avoid wearing shoes that are tight and rub my skin"

_____ H. "I will get help immediately for a headache that doesn't respond to acetaminophen."

Thinking Exercise 20-1

The nurse collaborates with the trauma team to admit and stabilize a 17-year-old male adolescent following a diving accident. According to the report from the emergency transport services, the client was at a lake with family and friends when he dove into the lake from the side of the boat but did not resurface. A family member rescued the adolescent from the water and began cardio-pulmonary resuscitation. The client was intubated en route and presents now for stabilization. The nurse collects the following assessment data for the client:

- Temperature = 97.6°F (36°C)
- Heart rate = 72 beats/min and irregular
- Respiratory rate = 16 breaths/min as set on ventilator, with no breathing over ventilator rate noted
- Oxygen saturation = 99% (on 20% Fio_2)
- Glasgow Coma Scale (GCS) score = 14 due to intubation
- Lung sounds = coarse with rhonchi in lower lobes bilaterally
- FLACC score = 3
- Large abrasion on top of head
- Responds to commands
- Voluntary movements in upper extremities
- No movements noted in lower extremities bilaterally
- Initial CT scan of the spinal column demonstrates a severe and complete compression injury at the 10th thoracic vertebrae (T10)

Based on the assessment findings, what **priority** actions would the nurse take to help stabilize the client at this time? **Select all that apply.**

_____ A. Use the log-roll method of repositioning and turning.

_____ B. Maintain endotracheal tube and manage the ventilator.

_____ C. Maintain a neutral thermal body temperature.

_____ D. Administer antibiotics as prescribed for a urinary tract infection.

_____ E. Perform neurologic checks every hour.

_____ F. Obtain health history and details of the accidental injury from family.

_____ G. Administer saline bolus as prescribed.

_____ H. Perform a thorough assessment of the scalp abrasion.

Thinking Exercise 20-2

Choose the *most likely* options for the information missing from the statements below by selecting from the lists of options provided.

The nurse recognizes that clients with spinal cord injury suffer both _____1_____ and
_____1_____. The **priority** desired outcomes of treatment for this client are to
_____2_____ the injury and prevent _____2_____ damage to

his spinal cord. Additional client outcomes include establishing a _____3_____ and _____3_____ regimen. Other outcomes include maintaining the greatest amount of _____4_____ as possible, monitoring the client's adaptation to his paralysis, and preventing _____5_____.

Options for 1	Options for 2	Options for 3	Options for 4	Options for 5
Physiologically	Primary	Sleep	Respiratory effort	Metabolic acidosis
Mental breakdowns	Decrease	Bowel	Cardiac function	Relapse
Rhabdomyolysis	Stabilize	Rest	Integrity	Pressure injury
Psychologically	Tertiary	Physical therapy	Mobility	Acute kidney injury
Acute kidney injury	Reduce	Bladder	Psychological integrity	Bladder spasms
Chronically	Secondary	Occupational therapy	Sensory perception	Rhabdomyolysis

Thinking Exercise 20-3

The nurse is developing a plan of care for a 17-year-old who was admitted to the hospital following a complete severing of the spinal cord at T10 resulting in paraplegia and necessitating mechanical ventilation for 24 hours; the client is now off the ventilator and breathing on his own. He was admitted to the neurosurgical unit after open reduction and internal fixation (ORIF) to stabilize his spine. **Use an X to indicate whether the nursing actions below are <u>Anticipated</u> (appropriate or likely necessary), <u>Contraindicated</u> (could be harmful), or <u>Non-Essential</u> (make no difference or are not necessary) for the client's postoperative care at this time.**

Nursing Actions	Anticipated	Contraindicated	Non-Essential
Monitor vital signs per facility standards.			
Encourage coughing and deep breathing exercises.			
Administer analgesic as prescribed.			
Reposition the client every 4 hours.			
Apply sequential compression devices.			
Keep NPO until the client voids and reports no nausea.			
Obtain a prescription for echocardiogram.			
Consult clergy or social worker for family support.			
Collaborate with respiratory therapy to maintain oxygenation as needed.			
Complete a dietary assessment.			
Obtain a prescription for an indwelling urinary catheter.			
Monitor the client's level of sensory perception every 4 hours.			
Collaborate with physical therapy to promote independence.			

Thinking Exercise 20-4

The 17-year-old male client with a complete thoracic spinal cord injury reports that he is grateful for his family and the emergency personnel who saved his life, but wonders how he will ever be able to go to college. What are the **best** therapeutic responses for the nurse to use when communicating with the client? **Select all that apply.**

_____ A. Assess the client's support system and encourage engagement with peers.

_____ B. Ask the client if he has any feelings of guilt.

_____ C. Encourage family to participate in physical therapy.

_____ D. Assist the client in self-reflection to identify his positive progress and potential.

_____ E. Respond by saying, "Tell me what you mean by that statement."

_____ F. Respond by saying, "You are concerned because you don't know how you will care for yourself at college."

_____ G. Refer the adolescent and family to local support groups for spinal cord injury.

_____ H. Ask the client to share some of the feelings that he has had as a result of the accident.

Thinking Exercise 20-5

The nurse is caring for a recently admitted 16-year-old female client with a complete cervical spinal cord injury (C7) for acute rehabilitation and recognizes the need to help prevent and/or manage common complications. **Indicate which nursing actions listed in the far-left column are appropriate for the potential complications associated with cervical spinal cord injuries. Note that not all actions will be used.**

Nursing Action	Potential Spinal Cord Injury Complication	Appropriate Nursing Action for Complication
1 Remove restrictive clothing and check for urinary distention.	Pneumonia	
2 Perform cough assist as needed.	Urinary tract infection	
3 Administer beta-blocking agent per agency protocol.	Autonomic dysreflexia	
4 Teach the client to do wheelchair push-ups hourly.	Joint contractures	
5 Facilitate frequent bladder emptying.	Pressure injuries	
6 Administer a daily rectal suppository.		
7 Perform frequent range-of-motion exercises.		
8 Apply cervical traction.		

Thinking Exercise 20-6

The nurse is evaluating the progress of a 15-year-old male client with a spinal cord injury to determine whether or not he is ready for transfer to a facility for ongoing rehabilitation and preparation for self-management. **For each assessment finding, use an X to indicate whether the nursing and health care team interventions were <u>Effective</u> (helped to meet expected outcomes), <u>Ineffective</u> (did not help to meet expected outcomes), or <u>Unrelated</u> (not related to the expected outcomes).**

Assessment Finding	Effective	Ineffective	Unrelated
Temperature = 98.5°F (36.9°C)			
Heart rate = 68 beats/min and regular			
Respiratory rate = 16 breaths/min			
Blood pressure = 114/58 mm Hg			
Oxygen saturation = 88% (on room air)			
Glasgow Coma Scale score = 15			
Level of sensory and function impairment has not progressed			
Client is able to assist physical therapy with transfers and exercises			
Adolescent cries easily and expresses a lack of hope			
Nonblanching redness noted on sacrum			
Pain score: 0/10 on a 0 to 10 pain intensity scale			
Lung sounds are clear bilaterally			
Client reports daily bowel movement is soft and brown			

Exemplar 21. Traumatic Brain Injury (Medical-Surgical Nursing: Older Adult and Young Adult)

Thinking Exercise 21-1

A 79-year-old male client with a recent hip open reduction and internal fixation (ORIF) is discharged to a skilled nursing facility for postsurgical rehabilitative therapy. While at the facility, the client has a witnessed fall and sustains a head injury. The nurse performs a head-to-toe assessment and notes no neurologic changes. Three days later, the client is difficult to keep awake, asks to miss school that day because he doesn't feel well, and equally squeezes the nurse's hands when asked. The nurse compares assessment findings from today with those from 3 days ago, as listed below.

	Day of Fall	3 Days After Fall
Vital Signs		
Temperature	98.5°F (36.9°C)	98.4°F (36.9°C)
Heart rate	75 beats/min	60 beats/min
Respirations	22 breaths/min	14 breaths/min
Blood pressure	135/85 mm Hg	160/90 mm Hg
Oxygen saturation	94% (on room air)	91% (on room air)
Physical Assessment Findings		
Glasgow Coma Scale score	15	13
PERRLA	Present	Present
Level of consciousness	Alert	Lethargic
Orientation	3/3	2/3 (oriented to person and place)
Heart sounds	S_1/S_2 present	S_1/S_2 present
Lung sounds	Clear bilaterally	Clear bilaterally
Pulses: radial	+2	+1
Bowel sounds	Present and active × 4	Present and active × 4
Edema	Absent	Absent
Pulses: pedal	+2	+1
Skin	Clean, dry, and intact	Clean, dry, and intact

Highlight or place a check mark next to the assessment findings that require follow-up by the nurse.

Thinking Exercise 21-2

A 79-year-old male client with a new hip open reduction and internal fixation (ORIF) is discharged to a skilled nursing facility for rehabilitation therapy and experiences a fall. Based on client assessment findings, the nurse contacts emergency medical services (EMS) for ambulance transport to the hospital and gives a report to the paramedics. On arrival at the emergency department (ED), the paramedics share the facility's report with the ED nurse. The following are the client's vital signs on admission to the hospital:

Vital Signs	
Temperature	98.5°F (36.9°C)
Heart rate	57 beats/min
Respirations	22 breaths/min
Blood pressure	165/100 mm Hg
Oxygen saturation	89% (on room air)

The nurse recognizes that actions are needed based on the client's current vital signs and neurologic changes. **Use an X to indicate whether the nursing actions below are <u>Indicated</u> (appropriate or necessary), <u>Contraindicated</u> (could be harmful), or <u>Non-Essential</u> (make no difference or are not necessary) for the client's care at this time.**

Nursing Action	Indicated	Contraindicated	Non-Essential
Apply supplemental oxygen.			
Conduct a head-to-toe assessment.			
Obtain an electrocardiogram (ECG).			
Obtain a comprehensive metabolic profile (CMP).			
Obtain a chest x-ray.			
Insert an indwelling urinary catheter.			
Assess pain intensity and quality.			

Thinking Exercise 21-3

A 79-year-old male client has been transferred to the emergency department from a skilled nursing facility because of changes in orientation and level of consciousness due to a fall. The nurse records the most current set of vital signs as listed below:

Vital Signs	
Temperature	98.5°F (36.9°C)
Heart rate	57 beats/min
Respirations	22 breaths/min
Blood pressure	175/100 mm Hg
Oxygen saturation	89% (on room air)

In addition to starting oxygen therapy, which of the following nursing actions are needed for the client at this time? **Select all that apply.**

_____ A. Obtain a CT scan of the head.

_____ B. Administer 500-mL IV bolus of normal saline.

_____ C. Draw blood for a complete blood cell count (CBC).

_____ D. Determine the National Institutes of Health Stroke Scale score.

_____ E. Administer alteplase (rtPA).

_____ F. Check the client's blood glucose level.

_____ G. Prepare to intubate the client.

_____ H. Check pupil size and responsiveness.

Thinking Exercise 21-4

A 24-year-old man is found on the floor at his home by his girlfriend, who calls 911. He has a known history of heroin use and no one is aware of when he lost consciousness. The police find that the client has a "low" pulse and shallow respirations and feels cool to the touch. One of the officers administers naloxone per protocol. The paramedics arrive and record the following vital signs:

Vital Signs	
Temperature	95.0°F (35.0°C)
Heart rate	58 beats/min
Respirations	10 breaths/min
Blood pressure	85/60 mm Hg
Oxygen saturation	84% (on room air)

The paramedics insert an endotracheal tube and transport the client to the hospital. After assessment in the emergency department, the client is admitted to the critical care unit for further monitoring. **Indicate which nursing action listed in the far-left column is appropriate for the potential complication. Note that not all actions will be used.**

Nursing Action	Potential Complication	Appropriate Nursing Action for Potential Complication
1 Apply and maintain sequential or pneumatic compression stockings or devices.	Increased carbon dioxide	
2 Apply continuous capnography.	Hypothermia	
3 Apply warm blankets.	Increased ICP and decreased gas exchange	
4 Elevate the head of the client's bed to more than 30 degrees.	Increased brain swelling and damage	
5 Insert an indwelling urinary catheter.	Venous thromboembolism (VTE)	
6 Perform mental status checks every hour.		
7 Monitor vital signs every 15 minutes.		

Thinking Exercise 21-5

A 24-year-old male client who sustained a severe traumatic brain injury was hospitalized for opiate overdose. After the client is transferred from the critical care unit to the general medical unit, the client becomes easily agitated, does not follow commands, is nonverbal, and is unable to perform ADLs. The care coordination team is determining the best plan for the client's discharge and rehabilitation. What health teaching will the nurse provide for the family about the expected rehabilitation process for the client? **Select all that apply.**

_____ A. "The client may be depressed and lonely."

_____ B. "The client may need constant supervision."

_____ C. "The client may fatigue and be irritated easily."

_____ D. "The client's primary caregiver may need respite care at times."

_____ E. "The client's family may feel anger toward the client."

_____ F. "The client's family should join a local support group."

_____ G. "The client is at an increased risk for seizure."

_____ H. "The client will benefit from a structured environment."

Thinking Exercise 21-6

A 33-year-old man was involved in a motor vehicle crash and sustained a severe head wound. When the paramedics arrived, they found that the client was comatose. The paramedics inserted an endotracheal tube on the scene. The client has not regained consciousness and has no reflexes. When inventorying the client's belongings, the nurse finds the man's driver's license, which indicates the client wished to be an organ donor. The client's family has questions about organ donation. The nurse understands there are required criteria for a client to be considered as a donor. **Use an X to indicate whether the criteria below are <u>Indicated</u> (appropriate or necessary) or <u>Non-Essential</u> (make no difference or are not necessary) when considering the client as an organ donor.**

	Indicated	Non-Essential
Screened for medical conditions		
Comatose as determined by a primary health care provider, diagnostic testing, and history		
Normal or near-normal core body temperature		
Normal systolic blood pressure (>100 mm Hg)		
Neurologic examination by a neurologist or intensivist		
Donation coordinated by a local organ-procurement organization		

Thinking Exercise 22-1

An 83-year-old woman is brought into the emergency department (ED) by her neighbor because of mentation changes. The neighbor states that the client "fell last week and bruised her ribs." Today the neighbor noticed that the client had not styled her hair or done her makeup and was wandering in pajamas looking for a cat. This was very unusual for the client, and the neighbor talked her into coming into the hospital. The triage nurse assesses vital signs and does a quick neurologic assessment. The assessment findings are listed below.

Vital Signs	
Temperature	101.2°F (38.4°C)
Heart rate	110 beats/min
Respirations	26 breaths/min
Blood pressure	96/65 mm Hg
Oxygen saturation	92% (on room air)
Neurologic Assessment Findings	
Orientation	2/3 (oriented to person and place)
PERRLA	Present; pupils 3 mm
HEENT	Normal gaze, no facial palsy, equal smile, no tongue deviation, productive cough
Motor	No drift, follows commands, equal strength × 4
Sensory	No sensory loss
Language	No aphasia, no dysarthria
Neglect	None

The triage nurse gives the report to the ED nurse. **Use an X to indicate whether the following nursing actions are <u>Indicated</u> (appropriate or necessary), <u>Contraindicated</u> (could be harmful), or <u>Non-Essential</u> (make no difference or are not necessary) for the client's care at this time.**

Nursing Action	Indicated	Contraindicated	Non-Essential
Administer a normal saline 1000-mL bolus.			
Administer oxygen via nasal cannula.			
Draw a comprehensive metabolic profile (CMP).			
Obtain a sputum sample.			
Position the head of the bed at 30 to 60 degrees.			
Prepare for central line insertion.			
Notify the imaging department of the need for emergent head CT.			

Thinking Exercise 22-2

An 83-year-old female client was brought into the emergency department (ED) by her neighbor because of mentation changes. After assessment, the nurse administered 1000 mL of normal saline and started the client on supplemental oxygen. Thirty minutes later the nurse reassesses the client, with findings as listed below.

	Admission	30 Minutes Later
Vital Signs		
Temperature	101.2°F (38.4°C)	101.2°F (38.4°C)
Heart rate	110 beats/min	115 beats/min
Respirations	26 breaths/min	28 breaths/min
Blood pressure	96/65 mm Hg	90/60 mm Hg
Oxygen saturation	92% (on room air)	88% (on 2 L O_2)
Physical Assessment Findings		
Orientation	2/3 (oriented to person and place)	1/3 (oriented to self only)
PERRLA	Present, pupils 3 mm	Present, pupils 3 mm
HEENT	Normal gaze, no facial palsy, equal smile, no tongue deviation, productive cough	Normal gaze, no facial palsy, equal smile, no tongue deviation, productive cough
Motor	No drift, follows commands, equal strength × 4	No drift, follows commands, equal strength × 4
Heart sounds	S_1/S_2 present	S_1/S_2 present
Lung sounds	Clear upper, crackles in lower lobes bilaterally	Clear upper, crackles in lower lobes bilaterally
Pulses	Present, but weak × 4	Present, but weak × 4
Capillary refill	3 sec	>3 sec
Bowel sounds	Present	Present
Edema	+1	+2
Skin	Clean, dry, and intact	Clean, dry, and intact

Highlight or place a check mark next to the assessment findings that require follow-up by the nurse.

Thinking Exercise 22-3

An 83-year-old female client was brought into the emergency department (ED) by her neighbor because of mentation changes. After assessment, the nurse administered 1000 mL of normal saline, started the client on supplemental oxygen, and obtained samples for the laboratory testing. Forty-five minutes later, the laboratory posted the following findings.

Laboratory Test Results	Current
Hemoglobin	12.5 g/dL (7.5 mmol/L)
Platelet count	221,000/mm³ (221 × 10⁹/L)
White blood cell count	4800/mm³ (4.8 × 10⁹/L)
Neutrophils	2200/mm³ (2.2 × 10⁹/L)
Serum lactate	40 mg/dL (4.4 mmol/L)
Serum magnesium	1.5 mEq/L (0.8 mmol/L)
Serum potassium	4.9 mEq/L (4.9 mmol/L)
Serum calcium	9.0 mg/dL (2.25 mmol/l)
Blood urea nitrogen	22 mg/dL (7.3 mmol/L)
Creatinine	1.3 mg/dL (124 mcmol/L)
Blood culture	Pending
Sputum culture	Pending
Urine culture	Pending
Urinalysis	Appearance: Clear Color: Yellow pH: 6.0 Specific gravity: 1.020 Nitrites: None Ketones: None Bilirubin: None Crystals: None Casts: None Glucose: None WBCs: 0 RBCs : 0

Highlight or place a check mark next to the assessment findings that require follow-up by the nurse.

Thinking Exercise 22-4

An 83-year-old woman was brought into the emergency department (ED) by her neighbor because of mentation changes. After assessment, the nurse administered 1000 mL of normal saline and started the client on supplemental oxygen. The nurse reviews pertinent assessment and laboratory findings as listed on the next page.

	Admission	30 Minutes Later
Vital Signs		
Temperature	101.2°F (38.4°C)	101.2°F (38.4°C)
Heart rate	110 beats/min	115 beats/min
Respirations	26 breaths/min	28 breaths/min
Blood pressure	96/65 mm Hg	90/60 mm Hg
Oxygen saturation	92% (on room air)	88% (on 2 L O_2)
Physical Assessment Findings		
Orientation	2/3 (oriented to person and place)	1/3 (oriented to self only)
Heart sounds	S_1/S_2 present	S_1/S_2 present
Lung sounds	Clear upper, crackles in lower lobes bilaterally	Clear upper, crackles lower lobes bilaterally
Pulses	Present and weak × 4	Present and weak × 4
Capillary refill	3 sec	>3 sec
Edema	+1	+2

Laboratory Test Results	Current
White blood cell count	4800/mm³ (4.8 × 10⁹/L)
Neutrophils	2200/mm³ (2.2 × 10⁹/L)
Serum lactate	40 mg/dL (4.4 mmol/L)
Blood culture	Pending
Sputum culture	Pending
Urine culture	Pending

The nurse is compiling an SBAR report for the primary health care provider. **Complete the following statements by choosing the *most likely option* for the missing information from the lists of options provided.**

When making recommendations, the nurse would be sure to include _____1_____ and IV _____2_____. The client weighs 70 kg; therefore the nurse estimates the client needs at least an additional _____3_____ mL of fluid volume resuscitation to support circulation. In addition, vasopressors are suggested in order to maintain a mean arterial pressure (MAP) of _____4_____.

Options for 1	Options for 2	Options for 3	Options for 4
Ampicillin	Dextrose 5%/0.45% normal saline (D5/½NS)	500	50
Ceftriaxone	Dextrose 5%/0.9% normal saline (D5/NS)	1000	55
Doxycycline	Dextrose 5%/water (D5W)	1100	60
Metronidazole	Lactated Ringer's (LR)	1500	65
Rifampin	Normal saline (NS)	2000	70
Vancomycin	Normal saline bicarbonate (NSHCO₃)	2100	80

Thinking Exercise 22-5

An 83-year-old woman was brought into the emergency department (ED) by her neighbor because of mentation changes. After assessment, the nurse administered 1000 mL of normal saline and started the client on supplemental oxygen. The nurse reviews and compares the pertinent physical assessment and laboratory findings listed below.

	Admission	30 Minutes Later	1 Hour Later
Vital Signs			
Temperature	101.2°F (38.4°C)	101.2°F (38.4°C)	100.5°F (38.1°C)
Heart rate	110 beats/min	115 beats/min	110 beats/min
Respirations	26 breaths/min	28 breaths/min	26 breaths/min
Blood pressure	96/65 mm Hg	90/60 mm Hg	90/50 mm Hg
Oxygen saturation	92% (on room air)	88% (on 2 L O_2)	92% (on 10 L O_2)
Physical Assessment Findings			
Orientation	2/3 (oriented to person and place)	1/3 (oriented to self only)	
Heart sounds	S_1/S_2 present	S_1/S_2 present	
Lung sounds	Clear upper, crackles in lower lobes bilaterally	Clear upper, crackles in lower lobes bilaterally	
Pulses	Present and weak × 4	Present and weak × 4	
Capillary refill	3 sec	>3 sec	
Edema	+1	+2	

Laboratory Test Results	Current
White blood cell count	4800/mm³ (4.8 × 10⁹/L)
Neutrophils	2200/mm³ (2.2 × 10⁹/L)
Serum lactate	40 mg/dL (4.4 mmol/L)
Blood culture	Pending
Sputum culture	Pending
Urine culture	Pending

The ED nurse shares the client's assessment findings with the critical care unit (CCU) nurse through face-to-face bedside report. The ED nurse also informs the CCU nurse that the client is receiving her second liter of normal saline (NS) and has received a dose of IV ceftriaxone. Which of the following actions are appropriate for the nurse to perform for the client? **Select all that apply.**

_____ A. Redraw lactate in 6 hours.

_____ B. Take vital signs every 15 minutes.

_____ C. Initiate vasopressors.

_____ D. Assist with central line insertion.

_____ E. Insert an indwelling urinary catheter.

_____ F. Perform frequent cardiac assessments.

_____ G. Perform frequent skin assessments.

_____ H. Insert a nasogastric tube.

Gas Exchange
Chest Trauma

Thinking Exercise 23-1

A 56-year-old woman lost control of her car and hit a tree. When paramedics arrived, the client was difficult to arouse and could not follow commands. The paramedics applied a cervical collar, inserted an endotracheal tube, stabilized an open fracture on her forearm, and transported her to the local critical access hospital. The paramedics used sedation in the ambulance because the woman was restless. The emergency department (ED) triage assessment yielded the following:

- Unable to answer questions or follow commands
- Responds to painful stimuli
- Multiple small lacerations on her forehead
- Mucous membranes pink and moist
- Bilateral chest bruising
- Breath sounds in all lung fields
- S_1/S_2 present
- Abdominal bruising
- Hypoactive bowel sounds $\times$ 4
- Pulses present in all four extremities
- Capillary refill = 3 seconds

Vital Signs	
Temperature	99.2°F (37.3°C)
Heart rate	110 beats/min
Respirations	16 breaths/min
Blood pressure	96/65 mm Hg
Oxygen saturation	92% (on manual bag-valve and 100% Fio_2)

Highlight or place a check mark next to the assessment findings that require follow-up by the nurse.

Thinking Exercise 23-2

A 56-year-old woman is brought into the emergency department (ED) after a motor vehicle accident. The triage nurse gives a report to the ED nurse, whose findings include:

- Unable to answer questions or follow commands
- Responds to painful stimuli
- Multiple small lacerations on her forehead
- Mucous membranes pink and moist

- Bilateral chest bruising
- Breath sounds present in all fields
- S_1/S_2 present
- Abdominal bruising
- Hypoactive bowel sounds $\times$ 4
- Pulses present in all four extremities
- Capillary refill $=$ 3 seconds

Vital Signs	
Temperature	99.2°F (37.3°C)
Heart rate	110 beats/min
Respirations	16 breaths/min
Blood pressure	96/65 mm Hg
Oxygen saturation	92% (on manual bag/valve and 100% Fio_2)

Use an X to indicate whether the nursing actions below are <u>Emergent</u> (immediately necessary), <u>Contraindicated</u> (not indicated at this time), or <u>Non-Emergent</u> (not immediately necessary) for the client's care at this time.

Nursing Action	Emergent	Contraindicated	Non-Emergent
Administer 2 units of blood.			
Contact respiratory therapy department for a mechanical ventilator.			
Draw a comprehensive metabolic profile (CMP).			
Get a chest x-ray to confirm endotracheal tube placement.			
Raise the head of the bed to 30 degrees.			
Prepare for central line insertion.			
Notify imaging department about need for emergent head and neck CT.			

Thinking Exercise 23-3

A 56-year-old woman is being transferred to the ICU after being involved in a motor vehicle accident. The nurse receives the report from the emergency department and learns the client is on mechanical ventilation and has bruising throughout the chest and abdomen. The client is slightly tachycardic and responds to painful stimuli. The nurse assesses for changes in the client's condition and provides interventions to help prevent common complications associated with chest trauma. **Match the most appropriate nursing action from the provided list with the potential complication. Note that not all of the nursing actions will be used.**

Nursing Action	Potential Complication	Appropriate Nursing Action for Each Potential Complication
1 Apply continuous oximetry.	Acute pain	
2 Assess mucous membranes.	Impaired oxygenation	
3 Administer prophylactic IV antibiotic therapy.	Hypovolemia	
4 Insert an oral-gastric tube.	Infection	
5 Take vital signs every hour.	Impaired tissue integrity	
6 Ensure continuous cardiac monitoring.	Aspiration	
7 Monitor intake and output.		
8 Monitor for low-grade fever.		
9 Perform oral care every 2 hours.		
10 Reposition the client every 2 hours.		
11 Titrate sedation per facility policy and administer analgesic.		

Thinking Exercise 23-4

The nurse is caring a 56-year-old female client who is on mechanical ventilation after a motor vehicle accident caused chest and abdominal trauma. The nurse is caring for another client when the assistive personnel (AP) informs the nurse of "alarms going off" in the other room. **Complete the following sentences by choosing the *most likely* options for the missing information from the lists of options provided.**

The first thing the nurse would check is the _____1_____ to determine the cause of the alarm. Then the nurse would check the _____2_____. The nurse determines the alarms are due to low client oxygenation, hypertension, tachycardia, and high peak inspiratory pressure (PIP). Consequently, the nurse _____3_____, which results in no clinical change. The nurse then double-checks the current ventilator settings against previous documentation and notes that there have been no changes to the previous settings. The nurse notifies the primary health care provider and gives an SBAR report. The provider prescribes a repeat bedside _____4_____. After reviewing the results of the bedside test, the nurse prepares for bedside chest tube insertion to relieve _____5_____ in the lower left thorax.

Options for 1 and 2	Options for 3	Options for 4	Options for 5
Bed linens	Administers albuterol	Abdominal x-ray	Hemothorax
Client	Arouses the client	Abdominal ultrasound	Pneumothorax
Urinary catheter	Boluses IV saline	Bladder scan	Pericarditis
Head of bed	Obtains an ECG	Chest CT	Infection
IV tubing	Performs range-of-motion exercises	Chest x-ray	Pleural effusion
Lead placement	Repositions the client	Head CT	Adhesion
Monitors	Suctions the client	Venipuncture	Tension

Thinking Exercise 23-5

The nurse is caring for a 56-year-old woman who has a new chest tube and drainage system in place. Which nursing actions would the nurse perform to ensure client safety? **Select all that apply.**

_____ A. Check the chest tube dressing to ensure it is clean, intact, and loose.

_____ B. Keep the client on bedrest and encourage shallow breaths to avoid pain.

_____ C. Keep the drainage system at the same level as the chest tube entry point.

_____ D. "Strip" the chest tube to dislodge clots and ensure patency.

_____ E. If the chest tube disconnects from the system, place the end in sterile water.

_____ F. Document the amount, color, and characteristics of drainage daily.

_____ G. Check to ensure vigorous and continuous bubbling in the water-seal chamber.

Elimination
Complex Health Problems

Thinking Exercise 24A-1

A 58-year-old male client with a history of diabetes mellitus type 2, hypertension, and peripheral neuropathy follows up with the primary health care provider to discuss his most recent glycosylated hemoglobin (A1c) result. During the visit, the client reports urinary frequency during the day and night. The nurse reviews the complete list of his laboratory test results.

Laboratory Test Results	Current	6 Months ago	1 Year Ago
Glycosylated hemoglobin (A1c)	8.9%	8.5%	9.0%
Blood glucose	140 mg/dL (7.8 mmol/L)	145 mg/dL (8.0 mmol/L)	138 mg/dL (7.7 mmol/L)
Blood urea nitrogen (BUN)	20 mg/dL (7.1 mmol/L)	18 mg/dL (7.0 mmol/L)	18 mg/dL (7.0 mmol/L)
Serum creatinine	2.0 mg/dL (177 mcmol/L)	1.8 mg/dL (159 mcmol/L)	1.6 mg/dL (141 mcmol/L)
Serum calcium	8.0 mg/dL (2 mmol/L)	8.0 mg/dL (2 mmol/L)	8.5 mg/dL (2.1 mmol/L)
Serum potassium	3.5 mEq/L (3.5 mmol/L)	3.8 mEq/L (3.8 mmol/L)	3.9 mEq/L (3.9 mmol/L)
Serum magnesium	1.3 mEq/L (0.74 mmol/L)	1.5 mEq/L (0.95 mmol/L)	1.7 mEq/L (1.0 mmol/L)
Serum sodium	135 mEq/L (135 mmol/L)	140 mEq/L (140 mmol/L)	143 mEq/L (143 mmol/L)
Serum phosphate	3.8 mg/dL (1.23 mmol/L)	3.8 mg/dL (1.23 mmol/L)	3.0 mg/dL (0.97 mmol/L)
Serum carbon dioxide	23 mEq/L (23 mmol/L)	26 mEq/L (26 mmol/L)	26 mEq/L (26 mmol/L)
Glomerular filtration rate (GFR)	65 mL/min	92 mL/min	95 mL/min

Highlight or place a check mark next to the findings that require follow-up by the nurse.

Thinking Exercise 24A-2

The nurse plans an education session for a 58-year-old man who has recently been diagnosed with stage 2 chronic kidney disease (CKD). He also has a long history of hypertension, diabetes mellitus type 2, and peripheral neuropathy. **Complete the following statement** by choosing the *most likely* options for the missing information from the lists of options provided.

The nurse understands that chronic kidney disease (CKD) management requires changes in _____1_____ and _____2_____ to slow or prevent progression of the disease. These changes are designed to lower _____3_____, balance _____4_____, and maintain appropriate _____5_____. If these changes are not successfully made, the client's CKD status can change to stage _____6_____ and result in the need for kidney replacement therapies such as dialysis and/or transplant.

Options for 1	Options for 2	Options for 3
Activity level	Breathing pattern	Blood pressure
Ambulation	Over-the-counter medication	Blood sugar
Cholesterol intake	Physical therapy	Cholesterol
Fiber intake	Prescribed medications	Osmolality
Nutrition	Protein intake	Potassium
Sodium intake	Smoking status	Serum bicarbonate
Weight control	Supplement use	Sodium

Options for 4	Options for 5	Options for 6
Blood pH	Bone density	1
Electrolytes	Creatinine	2
Heart rate	Cortisol	3
Hemoglobin	Fluid volume	4
Hormones	Muscle strength	5
Mobility status	Oxygenation	6
Weight	Skin integrity	7

Thinking Exercise 24A-3

A 58-year-old male client returns to the clinic for routine laboratory monitoring for his chronic kidney disease (CKD) stage 2 and diabetes mellitus type 2. He reports to the nurse that he thinks he's getting better because over the past few weeks he only urinates a few times a day and doesn't need to get up in the middle of the night to void. He also states that he is having shortness of breath with activity. The nurse reviews his laboratory results and finds that his glomerular filtration rate has decreased from 65 mL/min to 40 mL/min. What will the nurse include in a health teaching plan for this client? **Select all that apply.**

_____ A. Preparing for possible hemodialysis

_____ B. Preparing for possible peritoneal dialysis

_____ C. Recognizing signs and symptoms of electrolyte imbalance

_____ D. Recognizing signs and symptoms of myocardial infarction

_____ E. Maintaining a low-protein, low-fat, low-phosphate diet

_____ F. Participating in moderately intense daily exercise

_____ G. Achieving a body mass index (BMI) goal of 22 to 25 kg/m^2

_____ H. Limiting alcohol intake to one or two drinks daily

Thinking Exercise 24A-4

A 58-year-old male client with a history of hypertension, diabetes mellitus type 2, and chronic kidney disease (CKD) stage 3 is brought to the emergency department after falling at church. The primary health care provider has labs drawn and finds the client is experiencing an acute kidney injury in addition to his CKD stage 3. After consulting with the nephrologist, the provider prescribes insertion of a subclavian hemodialysis line to emergently dialyze the client. **Use an X to indicate whether the nursing actions below are <u>Indicated</u> (appropriate or necessary), <u>Contraindicated</u> (could be harmful), or <u>Non-Essential</u> (make no difference or are not necessary) for the client having dialysis.**

Nursing Action	Indicated	Contraindicated	Non-Essential
Administer oral medications during the dialysis treatment according to the client's home schedule.			
Perform a clean dressing change to the access site.			
Perform frequent assessments of mental status.			
Provide a low-stimulation environment during the dialysis treatment.			
Use the dialysis catheter for IV fluids after the treatment is completed.			
Weigh the client before and after dialysis.			

Thinking Exercise 24A-5

A 62-year-old female client with gout and end-stage kidney disease had a new peritoneal dialysis catheter inserted. The nephrologist prescribed an instillation of dialysate using the new catheter. During the dialysis treatment, the nurse monitors for complications. **Indicate which nursing action listed in the far-left column is appropriate for the potential peritoneal dialysis complication. Note that not all nursing actions will be used.**

Nursing Action	Potential Dialysis Complication	Appropriate Nursing Action for Dialysis Complication
1 Monitor the client's finger stick blood glucose.	Abdominal pain	
2 Monitor the client's vital signs frequently.	Catheter site infection	
3 Monitor the client's level of consciousness.	Hyperglycemia	
4 Apply a mask to both the nurse and client during dialysis catheter access and use.	Peritonitis	
5 Monitor the color and clarity of the effluent.	Perforated bowel	
6 Monitor for warmth and redness at catheter site.		
7 Warm the dialysate before infusion.		

Exemplar 24B. Intestinal Obstruction (Medical-Surgical Nursing: Young Adult; Older Adult)

Thinking Exercise 24B-1

A 25-year-old paraplegic female client is brought to the urgent care center by her caretaker. The caretaker reports the client has not had a bowel movement for 3 days. The nurse suspects an intestinal obstruction and begins assessing the client. **Complete the following statements by choosing the *most likely* options for the missing information from the lists of options provided.**

During the client interview, the nurse asks the client about whether she has had _____1_____ and _____2_____. The client states that those symptoms "come and go." During the focused physical examination, the nurse inspects the abdomen for _____3_____. Then the nurse auscultates the abdomen and expects that bowel sounds may be _____4_____ distal to the obstruction. The nurse anticipates a prescription for a _____5_____ to aid the primary health care provider in diagnosis. In addition to acute pain, if an intestinal obstruction is confirmed, the client is at risk for _____6_____.

Options for 1	Options for 2	Options for 3
Angina	Abdominal pain	Bruising
Cough	Anxiety	Discoloration
Fear	Dizziness	Distention
Headache	Hunger	PEG tube patency
Nausea	Numbness	Petechiae
Indigestion	Pelvic pain	Rash
Urinary retention	Shortness of breath	Wounds

Options for 4	Options for 5	Options for 6
Absent	Complete blood count (CBC)	Anaphylaxis
Borborygmi	CT scan	Dehydration
High-pitched	Fasting blood glucose	Infection
Hyperactive	Fecal occult study	Perforation
Normal	Liver enzyme panel	Limb loss
Tinkling	Sputum sample	Pressure injuries
Undulating	X-ray	Rapid weight gain

Thinking Exercise 24B-2

A 25-year-old paraplegic female client was brought to the urgent care clinic by her caretaker. The caretaker reported the client had not had a bowel movement for 3 days. The client was diagnosed with intestinal obstruction, was admitted to the hospital, and underwent an exploratory laparotomy to determine the location and cause of the obstruction. While the client is recovering on the surgical unit, the nurse performs a postoperative assessment, provides preventive interventions, and monitors for potential complications. **Indicate which nursing action listed in the far-left column is appropriate for the potential postoperative complication. Note that not all nursing actions will be used.**

Nursing Action	Potential Postoperative Complication	Appropriate Nursing Action for Postoperative Complication
1 Assess the incision site for dehiscence and drainage.	Acute kidney injury	
2 Ensure continuous cardiac telemetry monitoring.	Electrolyte imbalance	

Nursing Action	Potential Postoperative Complication	Appropriate Nursing Action for Postoperative Complication
3 Increase the intravenous fluid rate of infusion.	Respiratory depression	
4 Monitor the client's level of consciousness and vital signs.	Hypotension	
5 Maintain sequential or pneumatic compression devices.	Venous thromboembolism	
6 Monitor the client's oxygen saturation levels.		
7 Monitor the client's urine output.		
8 Recheck the client's blood glucose.		

Thinking Exercise 24B-3

A 25-year-old paraplegic female client is recovering on the surgical unit after an exploratory laparotomy to relieve an intestinal obstruction. The nurse provides health teaching for the client and her caregivers about preventing future fecal impaction. Which statements by the client and care team indicate that the health teaching was effective? **Select all that apply.**

_____ A. "I will be sure to eat raw fruits and vegetables."

_____ B. "I will drink six glasses of water a day."

_____ C. "I will use laxatives only if I really need to."

_____ D. "I will go to the pool more to exercise my core muscles."

_____ E. "I will try using prune juice to get my gut moving."

_____ F. "I will take a psyllium fiber supplement once a day."

_____ G. "I will watch for diarrhea and oozing soft stool."

_____ H. "I will avoid using the bedpan if at all possible."

Thinking Exercise 24B-4

The nurse is assessing a 75-year-old male client after implementing postoperative interventions following an open abdominal hernia repair. **For each assessment finding, use an X to indicate whether the intervention was <u>Effective</u> (helped to meet expected outcomes), <u>Ineffective</u> (did not help to meet expected outcomes), or <u>Unrelated</u> (not related to the expected outcomes).**

Assessment Finding	Effective	Ineffective	Unrelated
Staples missing and visible pink tissue at surgical site			
Reports mild pain at the incision site			
Voiding using a urinal			
Capillary refill is less than 3 sec			
Bilateral +1 pitting edema in ankles and feet			

Thinking Exercise 24B-5

A 68-year-old female client is being seen for follow-up wound care on her right lower leg. During her visit, the client states she hasn't had a bowel movement since her last visit a week ago. The client states she hasn't had much of an appetite in the past few days and says, "I figure I don't have anything in there to come out." The nurse auscultates the client's abdomen and hears hyperactive high-pitched bowel sounds in the upper left quadrant and hypoactive bowel sounds in the lower left quadrant. The nurse collaborates with the primary health care provider and the client is directly admitted to the hospital for possible intestinal obstruction. Before going to the hospital, the client asks the nurse what to expect. Which of these statements by the nurse (is) are most likely accurate? **Select all that apply.**

_____ A. "An abdominal x-ray will determine if you have an intestinal obstruction."

_____ B. "A nasogastric (NG) tube will be placed to relieve intestinal distention."

_____ C. "Surgery will be necessary to remove any obstruction."

_____ D. "You will not be able to get out of bed while hospitalized."

_____ E. "You should expect to stay in the hospital for a lengthy amount of time."

_____ F. "You will be placed on a mechanical soft diet."

_____ G. "You should drink lots of water to help move the stool out of your body."

_____ H. "Diarrhea is a sign you are passing stool adequately."

Metabolism
Complex Health Problems

25

Exemplar 25A. Diabetic Ketoacidosis (Pediatric Nursing: Adolescent)

Thinking Exercise 25A-1

A 15-year-old male client who has diabetes mellitus type 1 arrives at the emergency department with his mother, who states that her son's blood sugar level was 330 mg/dL (18.3 mmol/L) when he returned from a 3-day baseball camp. The mother administered 8 units of regular insulin subcutaneously an hour ago, but the adolescent progressively became more confused. Initial nursing assessment and findings include:

- Lethargic, but follows simple commands
- Pupils equal and reactive to light
- Heart rate = 120 beats/min
- Blood pressure = 88/42 mm Hg
- Lung fields clear throughout
- Deep rapid respirations
- Breath smells of rotting fruit
- Scratches present on bilateral knees
- No head wounds or facial bruising present
- Voided 100 mL yellow urine in a urinal

Highlight or place a check mark next to the assessment findings that require follow-up by the nurse.

Thinking Exercise 25A-2

A 15-year-old male client who has diabetes mellitus type 1 arrives at the emergency department with his mother, who states that her son's blood sugar level was 330 mg/dL (18.3 mmol/L) when he returned from a 3-day baseball camp. The mother administered 8 units of regular insulin subcutaneously an hour ago, but the child progressively became more confused. Ongoing assessment findings and laboratory tests include the following:

Assessment Findings	Laboratory Results

- Lethargic
- Follows simple commands
- Pupils equal and reactive to light
- Lung fields clear throughout
- Deep rapid respirations
- Breath smells of rotting fruit
- Scratches present on bilateral knees
- No head wounds or facial bruising present
- Abdomen distended
- Bowel sounds hypoactive
- Voided 100 mL yellow urine in urinal
	- Blood glucose = 360 mg/dL (20 mmol/L)
	- Arterial blood gas
	  - pH = 7.32
	  - HCO_3^- = 12 mEq/L (12 mmol/L)
	  - CO_2 = 33 mEq/L (33 mmol/L)
	- Urine ketones = Positive
	- BUN = 36 mg/dL (12.8 mmol/L)
	- Serum creatinine = 1.1 mg/dL (97 mcmol/L)
	- Anion gap = 12 mEq/L (12 mmol/L)
	- Serum potassium = 3.4 mEq/L (3.4 mmol/L)

Choose the *most likely* options for the information missing from the statements below by selecting from the lists of options provided.

Based on the assessment findings and laboratory results, the nurse suspects that the client is experiencing _____1_____ because his _____1_____ is very high and his other laboratory results indicate that he has _____1_____. The nurse anticipates that the client will need _____2_____ and _____2_____ as soon as possible to manage his diabetic complication.

Options for 1	Options for 2
Respiratory alkalosis	IV fluid replacement
Serum potassium	Enteral feedings
Arterial pH	IV long-acting insulin
Hyperglycemic hyperosmolar state	Hemodialysis
Metabolic acidosis	Parenteral nutrition
Serum glucose	IV regular insulin
Diabetic ketoacidosis	Fruit juice

Thinking Exercise 25A-3

A 15-year-old male client who has diabetes mellitus type 1 arrives at the emergency department with his mother, who states that her son's blood sugar level was 330 mg/dL (18.3 mmol/L) when he returned from a 3-day baseball camp. The mother administered 8 units of regular insulin subcutaneously an hour ago, but the child progressively became more confused. Ongoing assessment findings and laboratory tests include the following.

Assessment Findings	Laboratory Results
• Lethargic	• Blood glucose = 360 mg/dL (20 mmol/L)
• Follows simple commands	• Arterial blood gas
• Pupils equal and reactive to light	• pH = 7.32
• Lung fields clear throughout	• $HCO_3^- = 12$ mEq/L (12 mmol/L)
• Deep rapid respirations	• $CO_2 = 33$ mEq/L (33 mmol/L)
• Breath smells of rotting fruit	• Urine ketones = Positive
• Scratches present on bilateral knees	• BUN = 36 mg/dL (12.8 mmol/L))
• No head wounds or facial bruising present	• Serum creatinine = 1.1 mg/dL (97 mcmol/L)
• Abdomen distended	• Anion gap = 12 mEq/L (12 mmol/L)
• Bowel sounds hypoactive	• Serum potassium = 3.4 mEq/L (3.4 mmol/L)
• Voided 100 mL yellow urine in urinal	

The primary health care provider prescribes a treatment plan, which includes:
- 0.9% normal saline IV infusion at 500 mL/hr for 1 L followed by 0.45% normal saline IV infusion at 250 mL/hr until the client's blood glucose is less than 250 mg/dL (13.8 mmol/L)
- 0.1 unit/kg regular insulin IV bolus followed by regular insulin IV infusion at 0.1 mg/kg/hr

The nurse records the client's weight as 90.4 lb (41 kg) and implements prescribed care and nursing interventions. **Use an X to indicate whether the nursing actions below are <u>Indicated</u> (appropriate or necessary), <u>Contraindicated</u> (could be harmful), or <u>Non-Essential</u> (make no difference or are not necessary) for the client's care at this time.**

Nursing Action	Indicated	Contraindicated	Non-Essential
Initiate potassium replacement per hospital protocol.			
Check the client's blood glucose level hourly.			

Nursing Action	Indicated	Contraindicated	Non-Essential
Administer 4 units regular insulin subcutaneously.			
Help the client drink 120 mL of fruit juice.			
Insert an indwelling urinary catheter to closely monitor output.			
Monitor the client for postural (orthostatic) hypotension.			
Check the client's vital signs every 15 minutes.			

Thinking Exercise 25A-4

A 15-year-old male client who has diabetes mellitus type 1 arrives at the emergency department with his mother, who states that her son's blood sugar level was 330 mg/dL (18.3 mmol/L) when he returned from a 3-day baseball camp. The mother administered 8 units of regular insulin subcutaneously an hour ago, but the child progressively became more confused. Physical assessment findings and laboratory tests indicate the client is experiencing diabetic ketoacidosis. The primary health care provider prescribes a treatment plan, which is implemented. **For each assessment finding, use an X to indicate whether the interventions were <u>Effective</u> (helped to meet expected outcomes), <u>Ineffective</u> (did not help to meet expected outcomes), or <u>Unrelated</u> (not related to the expected outcomes).**

Assessment Finding	Effective	Ineffective	Unrelated
Blood glucose = 198 mg/dL (11 mmol/L)			
Yellow nasal drainage present			
Arterial pH = 7.33			
Serum creatinine = 1.1 mg/dL (97 mcmol/L)			
Bowel sounds hypoactive × 4			
Urine ketones = negative			

Thinking Exercise 25A-5

A 15-year-old male client who has diabetes mellitus type 1 was hospitalized after a 3-day baseball camp with a diagnosis of diabetic ketoacidosis. The client is alert and oriented and sharing his experience at baseball camp with his mother and the nurse. Which activities does the nurse identify as contributing to the client's episode of diabetic ketoacidosis? **Select all that apply.**

_____ A. Ate 16 slices of pizza and almost won the eating contest

_____ B. Wore different athletic shoes each day and assessed feet each evening

_____ C. Administered insulin doses in his favorite spot, although it showed scar tissue

_____ D. Took his long-acting insulin dose each morning as prescribed

_____ E. Exercised 6 hours daily on the field and in the weight room with team members

_____ F. Was embarrassed to administer insulin in the dining hall with his meals

_____ G. Was nicknamed "urine-boy" because he had to use the bathroom frequently

Thinking Exercise 25A-6

A 15-year-old male client who has diabetes mellitus type 1 was hospitalized after a 3-day baseball camp with a diagnosis of diabetic ketoacidosis (DKA). The client is alert and oriented and shared his experience at baseball camp with his mother and the nurse, which helped the nurse to identify factors contributing to the client's DKA. After providing health teaching to the client and his mother, the nurse assesses the client's understanding. **For each client response, use an X to indicate whether the nurse's teaching was <u>Effective</u> (response indicates that the client understands his care), <u>Ineffective</u> (response indicates that the client does not understand his care), or <u>Unrelated</u> (response is not related to the nurse's health teaching).**

Client's Response	Effective	Ineffective	Unrelated
"I will check my blood sugar levels every 4 hours when exercising and playing baseball."			
"I will hold my long-acting insulin doses when I choose not to take my short-acting insulin doses."			
"When exercising I will drink only water and not sugar-filled sports drinks."			
"I will wear protective sports equipment during baseball games and practice."			
"I will rotate injection sites because scar tissue slows the absorption of insulin administered."			
"I will contact my mother if my blood sugar level is ever more than 250 mg/dL (13.8 mmol/L)."			

Exemplar 25B. Cirrhosis (Medical-Surgical Nursing: Older Adult)

Thinking Exercise 25B-1

A 67-year-old male client has been living at home after he was diagnosed with end-stage cirrhosis following a lengthy methicillin-susceptible *Staphylococcus aureus* (MSSA) treatment regimen including amoxicillin/clavulanate. Today the client presents to the emergency department after noticing black tarry stools. Initial nursing assessment findings are:

- Is alert and oriented to person, place, and time
- Mucous membranes are pale and yellow
- Breath sounds clear in all fields
- Heart sounds = S_1/S_2 present
- Capillary refill = 4 sec
- Bowel sounds = hypoactive $\times$ 4
- Abdomen is distended and firm
- Skin is warm and dry
- Petechiae on lower arms and legs
- Pedal pulses = +1 bilaterally
- Client reports severe pruritus
- Oxygen saturation = 98% (on room air)

Highlight or place a check mark next to the assessment findings that require follow-up by the nurse.

Thinking Exercise 25B-2

A 67-year-old male client who had been living at home with end-stage cirrhosis presents to the emergency department today after having noticed black tarry stools. He was consequently diagnosed with GI bleeding, anemia, and ascites. The nurse is preparing to transfuse packed red blood cells. **Use an X to indicate whether the nursing actions below are <u>Indicated</u> (appropriate or necessary), <u>Contraindicated</u> (could be harmful), or <u>Non-Essential</u> (make no difference or are not necessary).**

Nursing Action	Indicated	Contraindicated	Non-Essential
Obtain consent for the transfusion.			
Bathe the client with warm soapy water.			
Draw type and screen for blood transfusion.			
Ambulate the client to the toilet.			
Position the head of the client's bed at between 45 and 60 degrees.			
Frequently check client vital signs.			
Educate the client about incentive spirometry.			

Thinking Exercise 25B-3

A 67-year-old male client with end-stage cirrhosis has been diagnosed with GI bleeding, anemia, and ascites. After a successful blood transfusion, the primary health care provider performs paracentesis to remove fluid from the abdomen. The nurse assesses for potential complications that commonly occur in clients who have cirrhosis. **Indicate which nursing action listed in the far-left column is appropriate for the potential complication. Note that not all nursing actions will be used.**

Nursing Action	Potential Complication	Appropriate Nursing Action for Complication
1 Monitor oxygen saturation.	Impaired comfort	
2 Assess mucous membranes for jaundice.	Paracentesis insertion site infection	
3 Administer IV morphine.	Hypervolemia	
4 Monitor level of consciousness.	Hepatic encephalopathy	
5 Maintain continuous cardiac monitoring.	Electrolyte imbalance	
6 Monitor intake and output.		
7 Monitor for a low-grade fever and check needle insertion site.		

Thinking Exercise 25B-4

A 67-year-old male client has a diagnosis of end-stage cirrhosis and understands he has no hope of his liver returning to normal function. He asks the nurse for information about liver transplantation as a possible option. Which of the following responses by the nurse are **appropriate**? **Select all that apply.**

_____ A. "You must have good heart health to be considered for liver transplantation."

_____ B. "Your lungs need to be free from disease or infection to get a transplant."

_____ C. "You must be able to follow a strict drug therapy regimen after a transplant."

_____ D. "Your new liver tissue may come from a living donor."

_____ E. "Your body may reject the new liver tissue even with proper management."

_____ F. "Your risk for cancer increases after a liver transplant."

_____ G. "You'd need to report fever or right upper quadrant pain quickly after a transplant."

_____ H. "You would need to follow the recommended vaccination schedule after a transplant."

Thinking Exercise 25B-5

A 67-year-old male client with end-stage cirrhosis is waiting for a liver transplant in the critical care unit. The nurse conducts a physical assessment and documents findings to determine the effectiveness of nursing and collaborative interventions. **For each assessment finding, use an X to indicate whether interventions were _Effective_ (helped to meet expected outcomes), _Ineffective_ (did not help to meet expected outcomes), or _Unrelated_ (not related to the expected outcomes).**

Assessment Finding	Effective	Ineffective	Unrelated
Is oriented to person, place, and time			
Reports mild abdominal pain			
Voided 150 mL in 8 hr using a urinal			
Capillary refill is less than 3 sec			
Oxygen saturation is 95% on room air			
Bilateral +1 pitting edema in both ankles and feet			

Exemplar 25C. Acute Pancreatitis (Medical-Surgical Nursing: Middle-Age Adult)

Thinking Exercise 25C-1

A 36-year-old male client is assessed in the emergency department. The nurse notes the client has generalized jaundice, is guarding his abdomen, and vomits bile-colored emesis. The client reports severe pain in the left upper quadrant. Which priority assessments will the nurse complete **at this time**? **Select all that apply.**

_____ A. Heart rate and blood pressure for hemodynamic status

_____ B. Light palpation of abdomen for rigidity

_____ C. Complete health history for precipitating factors

_____ D. Auscultation of lung fields for adventitious sounds

_____ E. Inspection of periorbital and abdominal flanks for gray-blue discoloration

_____ F. CAGE assessment for history of alcoholism

_____ G. Pain for location, severity, duration, and contributing factors

Thinking Exercise 25C-2

A 36-year-old male client experiencing generalized jaundice, bile emesis, and severe left upper abdominal pain is evaluated in the emergency department and diagnosed with acute pancreatitis. The primary health care provider prescribes intravenous fluids, morphine patient-controlled analgesia (PCA), and a proton pump inhibitor. **Use an X to indicate whether the nursing actions below are <u>Indicated</u> (appropriate or necessary), <u>Contraindicated</u> (could be harmful), or <u>Non-Essential</u> (make no difference or are not necessary) for the client's care at this time.**

Nursing Action	Indicated	Contraindicated	Non-Essential
Provide the client with a low-fat diet.			
Help the client into a side-lying position with knees flexed.			
Teach the client to use an incentive spirometer.			
Monitor vital signs every 15 minutes.			
Provide pain relief by pushing the client's PCA button.			
Assess glucose management with a hemoglobin A1c level.			
Provide an emesis basin and measure amount vomited.			
Assist the client in performing frequent oral care.			

Thinking Exercise 25C-3

A 36-year-old male client experiencing generalized jaundice, bile emesis, and severe left upper abdominal pain is evaluated in the emergency department and diagnosed with acute pancreatitis. The primary health care provider prescribes intravenous fluids, morphine patient-controlled analgesia (PCA), and a proton pump inhibitor. After initiating the prescribed treatment plan and implementing nursing interventions, the nurse reassesses the client. **For each assessment finding, use an X to indicate whether the implemented interventions by the nurse were <u>Effective</u> (helped to meet expected outcomes), <u>Ineffective</u> (did not help to meet expected outcomes), or <u>Unrelated</u> (not related to the expected outcomes).**

Assessment Finding	Effective	Ineffective	Unrelated
Blood pressure = 125/63 mm Hg			
Bilateral crackles present on auscultation			
Alert and oriented; denies anxiety			
Positive Chvostek sign			
Reports a personal history of alcoholism			
Bowel sounds active × 4			
Abdominal pain rated 3/10 on a 0 to 10 pain intensity scale			

Thinking Exercise 25C-4

A 36-year-old male client experiencing generalized jaundice, bile emesis, and severe left upper abdominal pain was evaluated 2 days ago and diagnosed with acute pancreatitis. The primary health care provider prescribed intravenous fluids, morphine patient-controlled analgesia (PCA), and a proton pump inhibitor. The client is experiencing complications and will remain NPO for several more days. Total parenteral nutrition (TPN) is prescribed. **Indicate which nursing action listed in the far-left column is appropriate to prevent potential complications of TPN. Note that not all nursing actions will be used.**

Nursing Action	Potential Complication	Appropriate Nursing Action for Each Complication
1 Weigh the client daily and report a significant increase from the previous day.	Hyperglycemia	
2 Have a second nurse check the prescription and solution prior to administration.	Fluid overload	
3 Assess finger stick blood sugars every 4 hours.	Infection	
4 Change the IV tubing every 3 days.	Hypoglycemia	
5 Adjust the infusion rate to ensure the entire TPN bag infuses within 24 hours.		
6 Assess the IV site daily and change the dressing per facility policy.		
7 Infuse 10% dextrose in water if TPN solution is temporarily unavailable.		

Thinking Exercise 25C-5

A 36-year-old male client who had an acute pancreatitis episode has been hospitalized for several days. The nurse prepares the client for discharge and provides health teaching to help the client avoid future episodes of acute pancreatitis and prevent progression to chronic pancreatitis. **Choose the *most likely* options for the information missing from the statements below by selecting from the lists of options provided.**

The nurse teaches the client to eat small, frequent meals that contain high-_____1_____, moderate-_____1_____, and low-_____1_____ foods. GI stimulants such as _____1_____ and _____1_____ should be avoided. The client is taught to abstain from drinking alcohol because if alcohol is consumed, acute _____2_____ will return and further _____2_____ of the pancreas may lead to chronic pancreatitis. In addition to nutritional teaching, the nurse teaches the client to contact the primary health care provider with symptoms of biliary tract disease including _____2_____, _____2_____, and/or _____2_____.

Options for 1	Options for 2
Caffeine	Autodigestion
Calorie	Bleeding
Carbohydrate	Clay-colored stools
Fat	Clotting
Glucose	Dark urine
Lactose	Hypoxia
Orange juice	Jaundice
Pickled foods	Pain
Protein	Scarring
Spices	Vomiting

Tissue Integrity
Burns

Exemplar 26. Burns (Medical-Surgical Nursing: Young Adult)

Thinking Exercise 26-1

A 28-year-old female client was admitted to the emergency department (ED) with recent burns on both arms. Her husband explained that when she was cooking dinner, she accidentally started a grease fire while he was downstairs in the basement watching football. She put on oven mitts to cover both hands and tried to smother the fire with a towel and a small fire extinguisher, which was quickly successful. The nurse notes that the client has superficial partial-thickness burns on most of the anterior surfaces of both arms, but her hands are not affected. She also has a few superficial burns on about half of the posterior aspects of both arms. **Use an X to indicate whether the nursing actions below are Indicated (appropriate or necessary), Contraindicated (could be harmful), or Non-Essential (make no difference or are not necessary) for the client's care at this time.**

Nursing Action	Indicated	Contraindicated	Non-Essential
Obtain a 12-lead ECG.			
Initiate an IV line.			
Administer oxygen therapy.			
Remove eschar to prevent infection.			
Manage the client's pain with analgesia.			
Administer tetanus toxoid for prophylaxis.			
Help the client take a shower.			

Thinking Exercise 26-2

A 28-year-old female client was admitted to the emergency department (ED) with recent burns on both arms. Her husband explained that when she was cooking dinner, she accidentally started a grease fire while he was downstairs in the basement watching football. She put on oven mitts to cover both hands and tried to smother the fire with a towel and a small fire extinguisher, which was quickly successful. The nurse notes that the client has superficial partial-thickness burns on most of the anterior surfaces of both arms, but her hands are not affected. She also has a few superficial burns on about half of the posterior aspects of both arms. **Choose the *most likely* options for the information missing from the statements below by selecting from the lists of options provided.**

Using the Rule of Nines, the nurse calculates that the client has burns on an estimated ___1___ of her body. The client is at risk for developing ____2____ and ____2____ as a result of her burns. The nurse applies a wound dressing after giving the client a(n) _____3_____.

Options for 1	Options for 2	Options for 3
3%	Shock	IV antibiotic
5%	Infection	Sedative
10%	Airway obstruction	Hypnotic
15%	Decreased GI motility	Antiepileptic drug
18%	Seizures	Analgesic
22%	Edema	Potassium

Thinking Exercise 26-3

A 22-year-old male client was drinking alcohol and smoking marijuana with friends in his parent's garage while they were away on vacation. After his friends left, the client fell asleep while smoking a cigarette and awakened to heavy smoke in the garage. Neighbors found the client and called 911. At admission to the emergency department (ED), the nurse noted that the client has a dry cough. What are the **priority actions** for the nurse to perform at this time? **Select all that apply.**

_____ A. Manage the client's pain.

_____ B. Perform a head-to-toe assessment.

_____ C. Assess for airway patency.

_____ D. Keep the client NPO.

_____ E. Monitor vital signs frequently.

_____ F. Initiate an IV line.

_____ G. Prepare to possibly intubate the client.

_____ H. Administer tetanus toxoid.

_____ I. Apply oxygen therapy.

Thinking Exercise 26-4

A 22-year-old male client was drinking alcohol and smoking marijuana with friends in his parent's garage while they were away on vacation. After his friends left, the client fell asleep while smoking a cigarette and awakened to heavy smoke in the garage. Neighbors found the client and called 911. After stabilization in the emergency department (ED), the client did not need to be intubated and was admitted to a private room on the medical unit. Today is his second hospital day. The nurse recognizes that the client is at risk for which complications for this phase of the burn injury? **Select all that apply.**

_____ A. Airway obstruction

_____ B. Increased weight due to edema

_____ C. Sepsis

_____ D. Respiratory infection

_____ E. Posttraumatic stress disorder

_____ F. Pulmonary edema

_____ G. Anemia

Thinking Exercise 26-5

A 22-year-old male client was drinking alcohol and smoking marijuana with friends in his parent's garage while they were away on vacation. After his friends left, the client fell asleep while smoking a cigarette and awakened to heavy smoke in the garage. Neighbors found the client and called 911. After stabilization in the emergency department (ED), the client did not need to be intubated and was admitted to a private room on the medical unit. Today is his third hospital day. The nurse reviews the following progress note written by the previous shift nurse.

Nurses' Notes

9/18/20 7 a.m. (0700) Client states that his pain is often a 4-5/10 on a 0 to 10 pain intensity scale. PT this a.m. to begin exercises to prevent joint contractures. States he always feels hungry, especially after working with the therapist. Has lost 10 pounds since admission 3 days ago even though he is on a high-calorie diet. Serum albumin and prealbumin this a.m. continue to be below normal limits. _____ K.S. Atkins, RN

Highlight the findings in the progress note above that would indicate that the client is <u>not</u> progressing as expected.

Thinking Exercise 27-1

The nurse assesses a 15-year-old male client who was brought to the emergency department by his parents because of severe abdominal pain. The nurse observes that he is "doubled over" in pain, holding his abdomen and not standing up straight, but also unable to walk without swaying and bumping into the wall. The adolescent talks with slurred words, has difficulty focusing, and falls asleep repeatedly during assessment. Results of the health history and initial assessment reveal the following data.

Client History	Vital Signs
• History of attention deficit hyperactivity disorder (ADHD) and asthma • Home medications: amphetamine/dextroamphetamine daily, acetaminophen and ibuprofen as needed • Immunizations are up-to-date • Mother's occupation is homemaker • Father's occupation is nurse • Siblings: brother, 17 years old; sister, 11 years old • Reports casual social acquaintances without any close friends • "Struggles" in school per parents • Rates severe abdominal pain as "15" on a 0 to 10 pain scale; slightly worse in left lower quadrant	• Heart rate = 78 beats/min • Blood pressure = 116/62 mm Hg • Respiratory rate = 10 breaths/min

Serum Laboratory Results	Physical Assessment Findings
• Amylase = 250 units/L • Lipase = 260 units/L • AST = 14 units/L • ALT = 40 units/L • Alkaline phosphatase = 360 units/L • Blood alcohol level = 236 mg/dL (51.2 mmol/L)	• Oriented to self, but somnolent • Conjunctiva pink • Regular heart rate and rhythm • Lung sounds are clear and equal • Distended abdomen with hypoactive bowel sounds and tender to palpation • Mildly diaphoretic, otherwise skin intact • Negative for swelling in extremities

Highlight or place a check mark next to the assessment findings that require follow-up by the nurse.

Thinking Exercise 27-2

The nurse assesses a 15-year-old male client who was brought to the emergency department by his parents because of severe abdominal pain. The nurse observes that he is "doubled over" in pain, but also unable to walk without swaying and bumping into the wall. The adolescent talks with slurred words, has difficulty focusing, and falls asleep repeatedly during assessment. Several hours later, the nurse is able to interview the client about his use of drugs and alcohol. Which are the most appropriate questions for the nurse to ask to facilitate accurate answers? **Select all that apply.**

_____ A. "Why are you here today?"

_____ B. "What kinds of alcohol and drugs did you take before coming to the hospital?"

_____ C. "Do your friends drink alcohol with you?"

_____ D. "How long have you been taking these substances?"

_____ E. "How often do you take these substances?"

_____ F. "When was the last time you took any substance?"

_____ G. "How do you obtain the substances that you take?"

_____ H. "Do you fight often with your parents or siblings?"

Thinking Exercise 27-3

The nurse assesses a 15-year-old male client who was brought to the emergency department by his parents because of severe abdominal pain. The nurse observes that he is "doubled over" in pain, unable to stand up straight but also unable to walk without swaying and bumping into the wall. The adolescent talks with slurred words, has difficulty focusing, and falls asleep repeatedly during assessment. Several hours later, the nurse is able to interview the client about his use of drugs and alcohol. Based on the nurse's interview, the client reveals a history of vaping since age 13, marijuana use, routine alcohol consumption, opioid use, and participation in "pharm parties." At his most recent pharm party, he took an unknown pill that caused him to climb furniture, act "like a gorilla," and exhibit other bizarre behavior according to his friends. He does not remember any details of this incident. What would the nurse identify as the desired outcomes for the client during the detox period? **Select all that apply.**

_____ A. The client will remain free from injury during the withdrawal period.

_____ B. The client will set a goal to abstain from substances.

_____ C. The client will identify various persons and organizations for support.

_____ D. The client will engage in counseling services.

_____ E. The client will report no absence from school.

_____ F. The family will attend an Ala-Teen meeting.

_____ G. The family will actively participate in the detoxification program with the client.

Thinking Exercise 27-4

The nurse is caring for a 14-year-old female client admitted for suicidal ideations and polysubstance use. The nurse anticipates the possibility of substance withdrawal and monitors the client closely for the clinical manifestations of withdrawal from various drugs. **Indicate which clinical manifestations listed in the far-left column are expected if the client experiences withdrawal from selected drugs. Note that not all clinical manifestations will be used and some will be used more than once.**

Clinical Manifestations of Drug Withdrawal	Drug	Expected Clinical Manifestations From Drug Withdrawal
1 Client reports insomnia or sleep disturbances.	Sedative-hypnotics	
2 Client experiences dulled thinking and lethargy.	Cocaine	
3 Client reports hallucinations.	Heroin	
4 Client reports muscle aches or bone pain.	Oxycodone	
5 Client demonstrates restlessness or depression.	Phencyclidine (PCP)	
6 Client reports cold flashes and goose bumps.	Flunitrazepam	
7 Client demonstrates extreme anxiety and irritability.		
8 Client reports vivid unpleasant dreams and/or increased appetite.		
9 Client exhibits seizure activity or delirium.		
10 Client reports nausea or vomiting or stomach cramping.		
11 Client demonstrates elevated pulse, hyperthermia, and blood pressure.		

Thinking Exercise 27-5

The nurse is developing a plan of care for a 13-year-old male adolescent who was admitted after making racial slurs and threatening violence toward other students at school. The client presented with an elevated blood alcohol level and was found to be positive for marijuana use, which the parents report has been an ongoing concern. **Use an X to indicate whether the nursing actions below are <u>Indicated</u> (appropriate or necessary), <u>Contraindicated</u> (could be harmful), or <u>Non-Essential</u> (make no difference or are not necessary) for the client's care during hospitalization.**

Nursing Action	Indicated	Contraindicated	Non-Essential
Monitor the client's respiratory rate every 4 hours.			
Complete the Clinical Institute Withdrawal From Alcohol (CIWA-Ar) scale every 4 hours and as needed.			
Encourage the client to use denial as a coping mechanism.			
Complete a search of the client's personal belongings.			
Schedule time for an initial family therapy session.			
Administer naloxone.			
Recognize that substance use disorder is a disease influenced by genetic factors.			
Arrange and encourage counseling.			
Redirect the client when he projects anger.			
Provide an empathetic, warm, and nonjudgmental environment.			
Require that the client participate in group activities.			
Administer acetaminophen as needed for headaches.			

Thinking Exercise 27-6

The nurse is evaluating the progress of a 15-year-old male client undergoing management of alcohol dependence in an alcohol and addictions treatment center. **For each assessment finding, use an X to indicate whether the interventions were <u>Effective</u> (helped to meet expected outcomes), <u>Ineffective</u> (did not help to meet expected outcomes), or <u>Unrelated</u> (not related to the expected outcomes).**

Assessment Finding	Effective	Ineffective	Unrelated
The client reports that he cannot stay sober without help.			
The client shares that his parents' "nagging" makes him want to drink.			
The client actively engages in and attends self-help groups.			
The client plans to look for a new group of friends.			
The client is able to express feelings of sadness.			
The client reports satisfaction with body image.			
The client denies experiencing flashbacks or hallucinations.			
The client expresses hopelessness that he will be able to stay sober.			
The client sings and dances in the unit hallway.			

28

Management of Care
Complex Health Problems

Thinking Exercise 28-1

The nurse is assigned to provide care this shift for five (5) hospitalized clients who are admitted to monitored beds in private rooms as follows:

- **Client #1:** A 72-year-old woman admitted yesterday for new-onset atrial fibrillation; has a history of diabetes mellitus type 2 (insulin controlled), hypertension, severe osteoarthritis, and late-stage rheumatoid arthritis.
- **Client #2:** A 67-year-old man admitted last night for severe hypokalemia receiving IV fluids with potassium supplements; has a history of late-stage Parkinson disease, dementia, and heart failure.
- **Client #3:** A 43-year-old man admitted early this morning for severe dehydration, hypernatremia, and metabolic acidosis receiving continuous IV fluids; has a history of chronic kidney disease and renal calculi.
- **Client #4:** A 56-year-old woman admitted last night for lower GI bleeding and anemia currently receiving a unit of packed red blood cells; has a history of double mastectomy for breast cancer last year and bipolar disorder.
- **Client #5:** A 34-year-old woman admitted 3 days ago for viral pneumonia and respiratory distress; has a long history of extrinsic asthma, migraine headaches, anorexia nervosa, and depression; scheduled for discharge to home today with her parents.

Choose the *most likely* options for the information missing from the statements below by selecting from the lists of options provided.

After report from the previous shift, the nurse most likely would assess Client # ___1___ as the priority because this client is at risk for _____2_____. The second client that the nurse would assess is Client # ___1___ because this client is at risk for _____2_____.

Options for 1	Options for 2
1	GI bleeding
2	Embolic stroke
3	Septic shock
4	Respiratory failure
5	Blood transfusion reaction

Thinking Exercise 28-2

The nurse is assigned to provide care this shift for five hospitalized clients who are admitted to monitored beds in private rooms as follows:

- **Client #1:** A 72-year-old woman admitted yesterday for new-onset atrial fibrillation; has a history of diabetes mellitus type 2 (insulin controlled), hypertension, severe osteoarthritis, and late-stage rheumatoid arthritis.
- **Client #2:** A 67-year-old man admitted last night for severe hypokalemia receiving IV fluids with potassium supplements; has a history of late-stage Parkinson disease, dementia, and heart failure.
- **Client #3:** A 43-year-old man admitted early this morning for severe dehydration, hypernatremia, and metabolic acidosis receiving continuous IV fluids; has a history of chronic kidney disease and renal calculi.

- **Client #4:** A 56-year-old woman admitted last night for lower GI bleeding and anemia currently receiving a unit of packed red blood cells; has a history of double mastectomy for breast cancer last year and bipolar disorder.
- **Client #5:** A 34-year-old woman admitted 3 days ago for viral pneumonia and respiratory distress; has a long history of extrinsic asthma, migraine headaches, anorexia nervosa, and depression; scheduled for discharge to home today with her parents.

Which client(s) could the nurse safely assign to a licensed practical nurse/licensed vocational nurse (LPN/LVN)? **Select all that apply.**

_____ A. Client #1

_____ B. Client #2

_____ C. Client #3

_____ D. Client #4

_____ E. Client #5

_____ F. None of these clients

Thinking Exercise 28-3

The nurse is assigned to provide care this shift for five hospitalized clients who are admitted to monitored beds in private rooms as follows:
- **Client #1:** A 72-year-old woman admitted yesterday for new-onset atrial fibrillation; has a history of diabetes mellitus type 2 (insulin dependent), hypertension, severe osteoarthritis, and late-stage rheumatoid arthritis.
- **Client #2:** A 67-year-old man admitted last night for severe hypokalemia receiving IV fluids with potassium supplements; has a history of late-stage Parkinson disease (ADL dependent), dementia, and heart failure.
- **Client #3:** A 43-year-old man admitted early this morning for severe dehydration, hypernatremia, and metabolic acidosis receiving continuous IV fluids; has a history of chronic kidney disease and renal calculi.
- **Client #4:** A 56-year-old woman admitted last night for lower GI bleeding and moderate anemia currently receiving a unit of packed red blood cells; has a history of double mastectomy for breast cancer last year and bipolar disorder.
- **Client #5:** A 34-year-old woman admitted 3 days ago for viral pneumonia and respiratory distress; has a long history of extrinsic asthma, migraine headaches, anorexia nervosa, and depression; scheduled for discharge to home today with her parents.

Indicate which nursing action listed in the far-left column is appropriate for each assigned client's care at this time. Note that not all actions will be used.

Nursing Actions	Assigned Client	Appropriate Nursing Action for Assigned Client
1 Administer prescribed antibiotic therapy.	Client #1	
2 Assess client's neurologic status frequently.	Client #2	
3 Review medications for home care follow-up.	Client #3	
4 Assess for orthostatic hypotension.	Client #4	
5 Monitor hemoglobin and hematocrit values.	Client #5	
6 Monitor for new-onset cardiac dysrhythmias.		
7 Consult with physical and occupational therapy providers.		

Thinking Exercise 28-4

The nurse is caring for a group of residents in a skilled nursing facility and is planning to assign/delegate selected nursing tasks and activities to nursing assistive personnel. Which tasks and activities would be appropriate for the nurse to assign/delegate? **Select all that apply.**

_____ A. Taking vital signs, including pulse oximetry

_____ B. Measuring and recording intake and output

_____ C. Assessing the residents' pain level

_____ D. Giving showers or baths as needed

_____ E. Changing peripheral IV line dressings

_____ F. Turning residents every 2 hours

_____ G. Administering tube feedings

_____ H. Teaching residents about dietary restrictions

Thinking Exercise 28-5

The nurse is caring for a group of residents in a skilled nursing facility. Which client care activities would the nurse safely assign to a licensed practical nurse/licensed vocational nurse (LPN/LVN)? **Select all that apply.**

_____ A. Changing peripheral IV line dressings

_____ B. Administering tube feedings

_____ C. Monitoring finger stick blood sugars

_____ D. Performing comprehensive health assessments

_____ E. Monitoring peripheral IV infusions

_____ F. Teaching residents about dietary restrictions

_____ G. Administering medications including subcutaneous insulin

PART 5

Pharmacology for Nursing

Pharmacology in Management of Common Health Problems

Exemplar 29A. Drugs That Affect Nutrition and Elimination (Medical-Surgical Nursing: Older Adult; Pediatric Nursing)

Thinking Exercise 29A-1

A 66-year-old female client with a history of gastroesophageal reflux disease (GERD) and penicillin allergy is diagnosed with *Helicobacter pylori* infection. Her primary health care provider prescribes clarithromycin-based triple therapy for 14 days. Her new drugs include:

- Clarithromycin 500 mg orally twice daily
- Metronidazole 500 mg orally twice daily
- Pantoprazole 40 mg orally once daily

What health teaching would the nurse include for the client related to her drug therapy? **Select all that apply.**

_____ A. "Take all of the drugs that are prescribed for the full 14 days."

_____ B. "Report new-onset prolonged diarrhea to your primary health care provider."

_____ C. "Report any feeling of fluttering or palpitations while on these drugs."

_____ D. "Take all of these drugs on an empty stomach before breakfast."

_____ E. "Be sure to get a bone scan before and after the drug therapy."

_____ F. "Have the magnesium level checked in your blood before and after taking these drugs."

_____ G. "Be aware that pantoprazole may make you more likely to develop pneumonia."

_____ H. "Avoid alcohol while you are taking these drugs to prevent interaction."

Thinking Exercise 29A-2

An 8-year-old male client was recently diagnosed with limb-girdle muscular dystrophy and has an appointment with his pediatric specialist. During today's follow-up visit, his mother states that he is having "a lot of problems going to the bathroom for number 2." On assessment, the nurse notes that his abdomen is slightly distended and tender when lightly palpated. The primary health care provider prescribes docusate sodium 100 mg/day and polyethylene glycol 0.8 g/kg of body weight once daily. **Choose the *most likely* options for the information missing from the following statements by selecting from the lists of options provided.**

The child weighs 57 lb today; therefore the nurse calculates his prescribed dose of polyethylene glycol to be _____1_____ g once daily. The nurse teaches the mother to give the child a(n) _____2_____ with each dose of docusate sodium and report adverse effects of his new drug therapy, including _____3_____, _____3_____, and _____3_____.

Options for 1	Options for 2	Options for 3
3	Banana	Severe nausea
8	Cracker and milk	Fluid retention
12	Full glass of water	Excessive diarrhea
17	Full glass of juice	Edema
21	Laxative	Increased abdominal bloating
26	Antacid	Flatulence
30	Antidiarrheal drug	Weight gain

Thinking Exercise 29A-3

A 72-year-old male client was recently diagnosed with beginning heart failure and has taken hydrochlorothiazide (HCTZ) 25 mg orally each day for the past 4 months. He also has a history of erectile dysfunction, for which he has been taking sildenafil 50 mg as needed. Today the client is scheduled for his annual physical examination. **For each assessment finding, use an X to indicate whether his treatment plan has been Effective (helped to meet expected outcomes), Ineffective (did not help to meet expected outcomes), or Unrelated (not related to the expected outcomes).**

Assessment Finding	Effective	Ineffective	Unrelated
Serum potassium = 3.2 mEq/L (3.2 mmol/L)			
Serum sodium = 136 mEq/L (136 mmol/L)			
Increased sexual desire and erection			
No chest pain or dyspnea			
Blood pressure = 118/66 mm Hg			
Frequent tearing eyes and sneezing when outdoors			
1+ to 2+ edema in both ankles			

Thinking Exercise 29A-4

A 72-year-old male client was diagnosed with beginning heart failure that has been controlled by hydrochlorothiazide (HCTZ) 25 mg orally each day for the past 11 months. Two days ago he was admitted to the telemetry unit for sinus bradycardia and increased peripheral edema. This morning his weight indicated that he gained 4 lb (1.82 kg) since admission. The client also reports new-onset shortness of breath. **Use an X to indicate whether the nursing actions below are Anticipated (appropriate or necessary), Contraindicated (could be harmful), or Non-Essential (make no difference or are not necessary) for the client's care at this time.**

Nursing Action	Anticipated	Contraindicated	Non-Essential
Draw a comprehensive metabolic panel (CMP).			
Carefully monitor the client's intake and output.			
Initiate oxygen therapy.			
Continue to carefully monitor daily weights.			
Prepare to administer IV push furosemide stat.			
Keep the client in a supine flat position.			
Monitor the client's vital signs frequently.			

Thinking Exercise 29A-5

A 72-year-old male client was diagnosed with beginning heart failure, which has been controlled by hydrochlorothiazide (HCTZ) 25 mg orally each day for the past 11 months. Two days ago he was admitted to the telemetry unit for sinus bradycardia and increased peripheral edema. This morning his weight showed that he gained 4 lb since admission, and the primary health care provider prescribed furosemide 20 mg IV push. **Complete the following statements by choosing the *most likely option* for the missing information from the lists of options provided.**

For safe medication administration, the nurse will administer the IV push furosemide over _____1_____ minutes. Within an hour of administration, the client would be expected to _____2_____. If needed, IV push furosemide may be repeated in _____3_____.

Options for 1	Options for 2	Options for 3
1 to 2	Have an increased blood pressure	15 to 20 minutes
2 to 3	Have a bounding pulse	20 to 30 minutes
3 to 4	Void a large amount	1 to 2 hours
4 to 5	Feel weak due to loss of sodium	2 to 3 hours
5 to 6	Experience dizziness	3 to 4 hours

Exemplar 29B. Drugs That Affect Clotting (Medical-Surgical Nursing: Middle-Age and Older Adult)

Thinking Exercise 29B-1

A 42-year-old female client was injured at work and had a right surgical knee repair 2 weeks ago. Today she presents to the emergency department with reports of severe right calf pain and tingling, right leg swelling, and shortness of breath. After a complete work-up, the client is diagnosed and admitted to an acute care unit with a right calf deep vein thrombosis and pulmonary embolus. The primary health care provider prescribes an unfractionated heparin IV bolus of 5000 units followed by a continuous heparin infusion of 1300 units/hr. Which laboratory test values would the nurse carefully monitor during the administration of this drug? **Select all that apply.**

_____ A. International normalized ratio (INR)

_____ B. Activated partial thromboplastin time (aPTT)

_____ C. Prothrombin time (PT)

_____ D. Platelet count

_____ E. Anti-factor Xa heparin assay

_____ F. Complete blood cell count

Thinking Exercise 29B-2

A 42-year-old female client was injured at work and had a right surgical knee repair 2 weeks ago. The client was diagnosed and admitted to an acute care unit with a right calf deep vein thrombosis and pulmonary embolus. The primary health care provider prescribed an unfractionated heparin IV bolus of 5000 units followed by a continuous infusion of 1300 units/hour. **Choose the *most likely* options for the information missing from the statements below by selecting from the lists of options provided.**

During IV heparin administration, the nurse would monitor the client for possible adverse drug effects, especially bleeding or hemorrhage. To monitor for this complication, the nurse would assess for common signs of blood loss, including _____1_____ blood pressure and _____1_____ pulse. Other indications of bleeding include _____2_____, _____2_____, _____2_____, and _____2_____.

Options for 1	Options for 2
Orthostatic	Decreased level of consciousness
Irregular	Hematuria
Increased	Angioedema
Fluctuating	Red or black stools
Decreased	Constipation
Hyperreflexic	Ecchymosis

Thinking Exercise 29B-3

A 42-year-old female client was injured at work and had a right surgical knee repair 2 weeks ago. The client was diagnosed and admitted to an acute care unit with a right calf deep vein thrombosis and pulmonary embolus. After several days of continuous IV heparin infusion, the primary health care provider prescribed warfarin while the client continued with the heparin infusion. What health teaching related to drug therapy would the nurse provide for the client in preparation for the client's discharge to home on warfarin? **Select all that apply.**

_____ A. "Let your primary health care provider know if you plan to get pregnant before you try to conceive."

_____ B. "Do not take other drugs that can cause bleeding, including NSAIDs like ibuprofen."

_____ C. "Report any unusual bleeding to your primary health care provider immediately."

_____ D. "Be sure to get all laboratory testing done as prescribed to monitor your clotting values."

_____ E. "Use a soft toothbrush and do not be too aggressive with brushing."

_____ F. "Use an electric razor to shave your legs rather than any other type."

_____ G. "Stop taking your warfarin if bleeding occurs until you contact your primary health care provider."

_____ H. "Inform any other health care professional, including your dentist, that you are taking warfarin."

_____ I. "Be sure to eat more foods high in vitamin K to prevent another blood clot."

Thinking Exercise 29B-4

A 65-year-old female client with a long history of acute coronary syndrome (ACS) had two cardiac stents placed via percutaneous coronary intervention. After this procedure, she was started on aspirin 325 mg orally once daily and clopidogrel 75 mg orally once daily. The nurse is preparing to provide education about each of these drugs. **For each health teaching statement below, use an X to indicate whether it is <u>Essential</u> (necessary or appropriate drug information) or <u>Unrelated</u> (not relevant or appropriate drug information) for the client.**

Health Teaching	Essential	Unrelated
"Report any unexpected bleeding to your primary health care provider."		
"Continue taking your newly prescribed medications until your prescriber tells you not to do so."		
"Drink a glass of water after each dose of your new drugs."		
"Eat foods high in vitamin K and calcium to help prevent clotting."		
"Avoid taking other medications that can cause bleeding, such as NSAIDs like ibuprofen."		
"Follow up with the prescribed laboratory testing needed to monitor your clotting values."		

Exemplar 29C. Drugs That Affect Perfusion (Medical-Surgical Nursing: Middle-Age and Older Adult)

Thinking Exercise 29C-1

A 65-year-old male client has had a history of essential hypertension since he was 54 years of age. He has been on a variety of antihypertensive medications, but does not have consistent blood pressure control, especially when he is stressed or visits his provider. His new primary health care provider prescribed losartan 100 mg orally once daily at night because his serum creatinine is slightly elevated and his diastolic blood pressure is ranging between 86 and 90 mm Hg. Which health teaching would the nurse provide for the client at this time? **Select all that apply.**

_____ A. "This drug will help protect your kidneys because it is often used for hypertension caused by kidney disease."

_____ B. "Be sure to change positions slowly, especially from sitting or lying to standing, to prevent dizziness or light-headedness."

_____ C. "This drug can cause wheezing or tightness in your chest, especially if you have asthma."

_____ D. "Call 911 immediately if you experience swelling or tightness in your throat, mouth, or lips."

_____ E. "Check your pulse twice a day because this drug can cause it to decrease dramatically."

_____ F. "Don't take this drug with any other antihypertensive drug or diuretic."

_____ G. "Follow up with all appointments with your primary health care provider to monitor your blood pressure."

_____ H. "Buy a home blood pressure device and take your blood pressure at least daily at different times of the day."

Thinking Exercise 29C-2

A 65-year-old male client has had a history of essential hypertension since he was 54 years of age. He has been on a variety of antihypertensive medications but did not have consistent blood pressure control, especially when he was stressed or visited his provider. Three months ago, his new primary health care provider prescribed losartan 100 mg orally once daily at night because his serum creatinine was slightly elevated and his diastolic blood pressure ranged between 86 and 90 mm Hg. A review of his blood pressure readings for the last month during his follow-up appointment showed that the client's blood pressure usually stays within normal range until late afternoon, around 4 p.m. (1600). The primary health care provider added amlodipine 5 mg orally once daily to his drug regimen. **Choose the *most likely* options for the information missing from the statements below by selecting from the lists of options provided.**

In view of the client's blood pressure pattern and the peak action of amlodipine, the nurse would recommend that the client take his amlodipine _____1_____. He should also avoid drinking _____2_____ because they/it interfere(s) with the drug's metabolism in the intestines.

Options for 1	Options for 2
At night with the losartan	Milk and milk products
Every other day	Caffeinated beverages
During midafternoon	Carbonated beverages
In early morning	Sports drinks
At around midnight	Grapefruit juice

Thinking Exercise 29C-3

A co-worker called 911 for a 52-year-old male client who was working at his construction job and who experienced sudden severe chest pain. After an evaluation at the local emergency department, the client was placed on verapamil ER 180 mg daily for angina pectoris and sent home for follow-up with his primary health care provider. What nursing actions are required related to this client's condition and his newly prescribed medication? **Select all that apply.**

_____ A. Teaching the client to drink plenty of fluids and engaging in daily exercise to prevent constipation.

_____ B. Conducting medication reconciliation to ensure that the client is not currently taking a beta-blocking agent or digoxin.

_____ C. Reminding the client to avoid grapefruit juice while on the medication.

_____ D. Teaching the client about the need to take the drug on an empty stomach at night.

_____ E. Teaching the client the importance of checking his pulse daily, especially if taking other cardiac medications.

_____ F. Reminding the client to make a follow-up appointment with his primary health care provider.

_____ G. Reminding the client to call 911 if there are any other episodes of chest pain.

Thinking Exercise 29C-4

A 48-year-old obese male client was recently diagnosed with essential hypertension and a history of two "silent" myocardial infarctions diagnosed by electrocardiography. The client was placed on lisinopril 10 mg orally once a day, but the dose was increased to 20 mg 3 months ago. The client is visiting his primary health care provider for a follow up today, and the medical assistant takes his history and vital signs. The nurse reviews the following data in the client's electronic health record:

- Temperature = 98°F (36.7°C)
- Pulse = 82 beat/min
- Respirations = 16 breaths/min
- Blood pressure = 128/78 mm Hg
- O_2 saturation = 97% (on room air)

- Denies chest pain, palpitations, shortness of breath
- Reports new dry "hacking" cough that occurs almost every day
- No ankle or feet edema
- Has replaced sodium-based salt with potassium-based salt in his diet

Highlight the findings in the client data listed above that would be of immediate concern to the nurse related to his drug therapy.

Thinking Exercise 29C-5

A 75-year-old female client was recently started on low-dose digoxin and hydrochlorothiazide (HCTZ) for heart failure. The nurse is assessing the client during the visit to her primary health care provider. **Complete the following statements by choosing the *most likely option* for the missing information from the lists of options provided.**

The nurse performs a focused cardiovascular assessment because the client is at risk for _____1_____ and _____1_____ because she takes both digoxin and HCTZ. In addition, the client is at risk for drug toxicity, which can be prevented by monitoring the client's _____2_____ and _____2_____ levels.

Options for 1	Options for 2
Dysrhythmias	Platelet
Hypermagnesemia	HCTZ
Hyponatremia	Sodium
Stroke	Digoxin
Hypokalemia	Creatinine
Myocardial infarction	Potassium
Decreased hearing	Hemoglobin

Exemplar 29D. Drugs That Promote Comfort and Metabolism (Medical-Surgical Nursing: Middle-Age and Older Adult)

Thinking Exercise 29D-1

A 66-year-old male client was driven by his wife to the emergency department because he injured his back at work and can hardly stand upright. After an evaluation of his back pain, the primary health care provider prescribed the following:

- Cyclobenzaprine 5 mg orally three times a day
- Naproxen 500 mg orally every 12 hours
- Use ice/heat applications as instructed
- Follow up with personal primary health care provider

What health care teaching would the nurse include for the client and his wife related to drug therapy? **Select all that apply.**

_____ A. "Take your medications on an empty stomach to help reduce GI distress."

_____ B. "Avoid drinking alcohol while you are taking these medications."

_____ C. "Report any unusual bleeding or bruising to your primary health care provider."

_____ D. "Be aware that you may feel a little drowsy after the first few doses of the cyclobenzaprine."

_____ E. "Report any blurred vision or urinary retention to your primary health care provider."

_____ F. "Try to eat more high-fiber foods and drink more water while on these drugs."

_____ G. "Follow up with the laboratory testing to monitor your liver while on these drugs."

_____ H. "Report any chest discomfort or palpitations to your primary health care provider."

Thinking Exercise 29D-2

A 53-year-old male client who has diabetes mellitus type 2 reported having foot pain and tingling for several months. After an evaluation by his primary health care provider, he was started on pregabalin for diabetic neuropathy in addition to the other drugs he was taking. The nurse conducts medication reconciliation. **Match each of the client's drugs (Column A) with its correct drug class (Column C) from the choices provided in Column B.**

A. Client's Drugs	B. Drug Class	C. Correct Drug for Drug Class
1 Simvastatin	Anti-epileptic drug	
2 Empagliflozin	HMG-CoA reductase inhibitor	
3 Pregabalin	5-Alpha-reductase inhibitor	
4 Glyburide	NSAID	
5 Finasteride	SGLT-2 inhibitor	
6 Celecoxib	Sulfonylurea	

Thinking Exercise 29D-3

A 62-year-old female client with a history of hypertension, gastroesophageal reflux, osteopenia, and osteoarthritis has been managed for cervical and lumbar back pain for the past 20 years with ibuprofen 800 mg orally once daily and hydrocodone/acetaminophen 10/325, 1 tablet every 6 hours as needed. She is admitted to the hospital today for possible lower GI bleeding and scheduled for a colonoscopy tomorrow morning. Her most recent nursing note is as follows:

Nurses' Notes

7/19/20 1915. Given hydrocodone/acetaminophen as prescribed an hour ago but reports 7/10 lower back pain on a 0 to 10 pain intensity scale. Pulse = 98, B/P = 164/88, which have increased since admission. No obvious blood in stool but sent to lab for occult blood testing. Waiting for lab results for CBC and BMP.

———————————————————————————————— D.L. Morgan, RNC

Highlight the findings in the note above that indicate that the client's drug therapy is not effective.

Thinking Exercise 29D-4

During her annual examination, a 75-year-old female client with a long history of osteoarthritis, rheumatoid arthritis, and diabetes mellitus type 2 reports that she is having too much pain to fall asleep most nights. The client asked the primary health care provider for zolpidem because her neighbor takes it and she has no problem sleeping. The primary health care provider prescribed tramadol ER 100 mg orally at bedtime as needed instead of the client's requested medication. The client seems very upset and asks the nurse why she could not get the drug she wanted. **Choose the *most likely* options for the information missing from the statement below by selecting from the lists of options provided.**

The nurse teaches the client that zolpidem is a commonly prescribed _____1_____ that promotes _____2_____ but does not reduce pain. Common side effects include _____3_____ and _____3_____, which could place the client at risk for injury. In addition, some people of all ages perform activities during their sleep that could be dangerous, including _____4_____. Tramadol is a(n) _____1_____ that will help promote comfort and allow the client to rest and sleep.

Options for 1	Options for 2
Selective serotonin reuptake inhibitor	Urinary elimination
NSAID	Anti-inflammation
Hypnotic	Comfort
Diuretic	Bone density
Nonopioid analgesic	Sleep
Sedative	Bowel elimination

Options for 3	Options for 4
Nausea	Sensory deprivation
Urinary retention	Nightmares
Drowsiness	Binge eating
Skin rash	Hallucinations
Dizziness	Restless legs syndrome
Constipation	Sleep driving

Thinking Exercise 29D-5

A 66-year-old male client was diagnosed with metastatic bone cancer last year and has been on a variety of opioid drugs to manage his severe pain. He is currently a resident in a long-term care setting under hospice care. Recently his opioid analgesic was changed to fentanyl 50 mcg/hr via a transdermal system, which seems to be managing his cancer pain. This morning he was transferred to the emergency department for evaluation after sustaining a fall. His admission assessment findings include the following:

Assessment Findings

Temperature = 97.6°F (36.1°C)
Pulse = 79 beats/min and regular
Blood pressure = 167/72 mm Hg
O_2 saturation = 95% (on room air)
Pain level = 8/10 (left groin and knee; no shortening or rotation; leg in alignment)
Neuro = Alert and oriented × 3
Resp = Breath sounds clear in all lung fields
CV = Pulses 2+ except for both pedal pulses at 1+

Comments

Grimacing when moved and grabbing his left hip. States that pain behind left knee is worse than groin pain.

Based on the nursing assessment findings, choose the *most likely* options for the information missing from the statement below by selecting from the list of options provided.

The nurse anticipates that the primary health care provider will prescribe a(n) _____ because the client has _____. However, he will continue to receive his fentanyl patches to help control his _____.

Options

Antihypertensive drug
Benzodiazepine
Chronic cancer pain
Chronic neuropathic pain
Acute pain
Analgesic

Exemplar 29E. Drugs That Manage Infection (Medical-Surgical Nursing [Young and Middle-Age Adult]; Pediatric Nursing)

Thinking Exercise 29E-1

An 8-year-old male client complained to his parents about right ear pain for 2 days. He has multiple allergies, for which he takes fluticasone propionate 50 mcg (1 spray per nostril) once daily. His father took him to the primary health care provider, where the child's temperature was 102.4°F (39.1°C). After an evaluation, the provider recommended symptomatic relief with ibuprofen for comfort and pseudoephedrine to decrease fluid congestion in the child's middle ear. Three days later the child's temperature increased to 104°F (40°C) and he woke up crying with severe right ear pain. The primary health care provider placed the child on amoxicillin for otitis media with a follow-up visit in 5 days. The nurse teaches the father about the child's drug therapy. Which statement(s) by the father indicates **a need for further teaching** about drug therapy for this child? **Select all that apply.**

_____ A. "Amoxicillin is a commonly prescribed penicillin drug for ear infections."

_____ B. "When his ear feels better, he can stop taking the amoxicillin."

_____ C. "I will watch for any skin rash that may occur when he takes this antibiotic."

_____ D. "I know that amoxicillin gave my child diarrhea the last time, so I'll give it with meals."

_____ E. "I will continue to give my child ibuprofen or acetaminophen for his fever."

_____ F. "I will discontinue his nose spray and decongestant while he is taking this antibiotic."

Thinking Exercise 29E-2

A 56-year-old female client with a 5-year history of diabetes mellitus type 2 visits her primary health care provider with report of an "itchy" skin rash that she has never had before. On inspection, the nurse notes that she has multiple raised reddened lesions of varying sizes located primarily on her legs and arms. The client reports that her diet has not changed and that she feels embarrassed about her skin problem. The nurse documents her current medications:

- Glipizide 5 mg orally once daily with breakfast for diabetes mellitus type 2
- Furosemide 20 mg orally once every other day for hypertension
- Lovastatin 40 mg orally once daily for high cholesterol
- Duloxetine 60 mg orally once daily for clinical depression
- Trimethoprim/sulfamethoxazole DS 1 tablet every 12 hours for acute urinary tract infection

Choose the _most likely_ options for the information missing from the statements below by selecting from the lists of options provided.

The nurse will instruct the client that she should not continue taking _____1_____ be-cause the drug likely caused the _____2_____. The nurse will instruct the client that she may not be able to continue taking _____1_____ because the drug is a _____2_____.

Options for 1	Options for 2
Glipizide	Selective serotonin reuptake inhibitor
Furosemide	Increased cholesterol
Lovastatin	Skin reaction to sulfa
Duloxetine	Sulfonylurea
Trimethoprim/sulfamethoxazole DS	Depression

Thinking Exercise 29E-3

A 33-year-old male client recently returned from international business travel and was diagnosed with active tuberculosis. His current weight is 185 lb (84 kg). The client is started on the following intensive drug regimen for at least 8 weeks:

- Isoniazid 300 mg orally once daily
- Rifampin 600 mg orally once daily
- Pyrazinamide 2 g orally once daily
- Ethambutol 1.2 g orally once daily

The nurse teaches the client about the new drug regimen. **Choose the *most likely* options for the information missing from the statements below by selecting from the lists of options provided.**

The nurse teaches the client that he needs to take ethambutol _____2_____ to prevent GI upset. The client should take the other prescribed antituberculosis drugs every day _____2_____. After the 8-week drug regimen to effectively manage the client's infection, he will likely continue taking some of these drugs for an additional _____1_____ weeks.

Options for 1	Options for 2
5	First thing in the morning
8	Mid-day
10	With meals or food
12	At bedtime
18	On an empty stomach

Thinking Exercise 29E-4

A 50-year-old female client is admitted to the hospital for a severe herpes zoster (shingles) infection and is prescribed acyclovir IV 10 mg/kg every 8 hours and gabapentin 300 mg orally every 6 hours. The client weighs 160 lb (72.6 kg). The nurse teaches the client about these medications. Which statements would the nurse include in the teaching related to drug therapy? **Select all that apply.**

_____ A. "Acyclovir works to resolve fungal infections like shingles."

_____ B. "We will be giving your acyclovir infusions quickly over 20 to 30 minutes every 8 hours."

_____ C. "We will be monitoring your kidney function while you are on acyclovir."

_____ D. "You'll need to stay in the hospital for 3 weeks because acyclovir is only given IV."

_____ E. "Gabapentin can cause sleepiness the first few times you take it."

_____ F. "You are taking gabapentin to help manage your burning nerve pain."

_____ G. "Gabapentin does not need to be taken with meals or food."

Pharmacology in Management of Complex Health Problems

Exemplar 30A. Drugs That Affect Perfusion and Gas Exchange (Medical-Surgical Nursing: Older Adult; Pediatric Nursing: Adolescent)

Thinking Exercise 30A-1

A 65-year-old female client went to the emergency department for a "sore throat," fever of 100.8°F (38.2°C), and general achiness that started 2 days ago. She also reported new-onset shortness of breath today. After an initial assessment, the client was admitted to the hospital and placed on oxygen (2 L/min via nasal cannula) and antibiotics for a streptococcal upper respiratory infection. Within the first 24 hours, her respiratory rate increased to 30 breaths/min even though her oxygen therapy was increased to 3 to 4 L/min. On the second hospital day, the client's blood pressure began to drop and her pulse rate increased. The client's urinary output was between 15 and 20 mL/hr and she was placed on a dopamine IV drip (continuous infusion) for septic shock. **Choose the *most likely* options for the information missing from the statements below by selecting from the lists of options provided.**

The nurse's primary responsibility for the client receiving dopamine will be to monitor her _____1_____ and titrate the infusion rate of the drug based on agency or primary health care provider protocol. During drug infusion, the nurse would also observe for adverse effects of dopamine including _____2_____ and _____2_____.

Options for 1	Options for 2
Oxygen saturation	Delirium
Breath sounds	Chest pain
Urinary output	Tachypnea
Level of consciousness	Dysrhythmias
Cognitive status	Hypotension

Thinking Exercise 30A-2

A 16-year-old female client has had intrinsic asthma since she was 8 years old. Currently she is receiving drug therapy required for Step 5 chronic asthma. The nurse reviews her medications with the client and family:

- Fluticasone/vilanterol dry powder inhaler (DPI) 200 mcg/25 mcg per inhalation: 1 inhalation once daily
- Formoterol DPI 12 mcg per inhalation: 1 inhalation every 12 hours
- Albuterol metered-dose inhaler (MDI) 90 mcg/inhalation: 2 inhalations every 4 to 6 hours PRN
- Atomoxetine 80 mg orally once a day

Choose the *most likely* options for the information missing from the statements below by selecting from the list of options provided.

If the client feels that she is having problems breathing, she would use _____ for quick relief. In addition to oxygen therapy, if she has a severe asthma attack, the drugs of choice would most likely include _____, _____, and _____.

Options
Fluticasone/vilanterol DPI
Theophylline
Albuterol MDI
Terbutaline
Systemic corticosteroids
Nebulized levalbuterol
Nebulized formoterol
Nebulized ipratropium

Thinking Exercise 30A-3

A 71-year-old male client was diagnosed with an ST-elevation myocardial infarction (STEMI) in the emergency department. The only drug that he was taking before his MI was tamsulosin for recently diagnosed benign prostatic hyperplasia (BPH). During transport to the ED, the client's chest pain did not respond to three doses of sublingual nitroglycerin. After the client was stable, he was admitted to the coronary care unit with the following medication orders:

- Oxygen at 6 L/min
- Nitroglycerin 5 mcg/min IV infusion
- Unfractionated heparin IV bolus of 5000 units followed by a continuous heparin infusion of 1300 units/hr for 24 hours
- Propranolol 20 mg orally every 6 hours
- Tamsulosin 0.4 orally once a day

The client's wife asks why he has to take so many drugs because he "hates to take medicine." What health teaching will the nurse include to help the client's wife understand the purpose for these medications? **Select all that apply.**

_____ A. "The oxygen therapy will supplement the air he is breathing to keep all of his major organs functioning well."

_____ B. "The nitroglycerin drip will constrict the small vessels attached to his heart so that it won't get congested."

_____ C. "The IV heparin infusion will help prevent further clotting in your husband's blood vessels."

_____ D. "Your husband will likely continue to be on an oral anticlotting drug after discharge from the hospital."

_____ E. "Propranolol will help to decrease chest pain and prevent further heart damage."

_____ F. "Your husband will likely continue to be on propranolol after discharge from the hospital."

_____ G. "Propranolol can make your husband's heart rate increase so he'll need to monitor his pulse."

Thinking Exercise 30A-4

A 71-year-old male client was diagnosed with an ST-elevation myocardial infarction (STEMI) in the emergency department (ED). The only drug that he was taking before his MI was tamsulosin for recently diagnosed benign prostatic hyperplasia (BPH). During transport to the ED, the client's chest pain did not respond to three doses of sublingual nitroglycerin. After the client was stable, he was admitted to the coronary care unit with the following medication orders:

- Oxygen at 6 L/min
- Nitroglycerin 5 mcg/min IV infusion
- Unfractionated heparin IV bolus of 5000 units followed by a continuous heparin infusion of 1300 units/hr for 24 hours
- Propranolol 20 mg orally every 6 hours
- Tamsulosin 0.4 orally once a day

Choose the *most likely* options for the information missing from the statement below by selecting from the lists of options provided.

The nurse would question the primary health care provider before administering _____ 1 _____ because it can interact with _____ 2 _____ and cause _____ 3 _____.

Options for 1	Options for 2	Options for 3
Oxygen	Propranolol	Atrial fibrillation
Nitroglycerin	Oxygen	Severe hypotension
Heparin	Nitroglycerin	Second-degree heart block
Propranolol	Tamsulosin	Ventricular tachycardia
Tamsulosin	Heparin	Pulmonary embolism

Thinking Exercise 30A-5

A 71-year-old male client was diagnosed with an ST-elevation myocardial infarction (STEMI) in the emergency department (ED). The only drug that he was taking before his MI was tamsulosin for recently diagnosed benign prostatic hyperplasia (BPH). During transport to the ED, the client's chest pain did not respond to three doses of sublingual nitroglycerin. After the client was stable, he was admitted to the coronary care unit with the following medication orders:

- Oxygen at 6 L/min
- Nitroglycerin 5 mcg/min IV infusion
- Unfractionated heparin IV bolus of 5000 units followed by a continuous heparin infusion of 1300 units/hr for 24 hours
- Propranolol 20 mg orally every 6 hours
- Tamsulosin 0.4 orally once a day

After the client's unfractionated heparin infusion was discontinued and converted to a saline lock at 11:00 a.m. (1100) on hospital day 2, the primary health care provider prescribed aspirin 325 mg orally once a day. At 12 noon (1200), the client told the nurse that he was "having trouble urinating." A bladder scan assessment showed 300 mL of retained urine. **Use an X to indicate whether the nursing actions below are <u>Indicated</u> (appropriate or necessary), <u>Contraindicated</u> (could be harmful), or <u>Non-Essential</u> (make no difference or are not necessary) for the client's care at this time.**

Nursing Action	Indicated	Contraindicated	Non-Essential
Teach the client to increase his oral fluid intake, especially water.			
Perform a urinary catheterization.			
Start an IV infusion of 1000 mL saline.			
Help the client stand to use the urinal or bathroom.			
Run water while the client is trying to void.			
Request a diuretic for the client to facilitate voiding.			
Review the client's serum electrolyte values.			

Exemplar 30B. Drugs That Affect Immunity (Medical-Surgical Nursing: Young Adult; Middle-Age Adult)

Thinking Exercise 30B-1

A 31-year-old female client was diagnosed with probable rheumatoid arthritis. After a thorough evaluation by the primary health care provider, the client was placed on hydroxychloroquine 200 mg orally once a day, methotrexate (MTX) 10 mg orally once a week, and folic acid 400 mcg orally once a day. Which health teaching related to the drug therapy will the nurse include for the client at this time? **Select all that apply.**

_____ A. "Take your new medications with food or milk."

_____ B. "Be sure to avoid large crowds in public places."

_____ C. "Be sure to have frequent eye examinations to detect any changes."

_____ D. "Avoid children and adults who have infections."

_____ E. "Follow up with all lab testing to detect any changes from baseline."

_____ F. "Take MTX the same day each week to ensure the needed serum drug level."

_____ G. "Expect to see improvement from these drugs in 3 to 6 weeks."

_____ H. "When you begin feeling better, you can discontinue the medications."

Thinking Exercise 30B-2

A 31-year-old female client was diagnosed with probable rheumatoid arthritis 3 years ago. Since that time, the client has been taking hydroxychloroquine 200 mg orally once a day, methotrexate (MTX) 10 mg orally once a week, and folic acid 400 mcg orally once a day. Today she visits her primary health care provider for her regular follow-up visit. The nurse reviews the note entered by the certified medical assistant as follows:

> **Office Progress Note**
>
> 12/20/19 1030 Client reports that she has had increasing episodes of fatigue for the past month and has noticed new inflammation in both wrists. Both wrists are reddened and swollen with right wrist worse than left wrist. Is right-handed. Has a good appetite and is able to function most days without major difficulty. Recently visited her eye doctor and no vision changes noted since she began hydroxychloroquine. Unintentionally lost 5 lb (2.3 kg) since last visit 6 months ago. Says she feels "down" and sad most days about her disease.————————————————————— M.J. Brown, CMA

Highlight the findings in the client's Office Progress Note above that would be of immediate concern to the nurse related to the effectiveness of her drug therapy.

Thinking Exercise 30B-3

A 31-year-old female client was diagnosed with probable rheumatoid arthritis 3 years ago. Since that time, the client has been taking hydroxychloroquine 200 mg orally once a day, methotrexate (MTX) 10 mg orally once a week, and folic acid 400 mcg orally once a day. As a result of a visit to her primary health care provider, the client's hydroxychloroquine was discontinued, but golimumab IV 2 mg/kg repeated at 4 weeks and then every 8 weeks for maintenance was added to her MTX regimen. The client currently weighs 163 lb (74 kg). **Choose the *most likely* options for the information missing from the statements below by selecting from the lists of options provided.**

The nurse recognizes that golimumab is a(n) _____1_____ that works to modify the _____2_____. The nurse would administer _____3_____ mg of golimumab via IV infusion for the first dose if the client does not have _____2_____.

Options for 1	Options for 2	Options for 3
Tumor necrosis factor antagonist	Immune response	52
B-lymphocyte-depleting agent	Disease flare-up	74
Interleukin-1 receptor antagonist	Organ damage	116
NSAID	Infection	148
Corticosteroid	Severe pain	163

Thinking Exercise 30B-4

A 58-year-old male client was recently diagnosed with hepatitis C genotype 4 based on laboratory results. He states that he can't understand how he got this disease because he has not had any major health problems. He admits that he was a "hippie" when he was much younger and took illicit drugs with his friends at a commune in New Mexico. Today his primary health care provider prescribed ribavirin and peginterferon alfa to manage his chronic liver infection. What health teaching will the nurse include related to his new drug therapy? **Select all that apply.**

_____ A. "Ribavirin is an antiviral agent that is administered subcutaneously once a week."

_____ B. "You will need to have frequent laboratory tests to monitor for severe anemia."

_____ C. "Be aware that flulike symptoms may occur after starting the drug but these symptoms will diminish over time."

_____ D. "Be aware that taking these drugs can cause fetal injury if you and your partner decide to become pregnant."

_____ E. "Report any feelings of depression or suicidal ideation to your primary health care provider immediately."

_____ F. "Peginterferon alfa is a short-acting drug that requires daily administration."

_____ G. "Peginterferon alfa is an antiviral agent that also modifies the immune response to effectively treat hepatitis C."

Exemplar 30C. Drugs That Manage Psychoses (Mental Health Nursing: Young Adult)

Thinking Exercise 30C-1

A 21-year-old male client was recently diagnosed with schizophrenia, for which he has was prescribed chlorpromazine, a first-generation antipsychotic (FGA) drug. After the client was on the drug for several weeks, his mother found the client in the basement having a seizure and called 911. In the emergency department, the nurse documented the following client assessment findings:

Assessment Findings

- Temperature = 104°F (40°C)
- Heart rate = 118 beats/min
- Respirations = 26 breaths/min
- Blood pressure = 174/102 mm Hg
- O_2 saturation = 91% on room air
- Muscle rigidity in all four extremities
- Drowsy at times
- States he is nauseated, but has not vomited
- Has abdominal pain 3/10 (on a 0 to 10 pain intensity scale)

Highlight the findings that are related to a major complication of FGA drug therapy and of immediate concern to the nurse and health care team.

Thinking Exercise 30C-2

A 21-year-old male client was recently diagnosed with schizophrenia, for which he has was prescribed chlorpromazine, a first-generation antipsychotic (FGA) drug. After the client was on the drug for several weeks, his mother found the client in the basement having a seizure and called 911. In the emergency department, the nurse documented the following client assessment findings including:

Assessment Findings

- Temperature = 104°F (40°C)
- Heart rate = 118 beats/min
- Respirations = 26 breaths/min
- Blood pressure = 174/102 mm Hg
- O_2 saturation = 91% on room air
- Muscle rigidity in all four extremities
- Drowsy at times
- States he is nauseated, but has not vomited
- Has abdominal pain 3/10 (on a 0 to 10 pain intensity scale)

Choose the *most likely* options for the information missing from the statements below by selecting from the lists of options provided.

Based on the nurse's assessment findings, the client mostly likely has _____1_____, a rare but potentially fatal complication of first-generation antipsychotic drugs. Management of this complication includes giving the client two major drugs: _____2_____ and _____2_____.

Options for 1	Options for 2
Hyperthermic syndrome	Risperidone
Neuroleptic malignant syndrome	Sertraline
Tardive dyskinesia	Bromocriptine
Progressive encephalopathy	Chlordiazepoxide
Peripheral neuropathy	Dantrolene

Thinking Exercise 30C-3

A 21-year-old male client was recently diagnosed with schizophrenia, for which he has was prescribed chlorpromazine, a first-generation antipsychotic (FGA) drug. The drug was discontinued as a result of the client experiencing a major complication. Two weeks later the client was started on haloperidol. He tells his mother that he is having problems holding down a job and wants to move in with her until he "can get his life together." Six weeks after starting haloperidol, the client began experiencing a variety of signs and symptoms, including constipation, resting tremors, urinary hesitancy, blurred vision, facial muscle spasms, muscle rigidity, very dry mouth, and dizziness when changing positions. **For each sign and symptom in the far-left column, use an X to indicate what drug therapy complication it may likely represent. Note that some signs and symptoms may indicate more than one of these three complications of antipsychotic drug therapy.**

Signs and Symptoms	Parkinsonism	Acute Dystonia	Anticholinergic Effects
Constipation			
Resting tremors			
Urinary hesitancy			
Blurred vision			
Facial muscle spasms			

Continued

Signs and Symptoms	Parkinsonism	Acute Dystonia	Anticholinergic Effects
Muscle rigidity			
Very dry mouth			

Thinking Exercise 30C-4

A 29-year-old male client was diagnosed 8 years ago with schizophrenia, for which he has been taking drug therapy, and has been living at home with his mother for support on disability insurance. For many years he has been taking first-generation antipsychotics (FGAs), including chlorpromazine and haloperidol. However, he developed several of the extrapyramidal symptoms (EPSs) that frequently result from long-term drug therapy. **Match each listed EPS (Column B) with the drug that may be used to manage the effects (Column C) from the drug choices provided in Column A.**

A. Drug Choice	B. Extrapyramidal Symptom (EPS)	C. Drug That May Be Used to Manage EPS
1 Propranolol	Acute dystonia	
2 Benztropine	Parkinsonism	
3 Clozapine	Akathisia	
4 Amantadine	Tardive dyskinesia	
5 Zolpidem		
6 Lorazepam		

Thinking Exercise 30C-5

A 29-year-old male client was diagnosed 8 years ago with schizophrenia, for which he has been taking drug therapy, and has been living at home with his mother for support on disability insurance. For many years he has been taking first-generation antipsychotics (FGAs), including chlorpromazine and haloperidol. However, he developed several of the extrapyramidal symptoms (EPSs) that frequently result from long-term antipsychotic therapy. Today his primary health care provider discontinued all of his medications owing to concern about major side/adverse effects and prescribed olanzapine 10 mg orally once daily. The client expresses concern that he is afraid he will experience the same EPS that he had when he took other drugs in the past. What health teaching will the nurse include for the client about olanzapine? **Select all that apply.**

_____ A. "This drug is a first-generation antipsychotic (FGA) drug that has a low risk of EPSs and other serious complications."

_____ B. "Some clients find that this drug can cause insomnia until they get used to taking it for a while."

_____ C. "Be aware that you may have urinary hesitancy, constipation, blurred vision, and very dry mouth like you did before on the other drugs."

_____ D. "You will need to have periodic laboratory testing because this drug can cause infection due to a decreased white blood cell count."

_____ E. "This drug can cause serious metabolic problems including weight gain and diabetes mellitus."

_____ F. "Be sure to eat a well-balanced diet with high fiber and adequate fluids to help reduce the onset of constipation."

_____ G. "Report depression or acute confusion to the primary health care provider immediately because the drug could be toxic to your brain."

Exemplar 30D. Drugs That Manage Emergencies (Medical-Surgical Nursing: Young Adult; Older Adult)

Thinking Exercise 30D-1

A 20-year-old female client was diagnosed with epilepsy at 13 years of age, which has been effectively controlled by valproic acid and lamotrigine. Today she is admitted to the emergency department with a diagnosis of generalized convulsive status epilepticus. **Use an X to indicate whether the nursing actions below are <u>Indicated</u> (appropriate or necessary), <u>Contraindicated</u> (could be harmful), or <u>Non-Essential</u> (make no difference or are not necessary) for the client's care at this time.**

Nursing Action	Indicated	Contraindicated	Non-Essential
Maintain the client's airway and ventilation.			
Place the client in a flat supine position.			
Establish an IV line immediately and administer a benzodiazepine such as IV lorazepam or diazepam.			
Document type and duration of each seizure.			
Monitor vital signs, especially temperature and heart rate, and cardiac rhythm.			
Draw labs to assess serum electrolyte values.			
Monitor the client's level of consciousness frequently.			

Thinking Exercise 30D-2

A 68-year-old female client has had a diagnosis of hypertension for 15 years, which has been controlled by medication and diet. This morning she awakened with a severe headache and drove herself to the emergency department. On admission, the nurse recorded her blood pressure as 210/124. The client reports a 9/10 headache that "hurts all over her head." The primary health care provider prescribes IV fenoldopam at 0.25 mcg/kg/min to begin infusion immediately. The client weighs 110 lb (50 kg). **Choose the *most likely* options for the information missing from the statements below by selecting from the lists of options provided.**

Before administering the drug, the nurse calculates that the hourly rate of the drug infusion should be _____1_____ mcg. During drug administration, the nurse monitors the client's _____2_____ , which should decrease, and _____2_____ , which may increase.

Options for 1	Options for 2
100	Heart rate
250	Oxygen saturation
500	Temperature
750	Blood pressure
1000	Respiratory rate

Thinking Exercise 30D-3

A 78-year-old male client has been diagnosed with diabetes mellitus type 2 and chronic heart failure for many years, for which he takes hydrochlorothiazide (HCTZ), digoxin, and metformin. After his wife died last year, his health declined and he was admitted to a local nursing home. For the past 6 months, he has experienced cognitive decline, most likely due to hypoxia and/or multi-infarct dementia. The nurse referred the client to the registered dietitian nutritionist because of a 10-lb (4.5-kg) weight loss in 2 weeks, anorexia, and increasing blood glucose levels. The registered dietitian nutritionist prescribed oral supplemental feedings, and his metformin dose was increased by the primary health care provider. Today the charge nurse receives the client's latest lab work as follows:

Laboratory Test Values

- Blood urea nitrogen (BUN) = 67 mg/dL (23.9 mmol/L)
- Creatinine (Cr) = 1.2 mg/dL (106.08 mmol/L)
- Fasting blood sugar (FBS) = 259 mg/dL (14.4 mmol/L)
- Sodium (Na) = 141 mEq/L (141 mmol/L)
- Potassium (K) = 4.6 mEq/L (4.6 mmol/L)
- Chloride (Cl) = 96 mEq/L (96 mmol/L)
- Calcium (Ca) = 5.0 mEq/L (50 mmol/L)
- Carbon dioxide (CO_2) = 22 mEq/L (22 mmol/L)

Highlight the findings in the client situation that are of immediate concern to the nurse.

Thinking Exercise 30D-4

A 78-year-old male client has been diagnosed with diabetes mellitus type 2 and chronic heart failure for many years, for which he takes hydrochlorothiazide (HCTZ), digoxin, and metformin. After his wife died last year, his health declined and he was admitted to a local nursing home. For the past 6 months, he has experienced cognitive decline most likely due to hypoxia and/or multi-infarct dementia. The nurse referred the client to the registered dietitian nutritionist because of a 10-lb (4.5-kg) weight loss in 2 weeks, anorexia, and increasing blood glucose levels. The dietitian prescribed oral supplemental feedings, and his metformin dose was increased by the primary health care provider. Today the charge nurse receives the client's latest lab work as follows:

Laboratory Test Values

- Blood urea nitrogen (BUN) = 67 mg/dL (23.9 mmol/L)
- Creatinine (Cr) = 1.2 mg/dL (106.08 mmol/L)
- Fasting blood sugar (FBS) = 259 mg/dL (14.4 mmol/L)
- Sodium (Na) = 141 mEq/L (141 mmol/L)
- Potassium (K) = 4.6 mEq/L (4.6 mmol/L)
- Chloride (Cl) = 96 mEq/L (96 mmol/L)
- Calcium (Ca) = 5.5 mEq/L (55 mmol/L)
- Carbon dioxide (CO_2) = 22 mEq/L (22 mmol/L)

Choose the *most likely* options for the information missing from the statement below by selecting from the lists of options provided.

Based on the physical assessment findings, medical diagnoses, and lab test values, the nurse suspects that the client most likely has _____1_____ , which requires emergency management with _____2_____ and _____2_____ .

Options for 1	Options for 2
Diabetic ketoacidosis	IV sodium lactate
Chronic kidney disease	IV dopamine
Hyperglycemic-hyperosmolar state	IV fluids
Hyperkalemia	IV magnesium sulfate
Severe hypoglycemic reaction	IV regular insulin
Respiratory acidosis	IV furosemide

CHAPTER 3 **Perfusion:** *Common Health Problems*

Answers With Rationales for Thinking Exercises

Exemplar 3A. Heart Failure (Medical-Surgical Nursing: Older Adult)

Thinking Exercise 3A-1

Answers

- Oriented to person only
- Has sinus tachycardia
- Respirations = 26 breaths/min
- Oxygen saturation = 90% (on room air)
- Breathing labored with use of accessory muscles
- Has productive cough with pink frothy sputum

Rationales

Coronary artery disease is a common risk factor for ventricular dysfunction and heart failure. Confusion or orientation to person only should alert the nurse to impaired cerebral perfusion, a complication of inadequate cardiac output. Although the client is an older adult, the nurse cannot assume that the client's impaired orientation is related to age and must complete additional assessments to identify the cause. Sinus tachycardia is a manifestation of compensation for inadequate cardiac output, infection, or other physiologic issue. The nurse must follow up on this symptom based on the client's previous cardiac disease, which increases the client's risk for hypoxemia. An increase in heart rate creates an increased demand for oxygen by the myocardium, which can lead to angina and cardiac arrest. The client's respiratory status also alerts the nurse to complications of heart failure. Tachypnea, decreased oxygen saturation, dyspnea and labored breathing, and pink frothy sputum are symptoms of pulmonary congestion. When these symptoms are present, the nurse must intervene early to prevent an acute pulmonary edema episode, which could lead to respiratory failure. Crepitus in bilateral knee joints and enlarged bony nodes on hands are manifestations of osteoarthritis, are not acute symptoms, and do not require follow-up at this time. The client's white blood count is a little high and is likely a manifestation of the client's chronic lymphocytic leukemia.

Cognitive Skill

Recognize Cues

References

Ignatavicius et al., 2018, pp. 306, 694–697, 817–820

Thinking Exercise 3A-2

Answers

Nursing Action	Potential Heart Failure Complication	Appropriate Nursing Action for Each Potential Heart Failure Complication
1 Reduce sodium intake to 1 g daily.	Acute pulmonary edema	**4** Administer furosemide 20 mg intravenous push.
2 Administer oxygen therapy.	Fatigue	**10** Consult a cardiac rehabilitation specialist.
3 Weigh the client each morning on the same scale.	Hypokalemia	**7** Administer potassium supplements.
4 Administer furosemide 20 mg intravenous push.	Cardiac dysrhythmias	**8** Monitor electrocardiogram, oxygen saturation and serum electrolyte levels.
5 Encourage the client to drink at least 3 L of fluid daily.	Hypoxemia	**2** Administer oxygen therapy.
6 Teach the client pursed-lip breathing techniques.		
7 Administer potassium supplements.		
8 Monitor electrocardiogram, oxygen saturation and serum electrolyte levels.		
9 Reposition every 2 hours while in bed.		
10 Consult a cardiac rehabilitation specialist.		

Rationales

Acute pulmonary edema is an emergent situation and requires the nurse to implement care immediately in order to prevent respiratory failure. Rapid-acting diuretics, such as furosemide, are administered via intravenous push to remove fluid from the body, specifically from the alveoli, to improve oxygenation and perfusion (Action #4). Fatigue is a common manifestation of heart failure, secondary to decreased cardiac output, impaired tissue perfusion, and anaerobic metabolism, and leads to activity intolerance. Consulting a cardiac rehabilitation specialist who can focus on balancing client activity with symptoms of exertion will help the client to begin rehabilitation activities while in the hospital (Action #10). Hypokalemia is a common side effect of diuretic treatments prescribed for clients experiencing pulmonary congestion. Monitoring serum electrolyte levels will assist the nurse in identifying hypokalemia, but the administration of potassium supplements is necessary to ensure that levels remain within normal ranges (Action #7). Irregular heart rhythms from premature atrial contractions, premature ventricular contractions, or atrial fibrillation are common in clients with heart failure. Cardiac dysrhythmias result from myocardial ischemia, pulmonary hypertension, valvular disease, sympathomimetic agents, and electrolyte imbalances, specifically hypokalemia and hypomagnesemia. The nurse would closely monitor serum electrolyte levels, oxygenation saturation, and other vital signs to identify potential causes of dysrhythmias early. The client would also have continuous electrocardiogram monitoring (Action #8). Hypoxemia is a complication of inadequate oxygen diffusion secondary to pulmonary congestion, and impaired cardiac output related to ventricular dysfunction. Providing supplemental oxygen increases the amount of oxygenated blood available to organs throughout the body. Oxygen should be administered via mask as needed to keep oxygen saturation levels greater than 90%. Repositioning the client every 2 hours while in bed improves gas exchange and prevents skin breakdown but does not address the client's oxygen needs nor the client's fatigue with ADLs (Action #2).

Cognitive Skill

Generate Solutions

References

Ignatavicius et al., 2018, pp. 676–684, 697–705

Thinking Exercise 3A-3

Answers

A, B, D, E

Rationales

Changes in weight over a short period of time indicate changes in the body's fluid volume. Clients who have heart failure are taught to weigh themselves every day to monitor for fluid changes, especially fluid retention. Clients are taught to contact the primary health care provider immediately if they experience a rapid weight gain of 3 lb in 1 week or 1 to 2 lb in 1 day, as this is a sign of recurrent heart failure (Choice A). Clients with heart failure are taught to contact the primary health care provider when experiencing cold symptoms including a cough that lasts more than 3 to 5 days. Symptoms that a client might associate with a cold may be a sign of worsening heart failure (Choice B). Clients with heart failure frequently experience dyspnea and may sometimes experience chest pain with activity and exertion. Both shortness of breath and chest pain should resolve with rest. Experiencing dyspnea or angina while at rest is a sign of heart failure exacerbation. The client must be taught to contact the primary health care provider if these symptoms occur (Choice D). Although the client may experience shortness of breath with activity, the client is encouraged to maintain independence when performing ADLs. Therefore the client's daughter should *not* be taught to perform activities for her mother. Decreasing salt intake will reduce fluid retention by the kidneys. Clients with heart failure are taught to avoid salty foods and table salt and how to read food labels for sodium content (Choice E). Heart palpitations are a complication of heart failure, and the client *should be taught* to contact the primary health care provider if this symptom occurs.

Cognitive Skill

Take Action

Reference

Ignatavicius et al., 2018, pp. 697–705

Thinking Exercise 3A-4

Answers

Assessment Finding	Effective	Ineffective	Unrelated
States she has had no shortness of breath since hospital discharge	X		
Has 2+ pitting edema in both ankles and feet		X	
Blood pressure = 134/76 mm Hg	X		
Has had no chest pain since hospital discharge	X		
Reports feeling like she has more energy now when compared with before her hospital stay	X		
Has new-onset fungal skin infection			X

Rationales

The client was admitted to the hospital with fluid overload, dyspnea, and fatigue, which are all common symptoms of heart failure. Now she reports that she has no shortness of breath and has more energy. Therefore the interventions worked to manage her disease. Her blood pressure is likely within usual parameters for her advanced age and she has no chest pain, indicating successful management of her health. However, she continues to have some fluid overload as evidenced by ankle and foot edema. Having a fungal skin infection is not related to the client's current or previous medical diagnoses.

Cognitive Skill

Evaluate Outcomes

Reference

Ignatavicius et al., 2018, pp. 697–705

Thinking Exercise 3A-5

Answers

Medication	Dose, Route, Frequency	Drug Class	Indication
aspirin	**325 mg orally once a day**	Salicylate	Prevention of platelet aggregation
atorvastatin	20 mg orally once a day	HMG-CoA reductase inhibitor	**Management of hyperlipidemia**
carvedilol	12.5 mg orally twice a day	Beta-adrenergic blocker	Management of hypertension and heart failure
ibuprofen	400 mg orally every 6-8 hr as needed	Nonsteroidal anti-inflammatory drug	**Management of extremity pain**
digoxin	0.125 mg orally once a day	Cardiac glycoside	Increase myocardial contractile force
lisinopril	2.5 mg orally once a day	**Angiotensin-converting enzyme inhibitor**	Management of heart failure

Cognitive Skill

Analyze Cues

References

Burchum & Rosenthal, 2019, pp. 485–488, 517–519, 536–541, 578–584, 853–863

Thinking Exercise 3A-6

Answers

- Blurred vision
- Sinus rhythm with preventricular contractions
- Bilateral basilar crackles
- Creatinine kinase 1200 U/L (1200 IU/L)
- Potassium 5.2 mg/dL (5.2 mmol/L)

Rationales

The client is prescribed digoxin. Signs of digoxin toxicity include anorexia, fatigue, blurred vision, and changes in mental status, especially in older adults. The nurse must complete additional assessments to determine if the client has toxic digoxin levels. The client's ejection fraction is 38%, indicating moderate heart failure. Dyspnea with exertion is a typical symptom of heart failure and would not alert the nurse. If the client reported dyspnea or chest pain at rest, the nurse would need to follow up. Irregular heart rhythm resulting from premature atrial contractions, premature ventricular contractions, or atrial fibrillation may occur in clients with heart failure and should alert the nurse to assess vital signs and serum electrolyte levels. Pulmonary crackles are a sign of pulmonary congestion and should be monitored closely. The nurse must follow up with frequent respiratory assessments and document the precise location of crackles to evaluate if fluid is progressing from the bases to higher levels in the lungs. The client's creatinine kinase and potassium levels are elevated, and the nurse must follow up on them to prevent kidney failure and cardiac arrest. Lower extremity stiffness and ambulating with crutches are postpoliomyelitis manifestations and do not need to be followed up on at this time. The client's cardiac murmur is a manifestation of aortic valve stenosis. This assessment finding would be documented, but there is no follow up needed at this time.

Cognitive Skill

Recognize Cues

References

Ignatavicius et al., 2018, pp. 694–697, 700

Thinking Exercise 3A-7

Answers

When caring for a client who has left ventricular dysfunction, the nurse assesses for confusion related to inadequate cerebral perfusion, chest pain related to inadequate myocardium perfusion, and oliguria related to inadequate renal perfusion. The nurse monitors a client who has heart failure closely for complications of pulmonary congestion when administering intravenous fluids. Manifestations of pulmonary congestion include dyspnea, crackles, and tachypnea. If the client experiences acute pulmonary edema, the nurse would place the client in a sitting position and administer supplemental oxygen and furosemide intravenous push.

Rationales

Lack of adequate perfusion due to an ineffective heart pump causes inadequate oxygen to the brain (causing confusion), heart (causing chest pain), and kidneys (causing oliguria). If the lungs become congested, the alveoli cannot function properly, causing dyspnea, crackles, and tachypnea. If pulmonary congestion progresses to acute pulmonary edema, the nurse ensures that the client is in a sitting position for gravity to help expand the thoracic cavity. Furosemide is a fast-acting diuretic that allows the kidneys to eliminate excess water from the body and alleviate pulmonary edema.

Cognitive Skill

Prioritize Hypotheses

References

Ignatavicius et al., 2018, pp. 691–695, 702–703

Exemplar 3B. Sickle Cell Disease (Pediatric Nursing: Adolescent)

Thinking Exercise 3B-1

Answers

- Reports shortness of breath, chest discomfort, fatigue, and fever for the last 3 days
- Both parents are sickle cell disease carriers, but the client has had no symptoms of the disease
- Reports feeling "lightheaded" at times
- Hemoglobin = 11.4 g/dL (114 g/L)
- Hematocrit = 36% (0.36)
- Red blood cell (RBC) count = $3.2 \times 10^6/\mu L$ ($3.2 \times 10^{12}/L$)

- White blood cell (WBC) count = 15,500/mm³ (15.5 × 10⁹/L)
- Serum bilirubin = 1.8 mg/dL (30.4 mcmol/L)
- Oral temperature = 101.6°F (38.7°C)
- Blood pressure = 98/48 mm Hg

Rationales

The client's parents are sickle cell disease (SCD) carriers, and the client's blood work shows anemia (low hemoglobin, hematocrit, RBC count). She also feels lightheaded at times, most likely because she has low blood pressure (below 100 systolic) and anemia. The client has signs and symptoms of infection as evidenced by a high WBC count and oral temperature. She also has had shortness of breath, chest discomfort, fatigue, and fever for the past 3 days, which could indicate a respiratory infection.

Cognitive Skill

Recognize Cues

Reference

Ignatavicius et al., 2018, pp. 808–813

Thinking Exercise 3B-2

Answers

Nursing Action	Indicated	Contraindicated	Non-Essential
Initiate oxygen therapy.	X		
Prepare to give several units of packed red blood cells stat.			X
Administer IV antibiotic therapy.	X		
Refer the client to a social worker to discuss end-of-life care.		X	
Withhold pain medication until she has a drug screening.		X	
Keep the head of the client's bed up to at least 30 degrees.	X		

Rationales

Clients who have pneumonia require respiratory support including leaving the head of the bed upright and oxygen therapy to help with breathing. Appropriate antibiotic therapy is required to treat the infection. The client's pain needs to be managed regardless of the client's drug usage, either legal or illicit. SCD is not a terminal disease for all clients, and the social worker should not be discussing end-of-life care. Blood transfusion is not needed at this point because the client's hemoglobin and other blood counts are not low enough to require the transfusion and it may not be effective in a client with SCD.

Cognitive Skill

Generate Solutions

References

Ignatavicius et al., 2018, pp. 601–605, 808–813

Thinking Exercise 3B-3

Answers

As a result of the client's diagnosis of sickle cell disease, the nurse is aware that she could have multiple complications including acute severe pain periods known as acute vaso-occlusive episodes. The nurse also monitors for other major SCD complications such as stroke, acute kidney injury, and sepsis.

Rationales

Acute vaso-occlusive episodes (VOEs) occur when the sickled-shaped red blood cells clump together and block blood flow to various parts of the body and major organs. As a result, severe pain and organ failure, such as acute kidney injury, occur. Strokes may occur owing to lack of blood flow to the brain (ischemic stroke) or hemorrhage (hemorrhagic stroke). Infection and sepsis are also common complications due to splenic and immune dysfunction that accompany SCD.

Cognitive Skill

Analyze Cues

Reference

Ignatavicius et al., 2018, pp. 808–813

Thinking Exercise 3B-4

Answers

A, B, D, E

Rationales

Hydroxyurea is not a cure for sickle cell disease but helps to manage events like sickle cell crises. However, the drug has several adverse effects including bone marrow suppression (Choice A), birth defects/fetal harm (Choice B), and cancer (Choice E). Clients taking this drug are also very susceptible to infection and sepsis, and therefore must avoid others with infection and public crowds (Choice D).

Cognitive Skill

Take Action

Reference

Burchum & Rosenthal, 2019, p. 1317

Thinking Exercise 3B-5

Answers

B, C, D, E, F, G, H

Rationales

The nurse would teach the client to maintain a healthy lifestyle and try to avoid stress and stressful situations. For example, engaging in low-impact, mild exercise three or four times a week (Choice D) and avoiding strenuous physical activities (Choice B) prevent stress on the body and promote health. Eating a well-rounded diet with plenty of fruits and vegetables for vitamins and minerals (Choice E) is also part of a healthy lifestyle. Avoiding tobacco and smoking, including vaping, helps prevent cancers and cardiopulmonary disease (Choice G). Avoiding temperature extremes (Choice C) and dressing appropriately for the temperature (Choice H) can help prevent stress to the body. Higher altitudes have less available environmental oxygen, which can cause the client with SCD to have difficulty breathing and a sickling and pain event (Choice F).

Cognitive Skill

Take Action

Reference

Ignatavicius et al., 2018, pp. 808–813

CHAPTER 4 Clotting: *Deep Vein Thrombosis*

Answers With Rationales for Thinking Exercises

Exemplar 4. Deep Vein Thrombosis (Medical-Surgical Nursing: Middle-Age Adult)

Thinking Exercise 4-1

Answers

- Reports pain in right calf
- Left leg is cooler than right leg
- Right lower extremity edema

Rationales

The nurse's initial assessment indicates that the client has clinical manifestations of a deep vein thrombosis (DVT). Classic signs and symptoms of a DVT include calf or groin tenderness or pain and sudden onset of unilateral swelling of the leg. Extremity redness and warmth and induration along blood vessels are additional signs of a DVT. Other clinical manifestations presented are normal for this client's medical history, the first day after bowel surgery, and bedrest for several days. The DVT findings indicate a change in the client's status, should concern the nurse, and indicate need to follow up.

Cognitive Skill

Recognize Cues

Reference

Ignatavicius et al., 2018, pp. 742–743

Thinking Exercise 4-2

Answers

Nursing Action	Indicated	Contraindicated	Non-Essential
Apply sequential compression devices to bilateral lower extremities.		X	
Teach the client to avoid foods high in vitamin K.			X
Plan to check the client's platelet count in the morning.	X		
Use ice packs and massage techniques to decrease leg swelling and pain.		X	

Nursing Action	Indicated	Contraindicated	Non-Essential
Assess for hematuria and blood in the client's stool.	X		
Place client's legs in a dependent position when sitting in a chair.		X	
Monitor the client's intake and urinary output.	X		

Rationales

Heparin-induced thrombocytopenia, a severe reduction in a client's platelet level, is a potential complication of heparin therapy. Therefore the nurse must monitor the client's platelet levels daily. Internal hemorrhage is another complication of heparin therapy. The nurse must monitor for bleeding in the gastrointestinal tract with fecal occult testing and assessing for visualization of dark and tarry stools, and the urinary tract by looking for visible or microscopic blood in the urine. The half-life of heparin is increased in clients with liver and kidney impairment because heparin undergoes hepatic metabolism and renal excretion. Closely monitoring the client's intake and urinary output as well as creatinine levels will help the nurse to identify if the client has any renal insufficiency, which could increase the client's risk for complications. For clients who have a moderate-to-high risk for a deep vein thrombosis (DVT), sequential compression devices should be administered to both lower extremities as a preventive measure. **When a client has a positive diagnosis for a DVT, the leg with the clot should not be massaged, nor should a sequential compression device be used, owing to the risk of dislodging the thrombus.** The client's legs should not be placed in a dependent position but instead should be elevated when in bed and a chair to improve venous return. Heparin activates antithrombin, which in turn inactivates thrombin and factor Xa. It has no impact on vitamin K synthesis, and therefore there is no reason for this client to avoid foods high in vitamin K.

Cognitive Skill

Generate Solutions

References

Ignatavicius et al., 2018, pp. 743–746; Burchum & Rosenthal, 2019, pp. 607–610

Thinking Exercise 4-3

Answers

Nurse's Responses	Client Questions	Appropriate Nurse's Response for Each Client Question
1 "There is an oral version of heparin called Coumadin. I will ask your provider about your request."	"My doctor said I needed to stop smoking. How does smoking have anything to do with my swollen leg?"	5 "Nicotine causes your blood vessels to constrict or narrow, which makes it easier for blood clots to become stuck in the vein."
2 "Heparin cannot be absorbed by your gastrointestinal tract. It has to be given via IV or injection to be effective."	"What can I do to help decrease the swelling in my leg?"	6 "Elevating your legs when in bed and the chair will help."
3 "The fecal occult test makes sure that you are not hemorrhaging."	"I read on the Internet that I should not move my leg because the clot will dislodge and go to my lungs. Is that true?"	8 "Increasing your activity slowly may decease your fear. Let's start with getting out of bed and then a short walk later today."

Continued

Nurse's Responses	Client Questions	Appropriate Nurse's Response for Each Client Question
4 "You have many risk factors for a DVT including smoking, oral contraceptive use, recent surgery with general anesthesia, and ongoing bedrest."	"Why are you testing my stool?"	**11** "Heparin is a blood thinner and can cause internal bleeding. This test helps us monitor for microscopic blood in your stool."
5 "Nicotine causes your blood vessels to constrict or narrow, which makes it easier for blood clots to become stuck in the vein."	"Why can't this blood thinning medication be given orally?"	**2** "Heparin cannot be absorbed by your gastrointestinal tract. It has to be given via IV or injection to be effective."
6 "Elevating your legs when in bed and the chair will help."		
7 "When a clot dislodges and moves to your lung it is called a pulmonary embolism. This is a serious complication of a deep vein thrombosis."		
8 "Increasing your activity slowly may decease your fear. Let's start with getting out of bed and then a short walk later today."		
9 "Swelling will decrease when the clot is gone, and the medication you are on will dissolve the clot."		
10 "If you have pain when I flex your foot then you should stay in bed until the swelling decreases."		
11 "Heparin is a blood thinner and can cause internal bleeding. This test helps us monitor for microscopic blood in your stool."		

Rationales

Nicotine causes vasoconstriction, which increases the client's risk for a thrombus occlusion. The nurse should take this moment to explain to the client the effects of nicotine on the cardiovascular system instead of simply stating that it is one of many risk factors (Response #5). The nurse should teach the client to elevate her legs (Response #6). Research shows that ambulation does not increase the risk for pulmonary embolus and therefore the client should be encouraged to walk. Increasing activity slowly will decrease the client's anxiety and fear about dislodging the clot (Response #8). The nurse should use nonmedical terms to explain why a fecal occult test is being done when a client is on heparin and what the test is testing (Response #11). There is not an oral version of heparin because the drug cannot be absorbed via the gastrointestinal tract owing to its polarity and large size. Warfarin is not an oral version of heparin (Response #2).

Cognitive Skill

Take Action

References

Ignatavicius et al., 2018, pp. 742–746; Burchum & Rosenthal, 2019, pp. 607–610

Thinking Exercise 4-4

Answers

When assessing a client for complications of a deep vein thrombosis, the nurse recognizes shortness of breath and chest pain as signs of pulmonary embolism, and hematuria and ecchymosis as signs of hemorrhage, which can occur as a result of heparin therapy.

Rationales

Clients who have a DVT are at high risk for the clot to dislodge and become an embolus, most often a pulmonary embolus. Because the clot travels to the lungs, respiratory symptoms such as shortness of breath and chest pain are common. Excessive bleeding (hemorrhage) can occur as an adverse effect of heparin, which is an anticoagulant. Common signs and symptoms of bleeding for which the nurse should assess include ecchymosis (bruising), gross or occult (microscopic) blood in the stool or urine (hematuria), and epistaxis (nosebleed).

Cognitive Skill

Prioritize Hypotheses

Reference

Ignatavicius et al., 2018, pp. 743–744

Thinking Exercise 4-5

Answers

A, B, C, F, H, I, K

Rationales

Choices A and B are correct statements; these actions will improve venous return and prevent chronic venous insufficiency. The client should be taught to elevate her legs when in bed and in a chair and to wear knee- or thigh-high sequential or graduated compression stockings for extended periods of time to prevent additional DVT. The client should also be taught the appropriate process for putting on and wearing compression stockings to prevent skin breakdown. Because the client is being discharged on warfarin, an anticoagulant, the nurse should teach the client about bleeding precautions including applying prolonged pressure over cuts and nosebleeds and when to seek medical attention when bleeding does not stop (Choice C). The nurse should also teach the client to monitor for signs of bleeding, which include increase in heart rate, decrease in blood pressure, black and tarry stools, and mental confusion (Choices I and K). Dizziness when changing positions may occur if the client is bleeding, and the client may still experience pain in the extremity; therefore the nurse should teach the client to rise slowly, increase activity as tolerated, and rest when needed (Choice F). The client also needs to follow up with a Coumadin (Warfarin) clinic for ongoing monitoring and adjustment of dose for a therapeutic effect, INR between 1.5 and 2.0 or higher as the primary health care provider prescribes (Choice H). The client should be taught to avoid foods high in vitamin K, to avoid medications that increase the client's risk of bleeding such as NSAIDs, and to take a missed dose of warfarin as soon as the client remembers the dose was missed. The client should never take two doses at one time, as this would greatly increase the client's risk of internal hemorrhage.

Cognitive Skill

Take Action

References

Ignatavicius et al., 2018, pp. 743–746; Burchum & Rosenthal, 2019, pp. 612–616

CHAPTER 5 Gas Exchange: *Common Health Problems*

Answers With Rationales for Thinking Exercises

Exemplar 5A. Asthma (Pediatric Nursing: School-Age Child)

Thinking Exercise 5A-1

Answers

- Child had shortness of breath during a soccer game
- Respirations = 32 breaths/min
- Oxygen saturation = 89% (on room air)
- Born at 30 weeks' gestation
- History of asthma
- Child is restless and refuses to lie down in bed
- Wheezing in both lungs
- Minimal air movement noted in lower lobes bilaterally
- Child only nods head "yes" or "no" to questions
- Peak flow meter results are <50% of child's baseline
- Moderate intercostal retractions

Rationales

An elevated respiratory rate, the child's restlessness and refusal to lie down, decreased air movement in the lungs, low oxygen saturation, retractions, and the inability to answer questions beyond nodding his head are all signs of impending respiratory failure and should be addressed by the nurse emergently. The fact that the child was born prematurely and has a history of asthma also indicate an increased risk of more severe exacerbations or adverse outcomes. Peak flow meter readings far below baseline are strongly indicative of asthma exacerbation that requires immediate intervention. Treatment of the child can still take place whether or not the trigger is known. A low-grade fever is to be expected and is not the priority.

Cognitive Skill

Recognize Cues

Reference

Hockenberry & Wilson, 2019, pp. 883–944

Thinking Exercise 5A-2

Answers

Nursing Action	Emergent	Not Emergent
Place nasal cannula to provide humidified oxygen in response to rescue treatment.		X
Administer methylprednisolone per the primary health care provider's prescription.	X	
Titrate oxygen to keep oxygen saturation >90%.	X	
Teach the child to use pursed-lip breathing technique.		X

Nursing Action	Emergent	Not Emergent
Administer albuterol per hospital protocol.	X	
Allow child to assume the most comfortable upright position.	X	
Insert a peripheral intravenous line.	X	
Enter the primary health care provider's NPO order into the electronic health record.		X
Encourage the family to change the child's clothing to promote comfort.		X

Rationales

Nursing Action	Rationale
Place nasal cannula to provide humidified oxygen in response to rescue treatment.	The child needs oxygen delivered in the least invasive, but most effective manner. Because the nurse notes that the child is a mouth breather, using a nasal cannula will not be as effective as a simple mask.
Administer methylprednisolone per the primary health care provider's prescription.	Resolving the child's respiratory distress caused by inflammation within the bronchioles requires a multimodal approach to treatment, including oxygen, beta$_2$ agonists, corticosteroids (either IV or oral) to decrease systemic inflammation, and IV fluids.
Titrate oxygen to keep oxygen saturation >90%.	The child needs oxygen delivered in the least invasive but most effective manner to maintain oxygenation saturation >90% in order to relieve anxiety and shortness of breath and to provide adequate oxygenation to vital organs.
Teach child to use a pursed-lip breathing technique.	Although this is a useful strategy for the child to use in the earliest stages of an acute asthma attack to ease anxiety and improve oxygenation, it is not as helpful to treat a moderate or severe attack, especially if the child has never used the technique.
Administer albuterol per hospital protocol.	Beta$_2$ agonists bind to smooth muscles of the airway to promote relaxation and decrease bronchospasms.
Allow the child to assume the most comfortable upright position.	Allowing the pediatric client to select his or her preferred upright position is critical in order to address the child's anxiety, which can cause escalation of respiratory distress if not handled appropriately.
Insert a peripheral intravenous line.	Emergent IV access allows administration of medications and fluids to promote adequate tissue hydration and resolve any acidosis.
Enter the primary health care provider's NPO order into the electronic health record.	The child in acute respiratory distress requires frequent or constant monitoring of the respiratory status until the child improves; adjusting the diet in the electronic medical record is not an emergent action for the nurse.
Encourage the family to change the child's clothing to promote comfort.	Although this activity might have a calming effect on the child, it is not emergent and can wait until the initial treatment is effective and the respiratory status has improved.

Cognitive Skill

Generate Solutions

References

Hockenberry & Wilson, 2019, pp. 927–944; Burchum & Rosenthal, 2019, p. 156

Thinking Exercise 5A-3

Answers

Assessment Finding	Effective	Ineffective	Unrelated
Oxygen saturation = 94%	X		
Child playing quietly on electronic device	X		
Heart rate = 121 beats/min		X	
Respirations = 26 breaths/min	X		
Blood pressure = 118/66 mm Hg			X
Temperature = 100.4°F (38.0°C)			X
Intermittent wheezing in lower lobes bilaterally	X		

Rationales

Data suggest that the initial stabilization of the child's respiratory status include an oxygen saturation greater than 90% with or without oxygen, a normalization or reduction of the respiratory rate, and improved lung aeration. The child's ability to play indicates that he is experiencing less shortness of breath, and therefore gas exchange is improving. Changes in the blood pressure or temperature are not relevant to evaluating the respiratory status. The increase in heart rate may be a compensatory mechanism related to decreased gas exchange, or it may be a side effect of albuterol administration.

Cognitive Skill

Evaluate Outcomes

Reference

Hockenberry & Wilson, 2019, pp. 939–940

Thinking Exercise 5A-4

Answers

Medication	Dose, Route, Frequency	Drug Action	Health Teaching
Methylprednisolone	0.5–1 mg/kg/dose IV every 6 hr	Reverses airflow obstruction by decreasing inflammation	**Do not schedule vaccines when your child is taking corticosteroids.**
Albuterol	0.025 mcg/kg/dose via nebulizer every 4 hr and every 2 hr PRN	**Reduces wheezing by dilating smooth muscles of the airways**	Monitor your child for increased heart rate and jitteriness.
Montelukast sodium	**5-mg chewable tablet once daily**	Reduces inflammation and bronchoconstriction	The drug is for long-term treatment, not for acute exacerbations; be aware that it can cause depression and suicidal thinking and behavior.
Acetaminophen	10 mg/kg/dose orally every 4–6 hr as needed for pain or temperature >101°F (38.2°C)	Decreases pain and fever	Do not exceed 75 mg/kg/day to prevent liver damage.

Cognitive Skill

Analyze Cues

References

Burchum & Rosenthal, 2019, pp. 149–150, 922–924, 931, 939; Hockenberry & Wilson, 2019, pp. 935–940

Thinking Exercise 5A-5

Answers

A, B, C, D, F

Rationales

Prevention or early identification of an impending asthma attack or exacerbation allows for preventive measures to avert the attack (Choices A and B). Triggers should be avoided, and a cough or poor sleep is often an early indicator of bronchospasm. The nurse would review home medications to prevent future asthma attacks (Choice C). Encouraging a calm environment helps to minimize air hunger and anxiety (Choice D). Currently there is no way to know for sure whether the child will outgrow his asthma symptoms or if it will be a chronic problem (Choice E). The need to continue with peak flow meter measurements should be part of the health teaching before discharge (Choice F).

Cognitive Skill

Take Action

Reference

Hockenberry & Wilson, 2019, pp. 940–944

Exemplar 5B. Chronic Obstructive Pulmonary Disease (Medical-Surgical Nursing: Middle-Age Adult)

Thinking Exercise 5B-1

Answers

Medication	Dose, Route, Frequency	Drug Class	Drug Action
Guaifenesin	200 mg orally every 4 hr	Mucolytic agent	**Reduces chest congestion**
Tiotropium	18 mcg as a dry powder inhalant once daily	Anticholinergic drug	**Maintains relief of bronchospasm**
Montelukast sodium	10-mg tablet orally once daily	**Leukotriene modifier**	Reduces bronchoconstriction and inflammation
Fluticasone propionate	100 mcg via inhalant twice daily	**Glucocorticoid**	Decreases inflammation
Albuterol	**2 puffs as an inhalation PRN every 4–6 hr**	Beta$_2$-adrenergic agonist	Reduces bronchoconstriction
Omeprazole	40 mg orally once daily	Proton pump inhibitor	Reduces acid reflux

Cognitive Skill

Analyze Cues

References

Burchum & Rosenthal, 2019, pp. 149–150, 922–924, 931, 939, 963–965

Thinking Exercise 5B-2

Answers

- Labored breathing
- Oxygen saturation = 88% (on room air)
- Leaning forward with hands on upper thighs
- Respirations = 26 breaths/min

Rationales

Based on the client's health history, the nurse would be on alert for clinical manifestations of COPD and would follow up on symptoms associated with an exacerbation of this disorder. Rapid shallow respirations, use of accessory muscles and orthopneic positioning are cues that the client is having trouble breathing. A client experiencing labored breathing for extended periods of time will become fatigued and oxygenation saturations will decrease, leading to hypoxemia. All of these are signs of an exacerbation of COPD. All the other assessment findings are normal including the client's arterial blood gas values. The nurse must assess for future acid-base imbalances if the client's breathing status does not improve.

Cognitive Skill

Recognize Cues

Reference

Ignatavicius et al., 2018, pp. 574–576

Thinking Exercise 5B-3

Answers

A, C, E, F, I

Rationales

Noticing that the client is breathless while sitting in a chair answering questions leads the nurse to assess the degree to which the client's dyspnea affects daily activities. Choices A and C assist the nurse in collecting information about the client's activity intolerance, and choice E supports the nurse in evaluating if the client experiences difficulty sleeping or orthopnea. Noticing that the client has a BMI of 17.6 leads the nurse to evaluate why the client is underweight. Choices F and I help the nurse to understand if weight loss occurred, whether or not it was planned, and what the client usually eats each day. Unplanned weight loss frequently occurs as the severity of COPD increases because the work of breathing increases metabolic needs and clients may experience dyspnea during meals that limits the amount of nutrition eaten.

Cognitive Skill

Analyze Cues

References

Ignatavicius et al., 2018, pp. 574–576, 1196

Thinking Exercise 5B-4

Answers

Nursing Action	Potential Complication	Appropriate Nursing Action for Each Complication
1 Teach pursed-lip breathing technique.	Respiratory infection	**12** Teach the client to drink at least 2 L of fluid daily.
2 Administer oxygen therapy.	Dysrhythmias	**5** Evaluate laboratory results for acid-base and electrolyte imbalances.
3 Assist the client with ADLs.	Activity intolerance	**7** Encourage paced self-care with periods of rest.
4 Provide five small meals each day.	Oral candidiasis	**9** Ask the client to rinse her mouth after administering corticosteroid inhalants.
5 Evaluate laboratory results for acid-base and electrolyte imbalances.	Hypoxemia	**2** Administer oxygen therapy.
6 Teach the client to swish and spit mouthwash three times a day.	Malnutrition	**4** Provide five small meals each day.
7 Encourage paced self-care with periods of rest.	Anxiety	**14** Help the client develop a plan for what she should do when symptoms occur.
8 Implement continued electrocardiographic monitoring.		
9 Ask the client to rinse her mouth after administering corticosteroid inhalants.		
10 Turn off the lights and ask the client to take slow, deep breaths.		
11 Provide protein shake after each meal.		
12 Teach the client to drink at least 2 L of fluid daily.		
13 Weigh the client each morning on the same scale.		
14 Help the client develop a plan for what she should do when symptoms occur.		

Rationales

Hypoxemia is a low level of oxygenation in the blood. Reduced gas exchange places a client who has COPD at risk for hypoxemia. Administering oxygen therapy (Action #2) to the client will improve the amount of oxygen exchanged with each breath and help prevent hypoxemia from occurring. Clients with COPD are at increased risk for respiratory infections due to pulmonary inflammation inducing thick and sticky mucus, which results in more bronchospasm. Hydration (Action #12) helps thin secretions so that the client can expectorate them. Dysrhythmias are common in clients with COPD and result from hypoxemia, acidosis, and electrolyte imbalances. Monitoring a client's cardiac rhythm (Action #8) will alert the nurse when a dysrhythmia occurs, but it will not prevent the dysrhythmia. Evaluating laboratory results for acid-base and electrolyte imbalances (Action #5) will provide the nurse with an opportunity to correct imbalances prior to the occurrence of dysrhythmias. Activity intolerance occurs because of respiratory fatigue and dyspnea. Encouraging independence with ADLs and teaching the client to rest periodically (Action #7) will help her to increase respiratory muscle strength, endurance, and activity tolerance. Malnutrition is a consequence of activity intolerance and increased metabolic needs. Although the client would be encouraged to eat high-calorie, high-protein foods including supplements, protein shakes after each meal (Action #11) would not lead to greater ingestion of nutrition. Providing four to six small meals throughout the day (Action #4) will provide opportunities for the client to eat more and rest between meals. Oral candidiasis is a side effect of corticosteroid inhalants. Rinsing the client's mouth after administering this medication (Action #9) limits the medication's ability to destroy normal flora, which is the body's natural defense again *Candida*. Clients with COPD become anxious during acute dyspneic episodes. Teaching the client what to do when symptoms begin and assisting the client in developing a writing action plan (Action #14) will help the client maintain control over the episode and decrease the client's anxiety.

Cognitive Skill

Take Action

Reference

Ignatavicius et al., 2018, pp. 573–581

Thinking Exercise 5B-5

Answers

Chronic obstructive pulmonary disease interferes with airflow and gas exchange leading to increased carbon dioxide levels, sputum production, and pulmonary pressure. These physiologic changes increase the client's risk for pulmonary infections, hypoxemia, and right-sided heart failure.

Rationales

In clients who have COPD, the client's alveoli become inflated, preventing an adequate amount of oxygen to diffuse into the bloodstream (hypoxemia) and preventing carbon dioxide as a waste product of cellular metabolism to be removed. As a result, serum carbon dioxide levels increase, leading to respiratory acidosis. Inflated alveoli also tend to collect mucus, which increases sputum production and makes the client susceptible to respiratory infection. Pressure within the cardiopulmonary system can lead in end-stage COPD to right-sided heart failure, also called *cor pulmonale*.

Cognitive Skill

Prioritize Hypotheses

Reference

Ignatavicius et al., 2018, pp. 573–574

Thinking Exercise 5B-6

Answers

Nursing Action	Indicated	Contraindicated	Non-Essential
Obtain sputum samples for culture and sensitivity.	X		
Administer humidified oxygen via Venturi mask.	X		
Provide the client with smoking cessation education.			X
Type and cross for blood products.			X

Nursing Action	Indicated	Contraindicated	Non-Essential
Perform pulmonary function tests after administrating bronchodilator.	X		
Administer 20 mEq oral potassium chloride.		X	
Administer albuterol nebulizer 15 minutes before each meal.	X		
Implement vibratory positive expiratory pressure therapy.	X		
Place the client on a 1200-mL fluid restriction.		X	

Rationales

Actions that are indicated focus on obtaining pertinent clinical information to make clinical judgments or interventions to ensure client safety and prevention of complications. Sending a sputum sample for culture and sensitivity will support the advance practice provider in prescribing appropriate anti-infective therapy, and performing pulmonary function tests before and after administering the client's bronchodilator assists the nurse and provider in judging whether treatments are effective. The client has thick, tenacious secretions that interfere with gas exchange and can cause airway obstruction. Administering humidified oxygen and vibratory positive expiratory pressure therapy thins mucous secretions and assists the client to expectorate unwanted mucus. The client should also be encouraged to drink 2 L of water daily to assist with the removal of thick, tenacious secretions. Oxygen administration is necessary to prevent or reverse hypoxemia. This client's current Pao_2 is 60 mm Hg and his oxygenation saturation is 84%. Oxygen up to 40% via Venturi mask may be necessary to maintain ideal oxygen saturations between 88% and 92%. The client's serum potassium level is normal, and administration of oral potassium chloride would be contraindicated at this time. The client has already quit smoking and has normal hemoglobin and hematocrit levels; therefore smoking cessation education and a type and cross for blood products are not essential.

Cognitive Skill

Generate Solutions

Reference

Ignatavicius et al., 2018, pp. 577–581

Thinking Exercise 5B-7

Answers

B, C, F, H

Rationales

This client's teaching focuses on self-care and management of his chronic pulmonary disorder. Chronic obstructive pulmonary disease is associated with activity fatigue and dyspnea; therefore the nurse teaches the client to build physical and respiratory endurance by walking daily for 20 minutes with periods of rest as necessary (Choice B). The nurse would also teach the client energy conservation strategies. Clients often experience orthopnea and anxiety related to dyspnea. The nurse encourages the client to sleep wherever he is comfortable, indicating that it is okay to be more relaxed in a chair or with multiple pillows supporting his back (Choice C). This helps the client sleep better and may reduce anxiety. Finally, the nurse teaches safety techniques related to prescribed medications. Fluticasone propionate is a corticosteroid, and gargling with water is necessary to minimize complications related to candidiasis (Choice F). Albuterol may be prescribed as a rescue inhaler, and the client must understand that waiting 1 minute between doses will ensure he obtains the greatest therapeutic effect (Choice H).

Cognitive Skill

Take Action

Reference

Ignatavicius et al., 2018, pp. 577–581

CHAPTER 6   Elimination: *Benign Prostatic Hyperplasia*

Answers With Rationales for Thinking Exercises

Exemplar 6. Benign Prostatic Hyperplasia (Medical-Surgical Nursing: Older Adult)

Thinking Exercise 6-1

Answers

Nursing Action	Indicated	Contraindicated	Non-Essential
Confirm that the client has a signed informed consent for the bladder sonography.			X
Refrigerate the urinalysis sample if it cannot be sent to the laboratory immediately.	X		
Ensure the client understands that a transducer will be inserted into his rectum to view the prostate and surrounding structures.	X		
Insert an indwelling urinary catheter to obtain a urine culture specimen.		X	
Ask the client to urinate prior to performing the bladder ultrasound.	X		
Collect the client's urine for a 24-hour period.			X

Rationales

Urine specimens become more alkaline when left at room temperature for more than an hour. If the sample cannot be sent to the laboratory immediately, the nurse must refrigerate it or the specimen will not provide accurate results. Urine culture specimens obtained from a clean-catch or urinary catheter are best. If the client cannot provide a clean-catch specimen, the nurse may insert a straight-catheter or in-and-out urinary catheter to obtain the sample. The nurse would not insert an indwelling urinary catheter with a urinary drainage system, which is designed to remain in the bladder for a period of time. Indwelling urinary catheters increase the client's risk for an infection and should not be used solely to obtain a urine specimen. A 24-hour urine collection is used to analyze urine levels of specific substances including creatinine, sodium, chloride, and catecholamine. A basic urinalysis requires only one sample and the best specimen is collected at the morning's first void. The primary health care provider prescribed a serum creatinine level, not a urine creatinine clearance test; therefore the 24-hour urine collection is not essential. Bladder sonography is used to measure residual urine in the bladder after the client voids, and therefore the client must urinate prior to the procedure. The bladder ultrasound is completed at the bedside by the nurse or an ultrasound technician. Informed consent is not needed for the procedure. The transrectal ultrasound is generally performed in the interventional radiology department and provides ultrasound images of the prostate and surrounding tissues via a transducer that is inserted into the rectum. The nurse would ensure that the client understands the procedure before it begins.

Cognitive Skill

Generate Solutions

References

Ignatavicius et al., 2018, pp. 1333, 1335–1337, 1476–1477

Thinking Exercise 6-2

Answers

B, C, E, F

Rationales

Terazosin is an alpha$_1$ blocker. Although it is a selective alpha blocker, the medication can cause orthostatic hypotension, tachycardia, and syncope, especially in older male clients. The client should be instructed to rise slowly to minimize hypotensive episodes and falls (Choice B). Nonsurgical interventions for clients with benign prostatic hyperplasia include decreasing urinary retention and preventing overdistention of the bladder. The client would be taught to avoid beverages that contain alcohol and caffeine as these increase diuresis, leading to more fluid in the bladder (Choice E). The client would also be encouraged to void as soon as he feels the urge to prevent bladder retention (Choice C). Anticholinergic and antihistamine medications can also increase urinary retention, so the client must follow up with his primary health care provider for these medications to be re-evaluated (Choice F).

Cognitive Skill

Take Action

References

Ignatavicius et al., 2018, pp. 1477–1479; Burchum & Rosenthal, 2019, pp. 162–163

Thinking Exercise 6-3

Answers

- Disoriented to place, time, and situation
- Temperature = 101.4°F (38.5°C)
- Reports lower back pain
- Reports needing to urinate multiple times each hour
- Urine output is less than 20 mL/hr
- Bladder ultrasound indicates 800 mL fluid in bladder

Rationales

The client's acute disorientation to place, time, and situation must be followed up, and the nurse would assess for potential neurologic events and cardiac dysrhythmias. The nurse would notice that the client is oriented to self and moves all extremities equally, eliminating key symptoms of a cerebral vascular accident. The nurse would also notice the client's heart rate is slightly elevated, most likely because of his pain; his blood pressure is within normal limits; and his oxygenation at 92% on room air is appropriate with his history of chronic obstructive pulmonary disease (COPD). These findings are within normal limits for a client who has COPD and do not need the nurse to follow up. The client's fever and report of dysuria would alert the nurse to a potential urinary tract infection, which in older adults often manifests with acute mental confusion. The nurse would therefore follow up and complete a more thorough investigation of the urinary tract and renal system. Although the client has a diagnosis of benign prostatic hyperplasia, his report of needing to void multiple times an hour and only urinating less than 20 mL each hour are manifestations of urinary retention. Lower back pain in addition to the urinary retention confirmed by bladder sonography and signs and symptoms of a urinary tract infection may indicate pyelonephritis (kidney infection). The nurse must take action to prevent acute kidney injury.

Cognitive Skill

Recognize Cues

References

Ignatavicius et al., 2018, pp. 1357–1359, 1372–1374, 1474–1477

Thinking Exercise 6-4

Answers

Nursing Action	Potential Postoperative Complication	Appropriate Nursing Action for Each Postoperative Complication
1 Maintain the rate of continuous bladder irrigation to keep the urine clear.	Urinary catheter obstruction	**5** Assess the three-way urinary catheter for kinks and blood clots.
2 Subtract the amount of irrigating solution that was instilled to determine actual urinary output.	Bladder spasm	**8** Keep the three-way urinary catheter attached to the client's thigh and encourage the client to relax his bladder muscles.
3 Discontinue the urinary catheter within 24 hours of the procedure.	Immobility	**6** Help the client to get out of bed, ambulate, and sit in a chair as soon as permitted after surgery.
4 Ask the client to contract his bladder muscle and attempt to void.	Urine blood clots	**1** Maintain the rate of continuous bladder irrigation to keep the urine clear.
5 Assess the three-way urinary catheter for kinks and blood clots.	Pain	**7** Assess for pain every 2 hours and administer pain mediation as needed.
6 Help the client to get out of bed, ambulate, and sit in a chair as soon as permitted after surgery.		
7 Assess for pain every 2 hours and administer pain mediation as needed.		
8 Keep the three-way urinary catheter attached to the client's thigh and encourage the client to relax his bladder muscles.		
9 Perform passive range-of-motion activities while client is in bed.		
10 Teach the client's wife to use the patient-controlled analgesia pump.		

Rationales

During the transurethral resection of the prostate surgery, a three-way urinary catheter is placed to provide irrigation of the bladder and drainage of urine. Clients may have the catheter in place with continuous bladder irrigation for several days after surgery to prevent urinary obstruction. When bleeding occurs in the bladder, it manifests as blood clots or red, ketchup-looking urine. The nurse must titrate the flow of the bladder irrigating solution to keep the urine clear and free of blood clots (Action #1). The urine catheter may put pressure on the bladder, causing the sensation of needing to void. Contracting bladder muscles and attempting to urinate around the catheter may cause bladder spasms. The nurse would keep the catheter secured to the client's thigh to minimize bladder pressure and irritation and encourage the client to relax his bladder muscles (Action #8). Clients, especially older adults, should be helped out of bed and assisted in performing active range-of-motion activities to decrease immobility complications after surgery (Action #6). Catheter kinks and blood clots can cause urinary catheter obstructions and should be monitored closely (Action #5). The client may experience pain after a transurethral resection of the prostate. The nurse would assess for pain every 2 to 4 hours and administer prescribed pain medications as needed (Action #7). If patient-controlled analgesia is prescribed, the nurse would teach the client how to use it, not his wife.

Cognitive Skill

Generate Solutions

Reference

Ignatavicius et al., 2018, pp. 1479–1481

Thinking Exercise 6-5

Answers

A, C, F, G

Rationales

Bright red or ketchup-like urinary drainage with numerous clots is a sign of arterial bleeding and is a medical emergency. The nurse would notify the surgeon immediately (Choice F) and manually irrigate the urinary catheter with normal saline solution until the drainage is light reddish-pink to clear (Choice A). The nurse would then restart the bladder irrigating solution at a higher rate and titrate to keep the urine clear and free of clots (Choice C). Since the client is actively bleeding, the nurse would also monitor vital signs, neurologic status, and lab results, specifically hemoglobin and hematocrit levels (Choice G). The surgeon may prescribe aminocaproic acid to control bleeding, or surgery may be needed if medical interventions are unable to clear the bladder of clots and stop the bleeding.

Cognitive Skill

Take Action

Reference

Ignatavicius et al., 2018, pp. 1479–1481

Thinking Exercise 6-6

Answers

Client's Statement	Effective	Ineffective	Unrelated
"I may still experience overflow incontinence due to ongoing urinary retention."		X	
"I will follow up with my primary health care provider if I experience erectile dysfunction."	X		
"I will drink at least 2000 mL of water daily to keep hydrated and my urine color clear."	X		
"Kegel exercises can only be performed by women and will not help me strengthen my sphincter muscle."		X	
"I may have temporary dribbling of urine and will wear an incontinence pad until I am confident that this has resolved."	X		
"I plan to walk for 30 minutes each day and rest if I experience pain or shortness of breath."			X

Rationales

Urinary retention and overflow incontinence are experienced by clients who have benign prostatic hyperplasia, but these symptoms should not continue after the client is treated with drug therapy and/or surgery. This client with no history of kidney or heart disease would be advised to drink 2000 to 2500 mL daily to decrease dysuria and keep the urine clear. He would also be instructed to perform Kegel exercises or frequent contraction and relaxation of his sphincter to re-establish urinary elimination control. Clients who undergo a transurethral resection of the prostate may experience temporary loss of control of urination or a dribbling of urine. The nurse would explain that these symptoms are temporary and encourage the client to wear an incontinence pad to keep his clothing dry. Sexual function should not be affected by surgery, but the client would be taught to contact his primary health care provider if he experiences erectile dysfunction. Exercising daily is healthy behavior but is not related to the recent hospitalization and surgery.

Cognitive Skill

Evaluate Outcomes

Reference

Ignatavicius et al., 2018, pp. 1479–1481

CHAPTER 7 Nutrition: *Common Health Problems*

Answers With Rationales for Thinking Exercises

Exemplar 7A. Cholecystitis/Cholecystectomy (Medical-Surgical Nursing: Middle-Age Adult)

Thinking Exercise 7A-1

Answers

Nursing Action	Indicated	Contraindicated	Non-Essential
Request a high-fiber, low-fat lunch tray from dietary services.		X	
Insert an intravenous catheter and initiate a normal saline infusion.	X		
Administer morphine 2 mg intravenously as needed to manage pain.	X		
Obtain blood and urine cultures for bacterial and viral testing.			X
Administer metformin 500 mg orally.		X	

Rationales

The client has been diagnosed with acute cholecystitis, but a treatment plan has not been determined. Additional testing including magnetic resonance cholangiopancreatography and/or hepatobiliary iminodiacetic acid (HIDA) scan may be completed. Treatment options include drug therapy, insertion of a biliary drain, or surgery. The nurse needs to anticipate potential diagnostic procedures and treatment plans so that there will be no delay in care. The nurse would not provide a lunch tray to the client because many of the procedures including the prescribed HIDA scan require the client to have nothing by mouth prior to the procedure. To ensure the client remains hydrated, the nurse would insert an intravenous catheter and initiate isotonic fluids. The nurse would also hold the client's metformin dose since the client is not eating and may be prescribed magnetic resonance cholangiopancreatography, which requires the administration of oral or intravenous contrast. Although clients who have diabetes mellitus often present with atypical symptoms of cholecystitis, the nurse would still manage the client's abdominal pain with opioid analgesia. The client's white blood count is elevated due to inflammation of the gallbladder. There is no indication of systemic or urinary infection and therefore blood and urine cultures are not essential.

Cognitive Skill

Generate Solutions

References

Ignatavicius et al., 2018, pp. 1192–1195, 1291–1292; Burchum & Rosenthal, 2019, pp. 276–281, 692–695

Thinking Exercise 7A-2

Answers

Nurse's Responses	Client Questions	Appropriate Nurse's Response for Each Client Question
1 "During surgery you will not be able to move. This device stimulates muscle contraction so that your legs do not become swollen."	"The surgeon said that he's removing my gallbladder. Will this surgery leave a large scar on my belly?"	**11** "It is a minimally invasive procedure requiring a couple of small incisions. I will ask the surgeon to speak with you again."
2 "A small midline incision at your umbilicus will be the one incision. This incision should not scar."	"The nursing assistant provided this machine that massages my legs. What is it for?"	**7** "That is an external pneumatic compression device that keeps blood from pooling in your legs during and after surgery."
3 "You have several other risk factors. You are taking simvastatin for your high cholesterol and orlistat to lose weight. Have you lost a lot of weight recently?"	"Will I need to be on a special diet after my gallbladder is removed?"	**4** "You will want to decrease or avoid fatty and fried foods."
4 "You will want to decrease or avoid fatty and fried foods."	"I have non–insulin dependent diabetes. Why are you giving me insulin?"	**9** "We can control your blood sugar levels more closely with insulin while you are taking nothing by mouth."
5 "The surgeon will attempt to remove your gallbladder through your belly button. If there are complications, then the surgeon will have to open your entire abdomen."	"I looked up cholecystitis on the internet, and it said I'm at risk because I'm female, 40, and fat. That sounds like every women I know. Why me?"	**3** "You have several other risk factors. You are taking simvastatin for your high cholesterol and orlistat to lose weight. Have you lost a lot of weight recently?"
6 "The metformin you used to take was not controlling your blood sugar levels. Therefore the primary health care provider prescribed insulin."		
7 "That is an external pneumatic compression device that keeps blood from pooling in your legs during and after surgery."		
8 "A diet high in protein will help you heal after surgery."		
9 "We can control your blood sugar levels more closely with insulin while you are taking nothing by mouth."		
10 "Diabetes mellitus also puts you at risk. Have your blood sugar levels been controlled appropriately?"		
11 "It is a minimally invasive procedure requiring a couple of small incisions. I will ask the surgeon to speak with you again."		
12 "When clients with diabetes mellitus type 2 are sick, they become insulin dependent."		
13 "You should follow a diabetic diet. I will consult a nutritionist to explain what that is."		
14 "I can understand why you are questioning this. Would you like to speak with a chaplain?"		

Rationales

It is the responsibility of the nurse to clarify facts that have been presented by the surgeon and to verify that an informed consent form is signed by the client. It is not the nurse's responsibility to provide detailed information about the surgical procedure. If the nurse believes that the client has not been adequately informed, the nurse must contact the surgeon and request that further clarification be provided. The client's question about a large scar indicates that she does not understand that the procedure will be laparoscopic and therefore the surgeon needs to speak with the client again (Action #11). External pneumatic or sequential compression devices are used to promote venous return and prevent deep vein thrombosis while the client is immobile because of surgery or bed rest. Explaining that the devices prevent blood from pooling in the lower extremities is correct. They do not keep the legs from becoming sore or swollen (Action #7). A client who has cholecystitis would be taught to follow a low-fat diet and decrease or avoid fried foods as well as "fast" foods (Action #4). Because this client also has diabetes mellitus type 2, the nurse would reinforce teaching related to a diabetic diet and may encourage protein to help with incisional healing, but neither of these responses appropriately answers the client's question. The client's metformin dose would be held prior to the surgical procedure owing to risks of lactic acidosis and acute kidney injury. The client would also be receiving nothing by mouth (NPO). The client's blood glucose levels should be monitored closely and a basal insulin dosage administered to maintain a baseline glucose level (Action #9). The nurse should help the client to understand that she has major risk factors for cholecystitis beyond her gender, age, and weight. Understanding all of her risk factors will assist her in coping with the disorder. Although diabetes mellitus is a risk factor, the nurse does not have adequate data indicating that the client's blood glucose levels have not been controlled appropriately (Action #3).

Cognitive Skill

Generate Solutions

References

Ignatavicius et al., 2018, pp. 239–241, 245–246, 1192–1197, 1291, 1302

Thinking Exercise 7A-3

Answers

Assessment Findings	Effective	Ineffective	Unrelated
Alert, oriented, and moving all extremities	X		
Stridor presented on auscultation		X	
Urine output of 100 mL/hr	X		
Incisional pain reported 6/10		X	
Client asks to use incentive spirometer			X
Denies nausea	X		

Rationales

The client's neurologic status, including being alert, oriented, and able to move all extremities, is a positive sign that consciousness and motor and sensory functions have returned after anesthesia. The presence of stridor, a high-pitched crowing sound, indicates airway obstruction resulting from tracheal or laryngeal spasm or edema, mucus in the airway, or blockage of the airway from edema or tongue relaxation. Although the client may be awake, this is a sign that anesthesia has not worn off and the client is at risk of respiratory failure. Urine output of 100 mL/hr indicates that the client remains well hydrated with intravenous fluids and her kidneys are functioning appropriately. Although there are only one or a few small incisions, the client may experience pain. While recovering from anesthesia, clients often experience nausea and vomiting, but this client does not have those symptoms. The client would be encouraged to use the incentive spirometer after surgery to decrease respiratory complications including atelectasis.

Cognitive Skill

Evaluate Outcomes

References

Ignatavicius et al., 2018, pp. 272–276, 280–281, 283–286, 1195–1196

Thinking Exercise 7A-4

Answers

- Oral temperature 101.4°F (38.5°C)
- Abdominal pain = 8/10
- Vomiting bile-colored emesis
- Urine dark yellow-orange

Rationales

Symptoms of postcholecystectomy syndrome, including abdominal or epigastric pain, vomiting, and diarrhea, must be identified and followed up by the nurse. Clients may experience incisional pain after a cholecystectomy, but should not experience abdominal pain, especially severe pain that the client rates at 8 out of 10 on a 0 to 10 pain intensity scale. Nausea and vomiting are also indications of complications after the cholecystectomy and must be evaluated. The nurse must follow up on the client's 101.4°F (38.5°C) temperature because it may indicate postoperative inflammation or infection. Although the client's urinary output is adequate, the dark yellow-orange urine should be evaluated as a potential sign of jaundice secondary to a common bile duct leak or liver dysfunction. The other findings are expected for a postoperative client.

Cognitive Skill

Recognize Cues

Reference

Ignatavicius et al., 2018, pp. 1196–1197

Thinking Exercise 7A-5

Answers

A, B, D, G, H

Rationales

Preprocedural care for a client undergoing endoscopic retrograde cholangiopancreatography (ERCP) includes being NPO for 6 to 8 hours before the procedure to minimize risk of aspiration (Choice A), ensuring intravenous access for moderate-sedation drugs during the procedure (Choice B), and verifying that an informed consent form has been signed, since the procedure is invasive (Choice H). The nurse would evaluate the client's allergies, especially to iodine, shellfish, and contrast media, because an iodine-based dye will be inserted through a cannula into the common bile duct during the procedure (Choice D). The client may be anxious about being NPO and should be taught that she will be able to eat and drink again once her gag reflex returns after the procedure (Choice G).

Cognitive Skill

Take Action

References

Ignatavicius et al., 2018, pp. 1071, 1196–1197

Exemplar 7B. Peptic Ulcer Disease (Medical-Surgical Nursing: Middle-Age Adult)

Thinking Exercise 7B-1

Answers

Medication	Dose, Route, Frequency	Drug Class	Indication
Warfarin	2.5 mg orally every day	Anticoagulant	**Atrial fibrillation**
Ibuprofen	400 mg orally every 6–8 hr as needed for pain	Nonsteroidal anti-inflammatory drug	Chronic back pain
Famotidine	20 mg orally twice a day	**H$_2$ antagonist**	Gastric acid reflux
Trimethoprim/ sulfamethoxazole	**160/800 mg orally twice a day**	Anti-infective agent	Urinary tract infection
Verapamil	40-mg oral extended release tablet once daily	Calcium channel blocker	**Angina pectoris**

Cognitive Skill

Analyze Cues

References

Burchum & Rosenthal, 2019, pp. 497–500, 612–616, 859, 962, 1072–1073

Thinking Exercise 7B-2

Answers

B, C, F, G

Rationales

When evaluating the client's health history and emergency department assessment findings, the nurse notices several medications that place the client at risk for peptic ulcers and GI hemorrhage, including warfarin. The nurse would ask questions about the use of these medications including dosage and frequency (Choice B). The nurse also notices that the client has a history of dyspepsia and presents with symptoms of gastrointestinal hemorrhage including hemoglobin and hematocrit levels on the lower end of the normal range, and positive occult blood in the client's stool. Asking questions about the client's GI upset and pain and their relationship to food intake and sleep patterns assists the nurse in identifying potential complications (Choice C). Changes in abdominal pain would also be assessed, including frequency, intensity, and location, because a change in the character of pain may be a sign of active ulcers or perforation (Choice F). In addition to evaluating symptoms related to peptic ulcer disease and its complications, the nurse would notice that the client has a history of atrial fibrillation, which affects cardiac output and perfusion of vital organs including myocardial and cerebral tissues. The nurse would ask about cardiac palpitations and chest pain recently experienced to evaluate cardiac involvement in the syncopal event (Choice G).

Cognitive Skill

Analyze Cues

References

Ignatavicius et al., 2018, pp. 306, 694–697, 817–820, 1108–1111

Thinking Exercise 7B-3

Answers

Massive bleeding from gastric or duodenal ulcers presents as hematemesis, and minimal bleeding from these ulcers can present as melena. If massive upper GI bleeding occurs, the client may experience dizziness secondary to hypotension and tachycardia. The nurse would administer oxygen and respiratory support as needed, start two large-bore intravenous lines for isotonic fluids and blood replacement, and monitor vital signs, hematocrit, and oxygenation saturation.

Rationales

Upper gastrointestinal (GI) bleeding is a medical emergency, especially if the bleeding is massive. Because of fluid volume loss through bleeding and hematemesis, the client is at risk for hypovolemic shock, which causes tachycardia and hypotension. The resulting hypoxia to the client's brain can lead to client reports of dizziness and lightheadedness. The nurse would provide oxygen and other respiratory support as needed and prepare for fluid volume replacement using an isotonic IV solution and blood transfusion. To determine if these interventions were effective, the nurse monitors the client's vital signs to observe an expected increase in blood pressure and decrease in pulse rate, hematocrit (which should increase), and an increased oxygen saturation.

Cognitive Skill

Prioritize Hypotheses

References

Ignatavicius et al., 2018, pp. 1108–1109, 1113

Thinking Exercise 7B-4

Answers

Client's Response	Effective	Ineffective	Unrelated
"The primary health care provider will explain the procedure to me and answer my questions before I sign the consent form."	X		
"I will not eat or drink anything for 6 to 8 hours before the procedure, but I will be able to drink water right after it is done."		X	
"During the procedure a small flexible tube will be inserted into my colon."		X	
"The procedure is short, so I don't have to worry about caffeine withdrawal."			X
"My vital signs and breathing will be monitored by a specialized endoscopy nurse during the procedure."	X		
"This test will allow the primary health care provider to see any ulcers inside of my esophagus, my stomach, and the upper part of my intestines."	X		

Rationales

The esophagogastroduodenoscopy (EDG) is a visual examination of the esophagus, stomach, and duodenum by means of insertion of a flexible fiberoptic endoscope (tube) through the client's mouth and down the client's throat. The client is administered moderate sedation during the procedure, and a specialized endoscopy nurse closely monitors the client's vital signs and respiratory status during and after the procedure. The procedure requires an informed consent form to be signed. The primary health care provider is required to discuss the procedure and answer the client's questions before the client signs the consent. The client would be NPO for 6 to 8 hours prior to the procedure and remain NPO until the client's gag reflex returns. Keeping the client NPO before and after the procedure is essential to minimize the risk of aspiration.

Cognitive Skill

Evaluate Outcomes

References

Ignatavicius et al., 2018, pp. 1070–1071, 1113

Thinking Exercise 7B-5

Answers

Nursing Action	Indicated	Contraindicated	Non-Essential
Administer throat lozenges as needed for throat discomfort.	X		
Keep the client NPO until the client's gag reflex returns.	X		
Discontinue intravenous fluids if the client becomes nauseated and vomits.		X	
Encourage the spouse to be at the bedside when the sedation is wearing off.			X
Monitor vital signs every 30 minutes until the client is fully wake and stable.	X		
Keep the client in a supine position with the head of the bed lower than 30 degrees.		X	

Rationales

After the esophagogastroduodenoscopy (EGD) the client will be monitored closely by a specialist endoscopy nurse who will assess vital signs every 15 to 30 minutes until the sedation wears off. The nurse will assess the client's gag reflex prior to administering any oral fluids and keep the client's head of the bed at greater than 30 degrees to prevent aspiration. The nurse will discontinue intravenous fluids when the client is fully awake, has a positive gag reflex, is able to drink fluids, and denies nausea or vomiting. The nurse may administer throat lozenges to decrease discomfort caused by the endoscope passing through the back of the throat. Although the client's spouse should be allowed at the bedside, this is not essential to the safety and care of the client.

Cognitive Skill

Generate Solutions

References

Ignatavicius et al., 2018, pp. 1070–1071, 1113

Thinking Exercise 7B-6

Answers

A, B, C, D, E, H

Rationales

Discharge teaching for a client with peptic ulcer disease would focus on recognizing complications and what to do if complications occur. Complications of peptic ulcer disease include gastrointestinal hemorrhage, perforation, and pyloric obstruction. The nurse would teach the client to contact the primary health care provider if she experiences sharp, sudden, persistent, and severe epigastric or abdominal pain, bloody or black stools, and vomit that looks bloody or like coffee grounds (Choice A). The client should not wait until the follow-up visit to report bloody or black stools. A journal would be useful to keep track of any changes in the client's stool (Choice C). In addition to complications, the nurse would teach the client to avoid substances that increase gastric acid secretion including caffeine-containing beverages, alcohol, tobacco, and certain foods including tomatoes, onions, fried food, and hot spices. Because the client drinks a large amount of carbonated drinks, decreasing intake would be the first step to avoiding all caffeinated beverages (Choices B and D). The NSAID that the client takes for chronic back pain increases the client's risk for future peptic ulcers. The client should talk with her primary health care provider about alternative treatments to decrease this risk while maintaining appropriate pain management (Choice H). Hypomagnesemia is a side effect of omeprazole. Therefore the client would be taught to identify symptoms of hypomagnesemia and contact the primary health care provider if they occur. Common symptoms of hypomagnesemia include tremors, muscle cramps, seizures, and dysthymias (Choice E).

Cognitive Skill

Take Action

References

Ignatavicius et al., 2018, pp. 1112–1115; Burchum & Rosenthal, 2019, pp. 963–965

Chapter 8 Mobility: *Common Health Problems*

Answers With Rationales for Thinking Exercises

Exemplar 8A. Fractured Hip/Open Reduction Internal Fixation (Medical-Surgical Nursing: Older Adult)

Thinking Exercise 8A-1

Answers

Nursing Action	Indicated	Contraindicated	Non-Essential
Remove traction weights when turning the client.		X	
Assess pin sites of external fixator for signs and symptoms of infection.	X		

Nursing Action	Indicated	Contraindicated	Non-Essential
Take the client's temperature every hour.			X
Check the cast to ensure that it is not too tight.			X
Manage the client's pain with analgesia.	X		
Assist the client when she is ambulating with her walker.		X	
Check all traction ropes and knots every shift for intactness.	X		

Rationales

The client is currently in skin traction (Buck) for which the nurse allows the weights to hang freely and not rest on the floor or be removed. All traction ropes and knots should be checked every shift for intactness. Clients in this type of traction do not ambulate because this action could be harmful. The client's fracture has not been stabilized, and additional damage would result if the client ambulates with or without assistance. Fractures are very painful and require analgesic medications. The pin sites of the external fixator may become infected, and therefore the nurse would assess the sites at least every shift for redness and drainage. It is not necessary to take the client's temperature every hour, and the client with these types of fractures do not have a cast.

Cognitive Skill

Generate Solutions

References

Ignatavicius et al., 2018, pp. 1040–1043, 1047–1048

Thinking Exercise 8A-2

Answers

Medication	Dose, Route, Frequency	Drug Class	Indication
Tramadol	100 mg orally once at bedtime	Nonopioid centrally acting analgesic	Moderate-to-severe back pain and osteoarthritis
Sofosbuvir/velpatasvir	400 mg/100 mg orally once daily	NS5A inhibitor	**Hepatitis C**
Risedronate	5 mg orally once daily	**Bisphosphonate**	Osteopenia/osteoporosis
Metoprolol	**100 mg orally once daily**	Beta blocker	Hypertension
Glipizide	20 mg orally twice daily	Second-generation sulfonylurea	Diabetes mellitus type 2

Cognitive Skill

Analyze Cues

References

Burchum & Rosenthal, 2019, pp. 168, 294, 695–696, 912, 1124–1126

Thinking Exercise 8A-3

Answers

A, B, C, E, G

Rationales

The client has several pressure injuries that the nurse would need to manage by teaching assistive personnel to turn the client frequently and avoid placing her on her back in a supine position (Choice A). The client should also not sit in a chair more than an hour at one time because she has a pressure injury on her coccyx (Choice B). Because the client's heels are bluish and feel "mushy," the client's heels should be kept off the bed at all times (Choice C). The nurse would also consult with the registered dietitian nutritionist to plan meals and supplements that are high in protein for tissue healing (Choice E) and apply a pressure-reducing mattress overlay onto the bed to help reduce pressure on the client's skin and underlying tissues (Choice G).

Cognitive Skill

Take Action

Reference

Ignatavicius et al., 2018, pp. 447–458

Thinking Exercise 8A-4

Answers

- Temperature = 100°F (37.8°C)
- Blood pressure = 96/52 mm Hg
- Redness around proximal end of left wrist incision
- Reports feeling unusually tired today
- Drowsy but easily awakened

Rationales

The client's elevated body temperature and low blood pressure are not within normal or usual limits. Her report of feeling very tired and being drowsy is also of concern for the nurse on the client's third postoperative day. She had been alert and oriented prior to today. The redness at the proximal end of her wrist incision could indicate infection that needs to be assessed by the primary health care provider for possible pharmacologic intervention.

Cognitive Skill

Recognize Cues

Reference

Ignatavicius et al., 2018, pp. 1032–1035

Thinking Exercise 8A-5

Answers

A, B, D, F

Rationales

This thinking exercise is to determine if you know the difference between acute and long-term chronic postoperative complications associated with fracture repair. Wound infection, venous thromboembolism (especially deep vein thrombosis), acute compartment syndrome due to neurovascular compromise, and fat embolism syndrome are acute postoperative complications that often occur during hospitalization (Choices A, B, D, F). Chronic osteomyelitis (bone infection), ischemic bone necrosis (cell death), and complex regional pain syndrome are all serious chronic complications that usually require long-term management.

Cognitive Skill

Recognize Cues

Reference

Ignatavicius et al., 2018, pp. 1032–1035

Thinking Exercise 8A-6

Answers

Nursing Action	Potential Postoperative Complication	Appropriate Nursing Action for Each Postoperative Complication
1 Administer long-term antibiotic therapy.	Acute compartment syndrome	**6** Remove the cause of the increased pressure, if possible.
2 Consult with a specialist to manage pain.	Deep vein thrombosis	**3** Administer IV sodium heparin.
3 Administer IV sodium heparin.	Fat embolism syndrome	**4** Initiate IV fluids and oxygen therapy.
4 Initiate IV fluids and oxygen therapy.	Complex regional pain syndrome	**2** Consult with a specialist to manage pain.
5 Prepare the client for a fasciotomy.	Chronic osteomyelitis	**1** Administer long-term antibiotic therapy.
6 Remove the cause of the increased pressure, if possible.		
7 Prepare to administer a blood transfusion.		

Rationales

Acute compartment syndrome occurs as a result of increased compartment pressure caused by either an internal (e.g., swelling) or external cause (e.g., bandage, cast). The nurse would remove the cause of the pressure if known (Action #6). As an anticoagulant, IV sodium heparin is an appropriate intervention to prevent a deep vein thrombosis (DVT) from becoming larger or to prevent additional thrombi (Action #3). Fat embolism syndrome (FES) occurs most often in clients who have fractures of long bones, but any fracture can result in release of fat cells from the yellow bone marrow into the bloodstream to cause FES. FES often affects the lungs and causes dyspnea and chest pain, and therefore oxygen therapy and IV fluids are appropriate interventions as part of client management (Action #4). Chronic regional pain syndrome is a chronic health problem that often leads to intractable pain and requires the expertise of a pain specialist (Action #2). Chronic osteomyelitis is a deep bone infection that requires long-term IV antibiotic therapy (Action #1).

Cognitive Skill

Take Action

Reference

Ignatavicius et al., 2018, pp. 1032–1046

Exemplar 8B. Fractured Radius and Medial Epicondyle (Pediatric Nursing: Preschool Child)

Thinking Exercise 8B-1

Answers

A, B, D, E

Rationales

The nurse needs to collect as much data as possible about the accident to determine whether the injury is due to intentional or unintentional causes (Choices A, B, D, and E). Parents of children with osteogenesis imperfecta are often suspected of abuse initially until testing is completed. Regardless of the medical history, abuse cases are often initially suspected based on whether or not the description of the accident is consistent or inconsistent with the injury. The age of the child and type of fracture also provide support or negate abuse.

Cognitive Skill

Analyze Cues

Reference

Hockenberry & Wilson, 2019, pp. 1239–1242

Thinking Exercise 8B-2

Answers

- Heart rate = 112 beats/min
- Child is crying inconsolably with parents at the bedside
- Right forearm is dirty, reddened, and swollen
- Child points to her right elbow to signify where she hurts the most
- Capillary refill of right fingers is <5 sec and left fingers is <3 sec
- Right hand is slightly warm to touch, left hand is very warm to touch
- Child reports that her right fingers feel like they are being poked with stickers

Rationales

A major concern with fractures includes neurovascular compromise and potential for circulatory or nerve impairment. The focus of the nurse's assessment is early identification of these possible complications, such as unequal pulses, decreased capillary refill, change in color of affected extremity (pallor), numbness or tingling in the affected extremity (paresthesia), uncontrolled pain or pressure, and decreased ability to move the affected extremity (paresis). The nurse needs to be aware and recognize age-appropriate interpretations of these assessment findings.

Cognitive Skill

Recognize Cues

Reference

Hockenberry & Wilson, 2019, pp. 1261–1266

Thinking Exercise 8B-3

Answers

Before the procedure, the nurse will protect the child from further injury by keeping both arms immobilized and providing pain medication to promote cooperation from the child. Parental presence throughout the preprocedure and postprocedure periods is an important aspect of providing client-centered care, and the nurse must instruct the parents on what to expect at every stage. The nurse will use puppets and pictures of the operating suite or procedure unit to provide age-appropriate education to the child. Baseline assessment provides a comparison for postprocedure assessment and should include level of consciousness and vital signs. The nurse would use the Wong-Baker FACES Scale to assess the child's pain level.

Rationales

Preventing additional injury to the child by keeping both extremities as immobile as possible is the priority intervention for the nurse. Providing adequate pain relief is not only client-centered but also helps promote cooperation of the child. The nurse should always include the parents or guardians of a child because they are the primary support and security for the child. Age-appropriate adaptations should be made in every aspect of client care, but especially when assessing pain and providing teaching that the child will understand.

Cognitive Skill

Take Action

References

Hockenberry & Wilson, 2019, pp. 679–686, 1259–1264

Thinking Exercise 8B-4

Answers

Potential Complication	Appropriate Nursing Action for Each Complication	Rationales
Circulatory impairment	**4** Assess for equality of pulses, color of extremities, difficulty moving fingers, inconsolable crying.	Evaluating the child's circulatory system involves assessing for the presence of the 6 *P*s: pulselessness, paresthesia, pressure, pain, pallor, and paralysis. These findings indicate lack of circulation and possible compartment syndrome, a life-threatening complication.
Nerve impairment	**7** Remove cast and obtain an arteriogram.	Cast removal may be indicated for both circulatory and nerve compression; an arteriogram is often used to determine arterial perfusion to the peripheral nerves.
Decreased muscle strength	**8** Reassure parents that with normal activity the child will regain all mobility.	Atrophy of the muscle happens quickly in a cast, but children have little trouble regaining full mobility without additional physical therapy. This is true for the child with OI as well.
Fracture nonunion	**1** Assess for signs of infection.	Infection in the bone is one cause of nonunion. Nonunion is an unexpected finding that is assessed for at follow-up visits, especially prior to cast removal.
Skin breakdown	**3** Place protective barrier around the sharp edges on the cast.	Casts often have very rough edges and can be sharp and uncomfortable for the child. Using moleskin to petal the ends of the cast will minimize or prevent skin breakdown.

Cognitive Skill

Take Action

Reference

Hockenberry & Wilson, 2019, pp. 1259–1266

Thinking Exercise 8B-5

Answers

C, D, F, G, I

Rationales

Most of the statements reflect that the parents understand the potential complications associated with a cast and appropriate cast care. Ibuprofen is a COX-2 inhibitor that has been associated with delayed union of the bone. Therefore this drug is discouraged for pain control associated with fractures (Choice C). Heat should never be applied to the exterior of the cast because it will cause the cast to soften. Heat also increases the risk of swelling. Only cool or cold should be applied to the outside of the cast (Choice D). Although more appropriate activities for the child with osteogenesis imperfecta is recommended, keeping any child in bed is contraindicated after cast placement (Choice F). Keeping the affected extremity elevated is appropriate for the first 24 to 72 hours, but not developmentally appropriate for a 3-year-old (Choice G). Synthetic casts are not waterproof but can tolerate moisture better than other types of casting materials (Choice I).

Cognitive Skill

Evaluate Outcomes

References

Hockenberry & Wilson, 2019, pp. 147, 1248–1253

Thinking Exercise 8B-6

Answers

Assessment Finding	Effective	Ineffective	Unrelated
Radiograph of right radius displays extensive callus formation.	X		
Child is easily consoled by mother, but still hesitant with health care workers.	X		
Denies difficulty with urination.			X
Radial pulses are 3+ and equal bilaterally.	X		
Difficulty bending right arm at the wrist and elbow.			X
Small reddened, blistered area on the inner aspect of the right upper arm.		X	
Capillary refill is <3 sec in lower extremities.	X		
Mother reports that pain is well controlled with hydrocodone/acetaminophen elixir.		X	

Rationales

Expected outcomes for the pediatric client following fracture reduction and cast placement are that the child is pain free, the fracture demonstrates adequate healing, and the child does not show any signs of circulatory or nerve complications. The x-ray demonstrates callus formation, which supports evidence of adequate bone healing. Equal pulses and capillary refill <3 sec indicate that treatment to prevent possible complications has been adequate. Although the child is now easily consoled by the child's mother, the report of having to use opioid pain medication at this stage indicates a concern for the nurse to follow up because the child should not have pain after 1 to 2 days following cast placement. The small reddened area above the cast indicates that the child's skin integrity has been compromised from the cast, and thus preventive actions were not effective. It is an expected outcome that the child will have limited mobility in the wrist and elbow of the affected extremity, especially after a long arm cast is removed. This difficulty will resolve with normal activity and very rarely requires physical therapy.

Cognitive Skill

Evaluate Outcomes

References

Hockenberry & Wilson, 2019, pp. 147, 150–153, 1251–1253, 1261–1264

Exemplar 8C. Osteoarthritis/Total Knee Arthroplasty (Medical-Surgical Nursing: Middle-Age Adult)

Thinking Exercise 8C-1

Answers

A, C, E, G

Rationales

Ice or other cold application constricts blood vessels, which decreases inflammation, including pain and swelling (Choice A). Heat application would dilate the blood vessels, which would bring more blood to the affected area and increase swelling. Elevating the affected leg increases venous blood return, which reduces swelling (Choice E). The client may benefit from a physical therapy consultation and possible follow-up for muscle-strengthening exercises, pain management, and joint mobility (Choice C). Obesity increases the weight-bearing function of the lower extremity joints, especially the hips and knees. Therefore the client may need to be referred to a registered dietitian nutritionist, who may refer her to a weight reduction plan or specialist (Choice G).

Cognitive Skill

Take Action

Reference

Ignatavicius et al., 2018, pp. 305–308

Thinking Exercise 8C-2

Answers

A, B, D, E, F, G

Rationales

To help prevent postoperative infection, the client will need to shower with a special solution at least the night before surgery, wear clean night clothes, and sleep on clean linen (Choice A). A surgical drain may be used, but this practice is becoming less common owing to the risk of introducing potential pathogens that can cause infection (Choice G). Taking postoperative anticoagulants will help prevent venous thromboembolism (VTE) (deep vein thrombosis and pulmonary embolism) (Choice D). The client is expected to be in the hospital for 2 to 3 days and will be prescribed analgesia, including pain medication and a cold application, during her stay (Choices E and F). After surgery the physical therapist will work with the client for at least 6 weeks to teach her how to perform leg muscle strengthening exercises and ambulation with a walker and possibly progressing to a cane (Choice B). A cane is used on the unaffected or nonsurgical leg, not the affected leg.

Cognitive Skill

Take Action

References

Ignatavicius et al., 2018, pp. 95, 314–316

Thinking Exercise 8C-3

Answers

- Reports left knee pain of 6/10 (on a 0 to 10 pain intensity scale)
- Drowsy but arouses easily
- Reports that her legs and feet feel "heavy and numb"
- Reports "frequent waves of nausea"

Rationales

A client who is receiving PCA should not have pain at a 6/10 level unless she is not using it correctly. However, she is drowsy and reports that both legs feel heavy and numb. The epidural anesthetic should wear off in 2 to 4 hours after surgery. The nurse would carefully monitor the client to ensure that the leg symptoms improve. Nausea is common after surgery, and the nurse would likely need to administer an antiemetic drug.

Cognitive Skill

Recognize Cues

References

Ignatavicius et al., 2018, pp. 275–276, 314–316

Thinking Exercise 8C-4

Answers

The nurse should monitor postoperative clients who have a total knee arthroplasty under epidural anesthesia for common complications that can occur during their hospital stay, including venous thromboembolism and urinary retention. Nursing interventions that can help prevent these complications are to encourage fluids, ambulate the client early, and administer an anticoagulant.

Rationales

Postoperative VTE is a common serious complication following a total joint arthroplasty. Urinary retention can result from the epidural anesthetic. To help prevent these complications, the nurse would encourage the client to drink plenty of fluids. Early ambulation and anticoagulation are interventions to help prevent VTE. The client would also wear sequential compression devices (SCDs) and/or compression stockings to promote venous blood return and prevent venous stasis.

Cognitive Skill

Prioritize Hypotheses

References

Ignatavicius et al., 2018, pp. 283–286, 742–745

Thinking Exercise 8C-5

Answers

Health Teaching	Indicated	Contraindicated	Non-Essential
"Use the prescribed ambulatory aid such as a walker."	X		
"Use assistive/adaptive devices as needed (e.g., sock aids, shoehorns, dressing sticks, extenders)."	X		

Health Teaching	Indicated	Contraindicated	Non-Essential
"Do not put more weight on your affected leg than allowed and instructed."	X		
"Use heat as needed to operative hip to decrease pain and promote healing."		X	
"Do not bend your hips more than 90 degrees."			X
"Follow up with all physical therapy appointments as prescribed."	X		
"Inspect your surgical incision every day for increased redness, heat, or drainage; if any of these are present, call your surgeon immediately."	X		

Rationales

To promote time for healing of the TKA, the client should carefully follow the instructions of the surgeon and physical therapist regarding weight bearing, ambulatory aid (such as a walker), and the use of assistive/adaptive devices to promote ADL independence. Teach the client to inspect the incision every day for indications of possible infection. If present, the client needs to notify her surgeon immediately for evaluation and possible treatment with antibiotic therapy. Heat application could be harmful to the surgical area because it could cause increased swelling. Cold applications are more commonly used to decrease the long-term swelling that is common in the surgical knee. There are no restrictions about flexing the client's hips after a total knee arthroplasty. It is more important to prevent hip hyperflexion for clients who have a total hip arthroplasty, depending on the surgical approach used.

Cognitive Skill

Generate Solutions

Reference

Ignatavicius et al., 2018, pp. 309–316

Thinking Exercise 8C-6

Answers

Assessment Finding	Effective	Ineffective	Unrelated
Incision shows no sign of infection.	X		
Reports increased pain in her right (nonsurgical) knee.			X
Surgical knee flexion is 110 degrees.	X		
Cannot straighten surgical leg.		X	
Reports having periods of insomnia.			X
Surgical knee is less bruised and mildly swollen.	X		

Rationales

The expected outcomes for the client who had a recent total knee arthroplasty include being free of complications such as infection and VTE. The client's knee flexion needs to be adequate for climbing steps, so 110 degrees of flexion meets that outcome. However, knee extension should be at least 0 degrees or straight. Not being able to straighten the surgical leg can be a problem and is not a desired outcome. Knee bruising and swelling occur for several months for most clients who have a TKA. The client's insomnia and right knee pain are unrelated to this surgery; however, these problems need to be addressed.

Cognitive Skill

Evaluate Outcomes

Reference

Ignatavicius et al., 2018, pp. 306–314

Exemplar 8D. Parkinson Disease (Medical-Surgical Nursing/Mental Health Nursing: Older Adult)

Thinking Exercise 8D-1

Answers

- Needs assistance with ADLs on days when his rigidity is worse
- Walks short distances in the house using a walker
- Has resting tremors in both arms and hands, but right hand is worse than the left (client is right-handed)
- Chokes at times when he eats
- Has fallen twice in the past week because of dizziness when he stands from a sitting or lying position
- Blood pressure = 100/64 mm Hg (in supine position)

Rationales

Parkinson disease is a chronic neurologic disease that causes rigidity and resting tremors that can affect the ability to independently perform ADLs. The disease and/or medications that are typically used for treatment can cause orthostatic hypotension, which makes the client feel dizzy and lightheaded. Both of these problems can lead to safety issues including a risk for falling. His history of previous falls puts him at high risk for more falls.

Cognitive Skill

Recognize Cues

Reference

Ignatavicius et al., 2018, pp. 868–873

Thinking Exercise 8D-2

Answers

Medication	Dose, Route, Frequency	Drug Class	Indication
Levodopa/carbidopa	200 mg levodopa/50 mg carbidopa 1 tablet 4 times a day orally	Dopamine replacement	**Parkinson disease**
Baclofen	20 mg 3 times a day orally	Centrally acting muscle relaxant	**Muscle spasticity**
Entacapone	200 mg 4 times a day orally	**COMT inhibitor**	Parkinson disease
Venlafaxine XR	**75 mg once a day orally**	Serotonin-norepinephrine reuptake inhibitor (SNRI)	Depression
Zolpidem	10 mg every evening before bed orally	Sedative-hypnotic	Insomnia/promotion of sleep

Cognitive Skill

Analyze Cues

References

Burchum & Rosenthal, 2019, pp. 188–198, 250–253, 361, 388–389

Thinking Exercise 8D-3

Answers

Because of the client's orthostatic hypotension and dysphagia, he is currently *most likely* at risk for fall-ing and aspiration. During his hospital stay, he is also *most likely* at risk for complications associated with impaired mobility, especially pressure injury and constipation.

Rationales

Orthostatic hypotension can cause dizziness and lightheadedness, which can cause a client to fall. Aspiration is common in clients who have dysphagia (difficulty swallowing). Because of the client's impaired mobility, he is also at risk for pressure injury and constipation.

Cognitive Skill

Prioritize Hypotheses

Reference

Ignatavicius et al., 2018, pp. 868–873

Thinking Exercise 8D-4

Answers

A, B, D, E, G, H

Rationales

The client is at risk for falling because of orthostatic hypotension. Reminding the client and his wife to call the nursing staff for help out of bed, placing the client on fall precautions, and performing ortho-static checks to determine if the problem is continuing are all appropriate nursing actions (Choices B, D, and H). The nurse would refer the client to physical and occupational therapy to evaluate and improve the client's ability to ambulate and perform ADLs (Choice E). The nurse also would consult with the speech-language pathologist owing to the client's dysphagia, to obtain a swallowing evaluation, and would remind the nursing staff to place the client in a sitting position during meals (Choices A and G). Liquids must be avoided unless they are thickened for any client who has dysphagia to prevent choking.

Cognitive Skill

Take Action

Reference

Ignatavicius et al., 2018, pp. 868–873

Thinking Exercise 8D-5

Answers

Nursing Action	Indicated	Contraindicated	Non-Essential
Focus on reality and not the hallucination experience.	X		
Place the client in the least restrictive restraints.		X	

Continued

Nursing Action	Indicated	Contraindicated	Non-Essential
Request a prescription for pimavanserin.	X		
Refer the client to a mental health professional.			X
Make eye contact if culturally appropriate.	X		
Document the client's report of hallucinations.	X		

Rationales

Many clients with Parkinson disease (PD) have hallucinations that are usually caused by the disease. Pimavanserin is the first drug to be approved for clients who have hallucinations as part of PD. Referring the client to a mental health professional is not necessary at this time because the cause of hallucinations in this client is known. When caring for someone who is having a hallucination, the nurse recognizes that he or she needs to focus on reality, maintain eye contact, and not dwell on the hallucination experience or content of the hallucination. Any client behaviors need to be documented by the nurse.

Cognitive Skill

Generate Solutions

Reference

Halter, 2018, pp. 208–209

CHAPTER 9 Metabolism: *Common Health Problems*

Answers With Rationales for Thinking Exercises

Exemplar 9A. Diabetes Mellitus (Medical-Surgical Nursing: Middle-Age Adult)

Thinking Exercise 9A-1

Answers

Medication	Dose, Route, Frequency	Drug Class	Drug Action
Metformin	500-mg oral extended-release tablet once daily with evening meal	Biguanide	Decreases glucose production by the liver and increases tissue response to insulin
Aspirin	**81 mg orally once daily**	Salicylate	Minimizes platelet aggregation
Metoprolol	25-mg extended-release tablet once daily	Beta-adrenergic blocker	**Reduces blood pressure**
Exenatide	5-mcg subcutaneous injection twice daily before breakfast and dinner	**Incretin mimetic**	Slows gastric emptying, stimulates insulin release, suppresses glucagon release, and reduces appetite
Glipizide	10 mg orally once daily with breakfast	Second-generation sulfonylurea	**Promotes insulin secretion by the pancreas**
Gabapentin	300-mg oral capsule, daily before bed	Antiepileptic	Relieves neuropathic pain

Cognitive Skill

Analyze Cues

References

Burchum & Rosenthal, 2019, pp. 128, 234–235, 240, 310, 621–622, 692–695, 701–702

Thinking Exercise 9A-2

Answers

- Serum blood glucose = 486 mg/dL (27.1 mmol/L)
- Reports urinating multiple times every hour
- Serum potassium = 3.5 mEq/L (3.5 mmol/L)
- Burning pain from bilateral toes to mid-calves

Rationales

The nurse's initial assessment indicates that the client has clinical manifestations of hyperglycemia. Classic signs of hyperglycemia include serum blood glucose greater than 250 mg/dL (13.9 mmol/L), polyuria, polydipsia, and polyphagia. The client's serum blood glucose is 486 mg/dL (27.1 mmol/L), and she reports urinating multiple times every hour. These are symptoms that the nurse must follow up on immediately to prevent neurologic changes as well as other complications of hyperglycemia. The client's serum potassium level is a low normal and needs to be monitored. The nurse would follow up on this laboratory value so that potassium replacement therapy is initiated to prevent cardiac dysrhythmias secondary to hypokalemia. The client's report of burning pain in her legs is most likely a result of peripheral neuropathy, a complication of diabetes mellitus. Although this may not be a new symptom, the nurse would follow up by completing a focused skin and safety assessment on the client's feet and toes. Other signs and symptoms presented are normal for this client's medical history and recent upper respiratory infection. The client's hemoglobin A1c is less than 7%, indicating that this client usually adequately manages her blood glucose levels.

Cognitive Skill

Recognize Cues

References

Ignatavicius et al., 2018, pp. 1282–1285, 1289–1290; Pagana & Pagana, 2018, pp. 227–230, 238–240; Pagana et al., 2019, pp. 269–272, 281–284

Thinking Exercise 9A-3

Answers

Priority treatment for hyperglycemic-hyperosmolar state is fluid replacement. When administering large volumes of fluids, the nurse assesses for complications. Cerebral edema results from a large fluid volume shift from extracellular to intracellular spaces faster than brain cells can adapt. It presents as changes in level of consciousness, changes in pupil size, shape, or reaction, and seizure activity. Clients who have heart failure are at risk for fluid overload, which manifests as pulmonary congestion.

Rationales

When administering fluids to a client with a hyperglycemic-hyperosmolar state (HHS), fluids need to be replaced fast enough to improve central venous pressure and blood pressure (preventing severe hypotension and shock) but slow enough to prevent complications. Determining the rate for fluid replacement is challenging and requires the nurse to monitor the client closely and recognize changes in status. Cerebral edema is caused by shifts in fluid volume within the brain and is a complication of HHS due to changes in tissue permeability secondary to hyperglycemia and dehydration. Because the skull does not allow for the expansion of tissues, clients will experience neurologic changes when cerebral edema occurs. The nurse would monitor for changes in level of consciousness, seizure activity, and pupil size, shape, or reaction. If the nurse notices any of these changes, the primary health care provider would be notified immediately. When a client who has heart failure needs fluid replacement for treatment of HHS, the nurse must also monitor for complications of fluid overload. Left heart failure occurs when the heart is unable to contract forcefully enough to eject adequate amounts of blood into the circulation. Preload increases, resulting in blood accumulation in the pulmonary vasculature. Administering intravenous fluids quickly will rapidly increase blood volume including accumulation in the pulmonary system. The nurse would be on alert for pulmonary congestion including bilateral crackles, pink frothy sputum, and respiratory distress.

Cognitive Skill

Prioritize Hypotheses

References

Ignatavicius et al., 2018, pp. 691–964, 1314–1316

Thinking Exercise 9A-4

Answers

Nursing Action	Potential Complication	Appropriate Nursing Action for Each Complication
1 Teach the client to rise slowly from the bed.	Injury secondary to visual disturbances	**4** Ensure the path to the bathroom is well lit.
2 Coordinate meal-time insulin with food delivery and consumption.	Orthostatic hypotension	**1** Teach the client to rise slowly from the bed.
3 Administer intravenous 5%D/NS at 200 mL/hr.	Diabetic chronic kidney disease	**7** Administer angiotensin-converting enzyme (ACE) inhibitor as prescribed.
4 Ensure the path to the bathroom is well lit.	Hypoglycemia	**2** Coordinate meal-time insulin with food delivery and consumption.
5 Assist the client in putting on nonslip socks.		
6 Administer 1 mg glucagon IM PRN for blood glucose 70–90 mg/dL (3.9–5.0 mmol/L)		
7 Administer angiotensin-converting enzyme (ACE) inhibitor as prescribed.		
8 Encourage the client to drink 240 mL of sugar-free liquids every hour.		

Rationales

The many complications associated with diabetes mellitus are due to microvascular and macrovascular changes. Nephropathy, neuropathy, and retinopathy result from microvascular changes. Macrovascular changes cause coronary artery disease, cerebral vascular disease, and peripheral vascular disease. To prevent injury secondary to visual disturbances caused by retinopathy, the nurse will ensure that the room has proper lighting so that the client can safety move around the unfamiliar space including ambulating to the bathroom (Action #4). Orthostatic hypotension, a result of cardiovascular autonomic neuropathy, increases the client's risk for lightheadedness and syncope. The nurse would educate the client to rise slowly from the bed or chair to prevent a fall (Action #1). Diabetic chronic kidney disease or nephropathy may be prevented and the progression to end-stage kidney disease delayed by maintaining optimal blood glucose levels, keeping blood pressure within normal limits, and using drugs that protect the kidneys. Angiotensin-converting enzyme (ACE) inhibitors are one of the drug classes used to protect the kidneys and decrease blood pressure (Action #7).

Hypoglycemia is caused by too much insulin or not enough food. Timing insulin administration with food consumption will assist in the prevention of hypoglycemic episodes. The nurse must understand the onset and peak of insulin preparations so that food may be provided at the appropriate times (Action #2).

Cognitive Skill

Take Action

Reference

Ignatavicius et al., 2018, pp. 1283–1286

Thinking Exercise 9A-5

Answers

Nursing Action	Indicated	Contraindicated	Non-Essential
Help the client to drink 120 mL of fruit juice.	X		
Obtain the client's blood glucose level.	X		
Administer subcutaneous insulin per the sliding scale.		X	
Notify the primary health care provider.	X		
Initiate oxygen therapy per nasal cannula.			X
Administer 1 mg intramuscular glucagon.		X	
Reassess glucose level 15 minutes after treatment.	X		

Rationales

The nurse's assessment indicates the client is experiencing a hypoglycemic episode. Symptoms of hypoglycemia include confusion, anxiety, blurred or double vision, tachycardia and palpitations, and cool, clammy skin. The nurse would complete a point-of-care test depending on agency policy to determine the client's current blood glucose level. Management of a hypoglycemic episode is based on blood glucose level and client symptoms. Because this client can follow simple commands, the nurse would administer 10 to 15 g of oral carbohydrates. A half cup or 120 mL of fruit juice is indicated and appropriate for the treatment of this client's hypoglycemic episode. The nurse would also continue to monitor the client, reassess the glucose level in 15 minutes, and notify the primary health care provider. As the client's glucose level improves, the nurse would provide the client with a small snack of carbohydrates and protein. The nurse would not administer insulin to this client, who is already hypoglycemic, because this would further decrease the blood glucose level. Intramuscular glucagon is not indicated for mild or moderate hypoglycemia. It is used to treat severe hypoglycemia when a client is unable to swallow and no intravenous access is present. Oxygen is not indicated at this time as it has no impact on the client's symptoms associated with hypoglycemia.

Cognitive Skill

Generate Solutions

Reference

Ignatavicius et al., 2018, pp. 1308–1311

Thinking Exercise 9A-6

Answers

Client's Statements	Effective	Ineffective	Unrelated
"I will wash my feet, dry them thoroughly, and wear clean socks every day."	X		
"My antidiabetic medications allow me to eat whatever I desire."		X	
"I will take my glyburide dose with my first bite of breakfast."	X		
"It is okay for me to walk barefooted while inside my home."		X	
"I will weigh myself at the same time and on the same scale each day."			X
"I will make sure that I take my antidiabetic medications even when I am sick."	X		

Rationales

This client who has peripheral neuropathy and vascular disease secondary to diabetes mellitus is at risk for injury, specifically foot injury. The nurse would teach the client to practice proper foot care and maintain intact skin on the feet. Behaviors demonstrating the client understands how to prevent foot injury include cleansing and inspecting feet daily, wearing clean socks and properly fitting shoes, avoiding walking in bare feet even inside the home, trimming toenails properly, and reporting non-healing breaks in the skin of the feet to the primary health care provider. The client's statement related to washing her feet and wearing clean socks indicates she correctly understood the teaching, but her comment that it is okay to walk barefooted while inside her home does not. Effective management of diabetes mellitus requires nutrition and diet therapy. Nutritional plans should be individualized for each client and developed with a registered dietitian nutritionist. The client's statement that she can eat whatever she desires because she is on antidiabetic medications indicates the client does not understand the important role nutrition has in her treatment plan. Glyburide is a sulfonylurea that acts primarily by stimulating the release of insulin from pancreatic islets. Because the pancreas will be producing more insulin, the client needs to coordinate food intake with medication administration to prevent hypoglycemia. Stating that she will take her glyburide dose with the first bite of breakfast indicates she understands this concern. Illness increases the client's risk of dehydration and hyper-glycemia. The client would be taught to manage sick days by checking her blood glucose level every 4 hours, eating regular meals, drinking adequate fluids, and taking her medications as prescribed. The client's statement indicates she understands what to do on sick days. There is no need for the client to weigh herself daily because her disease processes are not associated with fluid retention. The client's statement related to weighing herself is unrelated to her discharge teaching.

Cognitive Skill

Evaluate Outcomes

References

Ignatavicius et al., 2018, pp. 1299–1301, 1304–1307, 1314; Burchum & Rosenthal, 2019, pp. 692–700

Exemplar 9B. Hyperthyroidism/Thyroidectomy (Medical-Surgical Nursing: Middle-Age Adult)

Thinking Exercise 9B-1

Answers

B, D, G

Rationales

Clients diagnosed with hyperthyroidism have an overactive thyroid gland that secretes excessive amounts of thyroxin and other thyroid hormones that control body metabolism. Heat intolerance, diaphoresis, and insomnia occur in clients who have an increased metabolic rate (Choices B, D, and G). The client's heart rate, blood pressure, appetite, and deep tendon reflexes also increase.

Cognitive Skill

Recognize Cues

Reference

Ignatavicius et al, 2018, pp. 1265–1266

Thinking Exercise 9B-2

Answers

B, D

Rationales

Clients diagnosed with hyperthyroidism have an overactive thyroid gland that secretes excessive amounts of thyroxin and other thyroid hormones that control body metabolism. Therefore they have increased amounts of circulating serum thyroxin (Choice B). In clients who have non-Graves disease, the serum thyroid-stimulating hormone (TSH) is also elevated (Choice D).

Cognitive Skill

Recognize Cues

Reference

Ignatavicius et al., 2018, p. 1267

Thinking Exercise 9B-3

Answers

The nurse teaches the client about the common side effects of methimazole, which include signs and symptoms of infection. This drug can also cause adverse drug effects such as birth defects and therefore should not be prescribed for women who are pregnant.

Cognitive Skill

Prioritize Hypotheses

Reference

Burchum & Rosenthal, 2019, pp. 717–718

Thinking Exercise 9B-4

Answers

Nursing Action	Potential Postoperative Complication	Appropriate Nursing Action for Each Postoperative Complication
1 Increase IV fluids and call the Rapid Response Team.	Acute respiratory distress	**3** Start oxygen therapy immediately, suction if needed, and notify the Rapid Response Team.
2 Monitor the client every 2 hours and reassure the client that the problem is temporary.	Bleeding	**1** Increase IV fluids and call the Rapid Response Team.
3 Start oxygen therapy immediately, suction if needed, and notify the Rapid Response Team.	Parathyroid gland injury	**4** Assess for signs of calcium deficiency and give IV calcium gluconate if needed.
4 Assess for signs of calcium deficiency and give IV calcium gluconate if needed.	Laryngeal nerve damage	**2** Monitor the client every 2 hours and reassure the client that the problem is temporary.
5 Prepare the client for additional surgery.	Thyroid storm	**6** Administer propranolol and corticosteroids and apply a cooling blanket.
6 Administer propranolol and corticosteroids and apply a cooling blanket.		
7 Prepare to administer an albumin transfusion.		

Rationales

The client who has respiratory distress as a postoperative complication of thyroid removal surgery usually has neck swelling and/or excessive secretions. Therefore the nurse would place the client in a sitting position, start oxygen therapy, and suction the client if needed. The nurse would call for the Rapid Response Team if additional respiratory support is needed (Action #3). If bleeding occurs, the nurse would replace lost fluid by increasing the client's IV rate or establishing IV access after contacting the Rapid Response Team (Action #1). If the parathyroid glands were damaged during surgery, the client may have a decreased calcium level, which can lead to cardiac and skeletal muscle symptoms. Calcium gluconate or other approved calcium replacement may be needed (Action #4). During surgery the client's laryngeal nerve may be affected, causing laryngitis. This problem is usually short term and is monitored frequently for signs of improvement (Action #2). A thyroid storm is an emergent, life-threatening complication that must be treated immediately with drug therapy and rapid cooling (Action #6).

Cognitive Skill

Take Action

Reference

Ignatavicius et al., 2018, pp. 1269–1270

Thinking Exercise 9B-5

Answers

B, C, D, E, F

Cognitive Skill

Take Action

Reference

Burchum & Rosenthal, 2019, pp. 715–717

CHAPTER 10 Cellular Regulation: *Breast Cancer*

Answers With Rationales for Thinking Exercises

Exemplar 10. Breast Cancer (Medical-Surgical Nursing: Middle-Age Adult)

Thinking Exercise 10-1

Answers

A, C, D, E, F, G, H

Rationales

Older women are at the highest risk for breast cancer, especially those who never were pregnant or had their first child after 30 years of age (Choices A, D, and E). Women who took hormone replacement therapy (HRT) within the past 5 years and had a late menopause are also at increased risk (Choices G and H). Additional risk factors for breast cancer include being of Jewish heritage and alcohol consumption (Choices C and F).

Cognitive Skill

Recognize Cues

Reference

Ignatavicius et al., 2018, p. 1442

Thinking Exercise 10-2

Answers

The client should practice breast self-awareness and have annual mammography. A clinical breast examination should be performed by the primary health care provider as part of regular annual health examinations. Options for reducing the client's risk for breast cancer include prophylactic mastectomy, prophylactic oophorectomy, and antiestrogen drug therapy.

Rationales

The nurse would teach all women to promote breast health by practicing frequent breast self-awareness. Breast self-examination is no longer recommended as best practice because annual 3D mammography and clinical breast examination are more reliable in detecting breast cancer. For women at high risk for developing breast cancer, options to reduce their risk include a prophylactic mastectomy and/or oophorectomy or antiestrogen drug therapy. Each option has advantages and disadvantages, and women must make the best decision for their own health.

Cognitive Skill

Analyze Cues

Reference

Ignatavicius et al., 2018, pp. 1443–1444

Thinking Exercise 10-3

Answers

Nursing Action	Indicated	Contraindicated	Non-Essential
Apply oxygen therapy at 2 L/min.			X
Monitor the amount and color of the JP drainage.	X		
Teach the staff to avoid taking blood pressures or drawing blood in the affected arm.	X		
Keep the client's head of the bed flat at all times.		X	
Elevate the affected arm on a pillow.	X		
Assess the surgical dressing for bleeding.	X		
Keep the client in bed for at least 48 hours.		X	
Begin teaching the client about how to perform postmastectomy exercises.	X		

Rationales

The postoperative mastectomy client stays in the hospital for 1 to 2 days, depending on age, surgical complexity, and hospital and surgeon protocol. Therefore keeping the client in bed for 48 hours is contraindicated and could be harmful by causing complications of decreased mobility. Applying oxygen is not needed for most clients unless they have other cardiopulmonary health problems. The nurse would monitor the amount of JP drainage and assess the surgical dressing for bleeding. To prevent lymphedema, a serious postoperative complication, the nurse would teach the staff to keep the client's affected arm on the surgical side elevated and keep the client in a semi-Fowler or sitting position as tolerated. Keeping the head of the bed flat could cause lymphedema and cellular edema that could put stress on the incision closures. The nurse would also begin teaching postmastectomy exercises to increase mobility and reduce the risk of lymphedema.

Cognitive Skill

Generate Solutions

Reference

Ignatavicius et al., 2018, pp. 1448–1451

Thinking Exercise 10-4

Answers

Assessment Finding	Effective	Ineffective	Unrelated
Mastectomy and reconstruction incisions show no sign of infection	X		
Reports an inability to straighten her left elbow		X	
States that she occasionally feels sad	X		

Assessment Finding	Effective	Ineffective	Unrelated
Mastectomy and reconstruction incisions are healed without redness or drainage	X		
Left arm is very swollen and much larger than the right arm		X	
Reports frequent heart palpitations when she drinks caffeinated beverages			X

Rationales

The client who had a mastectomy with reconstruction 6 weeks ago should be able to straighten her arm and have healed surgical incisions without any sign of infection. The arm on the surgical side should not be swollen and much larger than the other arm, which suggests possible lymphedema. The client's report of palpitations is not related to her surgery and is likely due to an excess of caffeine. The nurse would teach the client to avoid caffeinated beverages and follow up with her primary health care provider for cardiac palpitations.

Cognitive Skill

Evaluate Outcomes

Reference

Ignatavicius et al., 2018, pp. 1448–1454

Thinking Exercise 10-5

Answers

B, C, D, E, G

Rationales

Any client receiving external radiation is not radioactive and is not a danger to anyone. The primary health teaching that the nurse would include is how to care for the radiation site skin. The client should avoid sun (Choice B). Lotions, powders, and creams on the irradiated area that have not been approved by the primary health care provider or radiation specialist should not be used. The client should be careful to not wash off any ink markings on the skin and clean the irradiated skin area gently with mild soap and water, being sure to pat the area dry (Choices C and D). Most forms of radiation can cause increased fatigue (Choice E) and may affect the client's appetite. The nurse also teaches the client to report esophageal burning or dysphagia to the primary health care provider (Choice G).

Cognitive Skill

Take Action

Reference

Ignatavicius et al., 2018, pp. 388–390

Thinking Exercise 10-6

Answers

The nurse would teach the client that doxorubicin, cyclophosphamide, and paclitaxel can cause cardiac toxicity. Therefore the client should report shortness of breath and edema to the primary health care provider immediately. In addition, all three chemotherapeutic drugs can cause bone marrow suppression, which places the client at risk for infection and bleeding.

Cognitive Skill

Take Action

References

Burchum & Rosenthal, 2019, pp. 1237–1238, 1240, 1247

CHAPTER 11 Inflammation: *Common Health Problems*

Answers With Rationales for Thinking Exercises

Exemplar 11A. Crohn's Disease (Medical-Surgical Nursing: Young Adult; Middle-Age Adult)

Thinking Exercise 11A-1

Answers

Nursing Action	Potential Complication	Appropriate Nursing Action for Each Complication
1 Administer blood or blood products via a large-bore IV catheter.	Enteroenteric fistula	**7** Administer antibiotic therapy.
2 Observe stool for undigested food or undissolved medication.	Small bowel obstruction	**6** Insert a nasogastric tube and connect to suction.
3 Administer IV sodium heparin.	Lower GI bleeding	**1** Administer blood or blood products via a large-bore IV catheter.
4 Monitor client for hematemesis.	Malabsorption	**2** Observe stool for undigested food or undissolved medication.
5 Monitor for signs and symptoms of irritable bowel syndrome.		
6 Insert a nasogastric tube and connect to suction.		
7 Administer antibiotic therapy.		

Rationales

An enteroenteric fistula (an opening between two or more portions of the small bowel) is a common complication of Crohn's disease and can cause infection. Therefore antibiotics are prescribed to prevent peritonitis. Small bowel obstruction, either partial or complete, can cause serious complications, including abdominal distention, fluid and electrolyte imbalance, and severe pain. The nurse would insert a nasogastric tube, most likely a Salem sump tube, and connect it to suction to remove excessive secretions that tend to accumulate during a bowel obstruction and to rest the GI tract. Lower GI bleeding due to severe inflammation from the disease often requires blood replacement. Inflammation can also cause malabsorption of vital nutrients. The presence of undigested food or medication indicates that nutrients and medications are not being absorbed in the small bowel. Severe malabsorption can cause weight loss requiring nutritional interventions, including enteral supplements or parenteral nutrition.

Cognitive Skill

Take Action

Reference

Ignatavicius et al., 2018, pp. 1156–1161

Thinking Exercise 11A-2

Answers

Correct answers are in **bold type**.

Assessment	Assessment Findings on Admission 24 Hours Ago	Current Assessment Findings
Temperature	**100°F (37.8°C)**	**101.8°F (38.8°C)**
Heart rate	78 beats/min	82 beats/min
Blood pressure	128/76 mm Hg	124/72 mm Hg
White blood cell count	**9200/mm³ (9.2 × 10⁹/L)**	**13,500/mm³ (13.5 × 10⁹/L)**
Sodium	**138 mEq/L (138 mmol/L)**	**133 mEq/L (133 mmol/L)**
Potassium	**3.6 mEq/L (3.6 mmol/L)**	**3.2 mEq/L (3.2 mmol/L)**

Rationales

The nurse would be concerned about the client's increased body temperature combined with her increase in white blood cell (WBC) count. The increase is above the normal range for a WBC count. These findings indicate probable infection, which needs to be treated. The client's sodium and potassium have both decreased to below the normal range for these electrolytes. As a result, the client is at risk for cardiac dysrhythmias, skeletal muscle weakness, and mental status changes. These electrolytes must be replaced to prevent these complications.

Cognitive Skill

Recognize Cues

References

Pagana & Pagana, 2018, pp. 368, 417–418, 466–467; Pagana et al., 2019, pp. 420, 479, 549

Thinking Exercise 11A-3

Answers

Nursing Action	Indicated	Contraindicated	Non-Essential
Monitor the client's hemoglobin and hematocrit levels.	X		
Prepare to administer a blood or blood product transfusion.	X		
Decrease the rate of the IV infusion.		X	
Prepare the client for a GI bleeding scan.	X		

Continued

Nursing Action	Indicated	Contraindicated	Non-Essential
Monitor pulse and blood pressure frequently.	X		
Document the number of the client's daily stools.			X

Rationales

The client has lower GI bleeding; this can cause decreased hemoglobin and hematocrit levels, which the nurse needs to monitor every 6 to 8 hours. To replace lost fluid volume, the nurse ensures that the client has IV access with two large-bore catheters for increasing IV fluids and transfusing blood and/or blood products. The client will have a scan to detect the site and severity of the GI bleeding. The number of the client's stools does not need to be monitored. However, the quality of stools, including observing for gross blood or testing for occult blood, should be monitored.

Cognitive Skill

Generate Solutions

Reference

Ignatavicius et al., 2018, p. 1156

Thinking Exercise 11A-4

Answers

A, B, C, E, F, G, H

Rationales

The client who has an enterocutaneous fistula is at risk for infection, including systemic sepsis. Therefore the nurse monitors for temperature and WBC elevation. A decreased blood pressure with an increased pulse indicates possible onset of septic shock (Choice C). IV antibiotic therapy is administered, usually with two or more drugs to prevent infection (Choice H). The client is also at risk for skin breakdown from the enzymatic drainage of the small intestine. Therefore, skin care and interventions to enhance healing include protecting the skin using a skin barrier and pouch system or negative-pressure wound therapy for copious drainage (Choices A and F). The client requires additional protein and calories for healing (Choice G). The nurse would consult with the registered dietitian nutritionist to increase these nutrients in the client's diet (Choice B). The nurse would carefully monitor the client's fluid and electrolyte status because the contents of the small intestine are rich in potassium and sodium (Choice E).

Cognitive Skill

Take Action

Reference

Ignatavicius et al., 2018, p. 1160

Thinking Exercise 11A-5

Answers

Medication	Dose, Route, Frequency	Drug Class	Indication
Sulfasalazine	2 g orally each day	5-ASA drug	**Decreases inflammatory response**
Infliximab	5 mg/kg IV at 0, 2, and 6 weeks followed by maintenance infusions of 5 mg/kg every 8 weeks	**Biologic response modifier**	Decreases inflammatory and immune response

Medication	Dose, Route, Frequency	Drug Class	Indication
Ciprofloxacin XR	500 mg orally each day	**Fluoroquinolone**	Manages infection
Methotrexate	**25 mg orally once weekly**	Immunosuppressant	Decreases disease activity
Metronidazole	750 mg orally 3 times a day	Antibiotic	Manages infection

Cognitive Skill

Analyze Cues

References

Burchum & Rosenthal, 2019, pp. 912, 991–993, 1097–1099; Ignatavicius et al., 2018, pp. 1152–1153, 1159

Thinking Exercise 11A-6

Answers

B, D

Rationales

All of the choices about the ostomy are expected *except for* the stoma being dark red-purplish (Choice B). This findings should be reported to the primary health care provider immediately. A healthy new colostomy stoma should be reddish pink and protrude about ¾ in (2 cm) from the abdominal wall. The nurse would also report the client's severe pain, which is not expected when PCA is used for pain control (Choice D).

Cognitive Skill

Analyze Cues

Reference

Ignatavicius et al., 2018, p. 1131

Exemplar 11B. Appendicitis/Appendectomy (Pediatric Nursing: Adolescent)

Thinking Exercise 11B-1

Answers

- Temperature = 102°F (40.2°C)
- Acute pain of 10/10 on a 0 to 10 pain scale
- Pain "a few days" ago, but then improved until today
- Parents are Spanish speaking
- Heart rate = 123 beats/min
- Respirations = 34 breaths/min
- CT scan with contrast = inflammation of the appendix with fecalith present; free fluid and a 3 mm × 5 mm area of localized fluid formation present
- WBCs = 18,800/mm³ (18.8 × 10⁹/L)
- CO₂ = 18 mEq/L (18 mmol/L)

Rationales

Appendicitis is highly prevalent in the school-age child and initially presents as colicky pain that will localize to the lower right quadrant of the abdomen but is commonly associated with a sudden absence of pain when the appendix ruptures. A low-grade fever is common, but anything over 101°F (38.3°C) is of concern, as well as tachycardia and tachypnea. CT results are suggestive of rupture and abscess formation, which are supported by the elevated white blood cell count. The carbon dioxide is suggestive of dehydration and acidosis. That the parents speak only Spanish indicates a need to obtain a translator to provide them with information and to obtain informed consent for surgery and other procedures that may be needed.

Cognitive Skill

Recognize Cues

References

Hockenberry & Wilson, 2019, pp. 585–586, 1078–1081; Pagana & Pagana, 2018, pp. 126, 171–172, 251–253, 362, 368, 468–469; Pagana et al., 2019, pp. 155–156, 549–550

Thinking Exercise 11B-2

Answers

The nurse recognizes that an elevated temperature and an elevated white blood cell count are factors that complicate the treatment of appendicitis and need to be closely monitored. Failure to treat this health problem can lead to bowel obstruction, peritonitis, and sepsis.

Rationales

A temperature over 101°F (38.3°C) is elevated and one of the factors that could complicate the management of appendicitis. Increased temperature is usually an indication of infection caused by a ruptured appendix. Complications associated with ruptured appendix or delayed treatment include partial or complete bowel obstruction, peritonitis, and sepsis, which could lead to death (in rare cases).

Cognitive Skill

Prioritize Hypotheses

References

Hockenberry & Wilson, 2019 pp. 585–586, 1078–1081; Pagana & Pagana, 2018, pp. 126, 171–172, 251–253, 468–469; Pagana et al., 2019, pp. 155–156, 549–550

Thinking Exercise 11B-3

Answers

B, E, H

Rationales

An inflammation of the appendix can lead to rupture and infection (Choices B and E). Clients who have infection typically have an elevated temperature leading to dehydration (Choice H). Children can become dehydrated more quickly than adults because they have less body fluid.

Cognitive Skill

Prioritize Hypotheses

References

Hockenberry & Wilson, 2019, pp. 585–586, 1078–1081

Thinking Exercise 11B-4

Answers

Potential Nursing Action	Appropriate Nursing Action
Administer piperacillin and tazobactam intravenously.	X
Monitor oxygen saturation and CO_2 levels.	
Encourage oral clear liquids.	
Give the child intravenous morphine IV push.	X
Encourage the child to share his concerns with his parents.	X
Maintain 5%D/0.45% NS with 20 mEq/L (20 mmol/L) of KCl at 66 mL/hr.	X
Administer ondansetron immediately.	X
Maintain accurate intake and output.	X
Encourage visitors to help manage pain.	
Monitor daily weight using the same scale at the same time.	X
Monitor stool count for the next 3 days.	
Explain to the child about how pain control and healing are interrelated.	X
Encourage the use of incentive spirometer every 2 hours.	

Rationales

Administering antibiotics to treat infection and the abscess is of high importance. Because the child is not tolerating food or fluids, which could be a sign of bowel obstruction, maintaining appropriate hydration is also essential. IV fluids (IVF) should contain saline and include potassium chloride to replace the loss of sodium through vomiting and the lack of dietary intake of potassium. The nurse would keep the client NPO and provide IV analgesics (such as morphine) and antiemetics (such as ondansetron). The pediatric client who is vomiting, has decreased oral intake, and is receiving IVF should have accurate intake and output measurements and a daily weight to evaluate fluid status. It is not uncommon for 10-year-old children to lie if they feel that it is what is wanted or supported by their parents, or if they believe that it will help them meet their parent's expectations (e.g., being able to go home sooner). Helping the pediatric client to understand why controlling his pain will help him heal is important. Soliciting parental support would be essential to achieve adequate pain control.

Cognitive Skill

Take Action

References

Hockenberry & Wilson, 2019, pp. 571, 585–586, 1078–1081; Burchum & Rosenthal, 2019, pp. 267–281, 474, 981–982, 1036

Thinking Exercise 11B-5

Answers

Correct answers are in **bold type.**

	Current	24 Hours Ago	48 Hours Ago
Serum Lab Results			
Hemoglobin	**9.8 g/dL (98 g/L)**	10.9 g/dL (10⁹ g/L)	11.7 g/dL (117 g/L)
Hematocrit	**35.1% (0.35)**	41.8% (0.42)	44.6% (0.45)
Platelet count	**148,000/mm³ (148 × 109/L)**	200,000/mm³ (200 × 10⁹/L)	211,000/mm³ (211 × 10⁹/L)
White blood cell count	**12,700/ mm³ (12.7 × 109/L)**	12,200/ mm³ (12.2 × 10⁹/L)	11,700/ mm³ (11.7 × 10⁹/L)
Bands	**11%**	3%	0
Potassium	**3.2 mEq/L (3.2 mmol.L)**	3.4 mEq/L (3.4 mmol/L)	3.6 mEq/L (3.6 mmol/L)
Sodium	**132 mEq/L (132 mmol/L)**	129 mEq/L (129 mmol/L)	134 mEq/L (134 mmol/L)
Glucose	**111 mg/dL**	102 mg/dL	99 mg/dL
CO_2	20 mEq/L (20 mmol/L)	19 mEq/L (19 mmol/L)	16 mEq/L (16 mmol/L)
Prealbumin	**18 mg/dL (180 mg/L)**	22 mg/dL (220 mg/L)	24 mg/dL (240 mg/L)
Blood urea nitrogen	**18 mg/dL (6.5 mmol/L)**	12 mg/dL (4.4 mmol/L)	11 mg/dL (4.0 mmol/L)
Creatinine	**1.02 mg/dL (89 mcmol/L)**	0.6 mg/dL (53 mcmol/L)	0.45 mg/dL (40 mcmol/L)
Vital Signs			
Temperature	**101.6°F (38.6°C)**	100.1°F (37.8°C)	99.1°F (37.3°C)
Heart rate (beats/min)	98	90	92
Respirations (breaths/min)	16	18	16
Pain score	**7**	4	5
Daily weight (lb [kg])	**53 (24.1)**	50 (22.7)	51

Rationales

The decrease in hemoglobin and hematocrit values is suggestive of possible internal bleeding. Although the WBC count appears somewhat stable, the decrease in platelets, elevated temperature, and increase in bands suggest a left shift, which is highly indicative that the client is experiencing an overwhelming infection. Elevation of the serum creatinine, BUN, and weight suggests possible acute kidney injury. Increased pain also supports the presence of severe infection. The client's serum potassium level is currently below the normal range and his sodium levels continue to be low, most likely due to vomiting. Although the prealbumin level is currently within normal range, the downward trend may indicate the initial stages of malnutrition.

Cognitive Skill

Recognize Cues

References

Hockenberry & Wilson, 2019, pp. 585–586, 1078–1081; Pagana & Pagana, 2018, pp. 126, 171–172, 227, 248, 251–253, 362, 368, 371–372, 468–469, 515, 962; Pagana et al., 2019, pp. 155–156, 205–207, 285–286, 299–300, 416, 424–425, 534–536, 549–550

Thinking Exercise 11B-6

Answers

Assessment Finding	Effective	Ineffective	Unrelated
Hemoglobin = 9.8 g/dL (98 g/L)		X	
Platelet count = 128,000/mm³ (128 × 10⁹/L)		X	
Bands = 11%		X	
Potassium = 3.2 mEq/L (3.2 mmol/L)		X	
Glucose = 111 mg/dL (6.2 mmol/L)			X
CO_2 = 20 mEq/L (20 mmol/L)	X		
Creatinine = 1.02 mg/dL (89 mcmol/L)		X	
Prealbumin = 18 mg/dL (480 mg/L)		X	
Tolerating clear liquid diet	X		
Temperature = 101.6°F (38.6°C)		X	
Heart rate = 98 beats/min	X		
Respirations = 16 breaths/min	X		
Pain = 7 on a 0 to 10 pain intensity scale		X	
Incision site intact, red, and edematous with serous drainage under transparent dressing		X	
Child Life Specialist reports that school tutor for home has been arranged			X
Client playing video game with sibling			X

Rationales

The client's hemoglobin, platelet count, and serum potassium levels are not within normal limits. His elevated temperature, increased bands, reddened incision, and unresolved pain indicate that infection is still present and therefore treatment has not been effective. Elevation of the serum creatinine suggests possible early acute kidney injury. The child's heart rate and respiratory rate are normal. Blood glucose results are unrelated to the client's condition. The normalization of the CO_2 and potassium indicates that treatment has been effective. Although providing appropriate play and addressing the educational needs of the pediatric client are part of nursing care, it is not relevant in determining whether or not the expected outcomes related to abscess and postoperative complications are being appropriately managed. Although the prealbumin level is currently within normal range, the downward trend may indicate the initial stages of malnutrition.

Cognitive Skill

Evaluate Outcomes

References

Hockenberry & Wilson, 2019, pp. 585–586, 1078–1081; Pagana & Pagana, 2018, pp. 126, 171–172, 227, 248, 251–253, 362, 368, 371–372, 468–469, 515, 962; Pagana et al., 2019, pp. 155–156, 205–207, 285–286, 299–300, 416, 424–425, 534–536, 549–550

CHAPTER 12 Infection: *Common Health Problems*

Answers With Rationales for Thinking Exercises

Exemplar 12A. Cellulitis (Medical-Surgical Nursing: Middle-Age Adult)

Thinking Exercise 12A-1

Answers

Based on the nurse's assessment findings, the client is at risk for complications as a result of her cellulitis and wound, especially neurovascular compromise and sepsis. Assessment findings for which the nurse should monitor include left arm tingling and numbness, diminished left radial pulse, increased temperature, and leukocytosis.

Rationales

The client's left upper arm is swollen and very inflamed. Excessive swelling could increase pressure on the nerves and blood vessels in the left arm causing dysfunction that would be evidenced by tingling and numbness and a diminished radial pulse. She is also at risk for systemic infection, which would manifest as increased body temperature and leukocytosis (increased white blood cell count).

Cognitive Skill

Prioritize Hypotheses

References

Ignatavicius et al., 2018, pp. 466, 1033–1034

Thinking Exercise 12A-2

Answers

Nursing Action	Indicated	Contraindicated	Non-Essential
Place the client on Contact Precautions.	X		
Apply cold compresses on her left upper arm.		X	
Elevate the client's left arm on a pillow.	X		

Nursing Action	Indicated	Contraindicated	Non-Essential
Take a wound culture every shift to determine if the infection is improving.			X
Initiate IV access for the client to receive fluids and antibiotic therapy.	X		
Administer subcutaneous sodium heparin every 12 hours.			X

Rationales

The client has an infectious draining wound and requires wound precautions to prevent transmission of infectious pathogens (MRSA). She will receive IV fluids to prevent dehydration until she is taking adequate oral fluids and needs the IV access for antibiotic therapy. Her arm should be elevated on a pillow to decrease arm swelling, and heat rather than cold compresses would be used to improve blood flow to the wound and promote healing. She will not need multiple wound cultures and will not have to stay in bed. Therefore there is no need for administration of heparin to prevent venous thromboembolism.

Cognitive Skill

Generate Solutions

References

Ignatavicius et al., 2018, p. 466; also see Chapter 23

Thinking Exercise 12A-3

Answers

A, B, C, D, E, F, G

Rationales

Daptomycin is a cyclic lipopeptide antibacterial drug that is generally well tolerated. Rare adverse effects include myopathy (muscle injury) and eosinophilic pneumonia (Choice D). Tobramycin is an aminoglycoside that can be ototoxic (causing tinnitus) (Choice B) and nephrotoxic (causing kidney dysfunction) (Choice C). Any antibiotic can cause GI symptoms such as nausea and diarrhea (Choice A). Peak and trough levels of the drugs may be drawn (Choice E) and the IV site will likely be changed frequently (every 48 to 72 hours as tolerated) to prevent vein irritation if the client has other venous options (Choice F). If or when the client has no GI signs and symptoms, the IV can be converted to a saline lock for administering IV drugs only (Choice G).

Cognitive Skill

Take Action

References

Burchum & Rosenthal, 2019, pp. 1063–1065, 1099–1100

Thinking Exercise 12A-4

Answers

Based on the nurse's assessment, the client most likely has *Clostridium difficile* infection as a result of antibiotic therapy. The most common drugs used to treat this problem are vancomycin and metronidazole. The nurse should remind the nursing staff to use strict hand hygiene measures and use strict Contact Precautions to prevent transmission to other clients on the hospital unit.

Cognitive Skill

Prioritize Hypotheses

Rationales

C. difficile infection (CDI) is a highly contagious disease and must be contained in the hospital by using Contact Precautions and careful handwashing. Alcohol-based hand rubs are not effective against the pathogen's spores and should not be used when caring for clients with this infection. Metronidazole is recommended as the first-line drug for mild-to-moderate cases of CDI, but vancomycin is used for more severe infection.

References

Burchum & Rosenthal, pp. 1046–1047; Ignatavicius et al., 2018; also see Chapter 23

Thinking Exercise 12A-5

Answers

Assessment Finding	Effective	Ineffective	Unrelated
Client's oral temperature this a.m. is 98°F (36.7°C).	X		
Client reports mild pain in upper left arm at 2/10 on a scale of 0 to 10.	X		
Client reports that she has had less diarrhea today than the past 2 days.	X		
Client's early morning finger stick blood glucose (FSBG) was 97 mg/dL (5.4 mmol/L).	X		
Client's left upper arm slightly reddened when compared with the right upper arm.		X	
Client reports that her back is more achy since she came to the hospital.			X

Rationales

The client demonstrates signs and symptoms of wound healing, including a normal temperature and decreased arm pain, but there is a slight amount of redness around the wound. Her blood glucose is within normal limits. When a diabetic client has an infection, he or she usually has an increased blood glucose level. The client's diarrhea has decreased, which indicates that the *C. difficile* infection is improving. Having an achy back due to being in the hospital is not related to her diagnoses.

Cognitive Skill

Evaluate Outcomes

References

Ignatavicius et al., 2018, Chapter 23

Thinking Exercise 12A-6

Answers

C, D, E, F, G

Rationales

The wound is infected and does not require sterile technique for a dressing change. The client needs to take all of the prescribed antibiotics. The nurse would teach the client and her daughter to notify the primary health care provider if diarrhea increases or if cellulitis symptoms return (Choices C, D, and G). The client should rest frequently and avoid strenuous activity to allow the infection to resolve completely (Choices E and F).

Cognitive Skill

Take Action

Reference

Ignatavicius et al., 2018, pp. 457–458

Exemplar 12B. Respiratory Syncytial Virus (RSV) (Pediatric Nursing: Infant)

Thinking Exercise 12B-1

Answers

- Born at 32 weeks' gestation via spontaneous vaginal delivery
- Uncomplicated NICU stay for 5 weeks
- Mother reports that 7-year-old sibling has a "cold"
- Mother reports that the infant has not eaten well today
- Temporal temperature = 99.0°F (37.2°C)
- Heart rate = 156 beats/min
- Respirations = 66 breaths/min
- Nasal flaring
- Making soft sounds with each exhalation
- Substernal retractions
- Pale pink mucous membranes
- Quiet and arouses slightly during assessment

Rationales

The infant presents with several clinical manifestations of respiratory distress, including mild tachypnea and tachycardia. Cardinal signs of respiratory distress in an infant are grunting, flaring, and retracting. As the respiratory distress progresses, listlessness and poor feeding are signs of severe distress. The preterm infant is at higher risk for many complications, especially infection. An ill sibling increases the risk and possibility of infection.

Cognitive Skill

Recognize Cues

References

Hockenberry & Wilson, 2019, pp. 365, 371, 413, 416, 1188, 1675

Thinking Exercise 12B-2

Answers

Nursing Action	Indicated	Contraindicated	Non-Essential
Provide parents with consent forms for immunizations.		X	
Obtain oxygen saturation level.	X		
Complete the growth chart.			X

Continued

Nursing Action	Indicated	Contraindicated	Non-Essential
Assess for presence or history of rhinorrhea.	X		
Obtain manual blood pressure.			X
Administer *Haemophilus influenzae* type b (Hib) vaccine.		X	
Administer varicella vaccine.		X	
Provide anticipatory guidance education for car seat safety.			X
Provide parents with injury prevention education for infants.			X
Suction infant to clear nasal passages.	X		
Provide oxygen for O$_2$ saturation less than 90%.	X		
Obtain a nasopharyngeal swab for culture.	X		

Rationales

Indicated nursing actions address the infant's respiratory status first; monitoring and administering oxygen and maintaining nasal patency are extremely important because infants are obligatory nose breathers. Obtaining a nasopharyngeal swab is important to identify the source of infection and to determine if the source of infection is bacterial or viral. All vaccines are contraindicated at this time because the infant is showing signs of infection, so obtaining consent is also contraindicated. The varicella vaccine is contraindicated until age 12 months. Providing anticipatory guidance, health promotion teaching such as car seat safety, and evaluating the growth and development of the infant are certainly appropriate for the well-child visit, but not essential at this time. Manual blood pressures on an infant are very difficult to obtain and in general are not part of the routine well-child check until 3 years of age.

Cognitive Skill

Generate Solutions

References

Hockenberry & Wilson, 2019, pp. 365, 371, 413, 416, 1188, 1675

Thinking Exercise 12B-3

Answers

To ensure accurate dosages of medications, the nurse will practice safe medication administration principles. Per the primary health care provider's prescription, the nurse will give acetaminophen for fevers higher than 100.5°F (38°C) as needed. To provide an accurate dose, the nurse will calculate that to give 10 mg/kg per dose of acetaminophen with a 90 mg/0.9 mL solution, the nurse will administer 0.35 mL using a 1.0 mL oral syringe, or 35 mg of acetaminophen.

Rationales

The nurse's priority during medication administration is to keep the client safe. Therefore the nurse must use safe medication administration principles, which include accuracy, to maintain client safety. Acetaminophen is the only medication approved for a 2-month-old infant. A safe dose of acetaminophen is 10 mg/kg per dose with a maximum dosage of 75 mg/kg per day. All medications given orally should be given only in an oral syringe using the smallest available size to measure the medication to the nearest hundredth. Oral syringes are unable to calculate to the thousandths place.

Cognitive Skill

Take Action

References

Hockenberry & Wilson, 2019, pp. 365, 371, 413, 416, 1188, 1675; Burchum & Rosenthal, 2019, pp. 64–65, 864–866

Thinking Exercise 12B-4

Answers

Nursing Action	Indicated	Contraindicated	Non-Essential
Administer antibiotics.		X	
Monitor oxygen saturation and CO_2 levels.	X		
Encourage oral clear liquids.		X	
Maintain Contact and Droplet Precautions.	X		
Perform frequent nasal and oral suctioning.	X		
Perform deep suctioning two times daily.	X		
Administer albuterol.			X
Maintain accurate intake and output.	X		
Encourage visitors.		X	
Administer opioid pain medication.		X	
Instruct the infant's mother to pump and store breast milk.	X		
Maintain 5%D/0.45% NS with 20 mEq of KCl per liter at 14 mL/hr.	X		

Rationales

Indicated nursing actions include all actions that maintain airway patency and support breathing and oxygenation. Treating a viral infection with an antibiotic is contraindicated. Opioids are not given to infants with RSV. Oral fluids of any kind are also contraindicated until the respiratory rate is below 60 breaths/min due to the increased risk of aspiration; therefore it is important to have breast-feeding mothers pump and store breast milk to maintain a milk supply. Visitors are discouraged because RSV is highly contagious and dangerous for the very young and the very old. IV fluids are appropriate for the infant who is unable to take oral fluids; it is also indicated to thin mucous secretions and facilitate the evacuation of mucus during suctioning. The use of albuterol (orally or inhaled) in the absence of wheezing and corticosteroids is controversial and has not been shown to be effective in the treatment of RSV.

Cognitive Skill

Generate Solutions

References

Hockenberry & Wilson, 2019, pp. 365, 371, 413, 416, 1188, 1675; Pagana & Pagana, 2018, pp. 248–249, 251–254, 362–364; Pagana et al., 2019, pp. 295–298, 299–300, 416–418

Thinking Exercise 12B-5

Answers

Assessment Finding	Effective	Ineffective	Unrelated
Oxygen saturation 94% on ¼ L/min via nasal cannula	X		
<2nd percentile for height			X
Temperature 99.0°F (37.2°C)			X
Heart rate = 116 beats/min	X		
Respirations = 46 breaths/min	X		
Baby is awake and fussy		X	
17¾ inches or 45.4 cm in length			X
Baby is breast-feeding every 2–3 hr	X		
Weight is 3.41 kg (7 lb 5 oz)		X	

Rationales

Nursing actions that demonstrate effectiveness or improvement of the respiratory status include lower respiratory and heart rates, improved feeding, and maintaining oxygen saturation with supplemental oxygen. Weight loss, especially with IV fluids, suggests that the infant's hydration and nutritional needs are not being met. Fussiness is an indication of respiratory distress, and therefore the infant should be closely monitored by the nurse. Outcomes related to growth and development are unrelated to RSV desired outcomes. Low-grade fever is expected in a viral illness and is an unrelated response to the nursing actions presented.

Cognitive Skill

Evaluate Outcomes

References

Hockenberry & Wilson, 2019, pp. 365, 371, 413, 416, 1188, 1675

Thinking Exercise 12B-6

Answers

A, C, D, F, H, I

Rationales

Discharge instructions should include maintaining adequate nasal patency to promote adequate gas exchange and oxygenation (Choice C). Maintaining adequate nutrition and using good hand hygiene are the best ways to minimize the spread of the illness (Choices A and I). Although keeping the infant isolated from actively sick family members is recommended, keeping them away from all family members is not realistic. It is always recommended to keep children away from secondhand and thirdhand smoke, but especially preterm infants and infants with respiratory illness (Choice F). Discharge teaching should always include when to call the primary health care provider (Choice D). Palivizumab is a monoclonal antibody infusion that is indicated for preterm infants born at less than 32 weeks' gestation to prevent RSV infection and not to treat RSV. Using ambulatory care clinics to provide aggressive suctioning is one method used to decrease the incidence of admission or readmission.

Cognitive Skill

Take Action

References

Hockenberry & Wilson, 2019, pp. 365, 371, 413, 416, 1188, 1675

CHAPTER 13 Sensory Perception: *Cataracts*

Answers With Rationales for Thinking Exercises

Exemplar 13. Cataracts (Medical-Surgical Nursing: Older Adult)

Thinking Exercise 13-1

Answers

A, B, D, E, G

Rationales

As people get older, they develop presbyopia (nearsightedness due to aging) and often an inability to drive at night due to bright lights. This client is at risk for these visual changes in addition to his long history of decreased vision. As a result he has trouble walking to the bathroom in the dark and has sustained minor injuries. Therefore, increasing light (Choice B), moving obstacles out of the walking path (Choices E and G), and ensuring a nonskid floor will keep him safe at night at home (Choice D). The nurse would teach the client not to drive at night and instead ask someone else to drive him to where he needs to go (Choice A). This alternative would hopefully prevent a potential accident for the client.

Cognitive Skill

Generate Solutions

Reference

Ignatavicius et al., 2019, p. 974

Thinking Exercise 13-2

Answers

Medication	Dose, Route, Frequency	Drug Class	Indication
Apremilast	30 mg orally twice daily	Phosphodiesterase type 4 (PDE-4) inhibitor	**Psoriasis**
Cetirizine	5–10 mg orally every 24 hr	Second-generation H$_1$ antagonist	Seasonal allergic rhinitis
Pantoprazole	**40 mg orally once daily**	Proton pump inhibitor	GERD
Sildenafil	50 mg orally PRN	Phosphodiesterase type 5 (PDE-5) inhibitor	**Erectile dysfunction**
Rivaroxaban	20 mg orally once daily with the evening meal	**Direct factor Xa inhibitor**	Nonvalvular atrial fibrillation

Cognitive Skill

Analyze Cues

References

Burchum & Rosenthal, 2019, pp. 619–620, 797–802, 950, 966

Thinking Exercise 13-3

Answers

A, B, C, E, F, G, H

Rationales

Although the surgery will be performed in the ophthalmologist's office, someone will need to drive the client to the office and back home after the procedure (Choice C). Several types of eyedrops and ointments will be needed before and after surgery that will impair the client's ability to see out of the operative eye and drive (Choices B, E, and H). Rivaroxaban affects blood clotting and will need to be discontinued most likely for 5 to 7 days prior to surgery (Choice A). The operative eye will be red for some time during the healing process (Choice F). After healing, glasses or contact lenses will likely still be needed for this client who had severely impaired vision prior to the procedure unless he also has LASIK or other additional procedures (Choice G).

Cognitive Skill

Take Action

Reference

Ignatavicius et al., 2019, pp. 969–975

Thinking Exercise 13-4

Answers

Health Teaching	Potential Postoperative Complication	Appropriate Health Teaching for Each Potential Postoperative Complication
1 "Report increased swelling or redness of the operative eyelid."	Increased intraocular pressure	3 "Remind the client to avoid coughing, sneezing, lifting, and sexual intercourse until after his follow-up visit."
2 "Encourage the client to eat high-protein foods to promote healing."	Infection	8 "Contact the surgeon immediately if there is yellow or green discharge on the eye dressing when you change it."
3 "Remind the client to avoid coughing, sneezing, lifting, and sexual intercourse until after his follow-up visit."	Hemorrhage	5 "Observe the eye bandage for any signs of bleeding."
4 "Have the client sleep in a sitting position at all times until after the follow-up visit."	Eyelid swelling	1 "Report increased swelling or redness of the operative eyelid."
5 "Observe the eye bandage for any signs of bleeding."	Detached retina	6 "Contact the surgeon immediately if the client has severe pain or sees floating particles in the operative eye."
6 "Contact the surgeon immediately if the client has severe pain or sees floating particles in the operative eye."		

Health Teaching	Potential Postoperative Complication	Appropriate Health Teaching for Each Potential Postoperative Complication
7 "Be sure the client takes his oral antibiotic for 14 days."		
8 "Contact the surgeon immediately if there is yellow or green discharge on the eye dressing when you change it."		

Rationales

Increased intraocular pressure can cause damage to the operative eye and must be prevented by avoiding activities such as coughing, sneezing, lifting, and sexual intercourse. Infection is indicated by a yellowish or green discharge that often has a foul odor. Hemorrhage or bleeding would be obvious by observing the dressing covering the operative eye. Eyelid swelling and redness are also easily observed. If the client reports seeing floating particles or flashes of light and/or reports sudden severe pain, he may be experiencing a detached retina, which can result from the surgery. This is a medical emergency!

Cognitive Skill

Take Action

Reference

Ignatavicius et al., 2019, pp. 969–975

Thinking Exercise 13-5

Answers

Assessment Finding	Effective	Ineffective	Unrelated
Has no bleeding or discharge from the operative eye	X		
Operative eyelid is swollen but not reddened		X	
Vision in operative eye is improved	X		
Reports new-onset constipation			X
Reports no sharp or sudden episodes of pain	X		
Reports no flashes of light or floating shapes	X		
Tearing eyes and nose from allergic response to pollen			X
Reports frontal sinus headache			X

Rationales

Most of the eye assessment findings indicate that the operative eye is healing well without complications. The only concern is that the operative eyelid is swollen, although it is not reddened. The primary health care provider would need to determine the cause and possibly treat that problem. Reports of constipation or having allergic rhinitis symptoms and headache are not related to the cataract surgery.

Cognitive Skill

Evaluate Outcomes

Reference

Ignatavicius et al., 2019, pp. 969–975

CHAPTER 14 Cognition: *Common Health Problems*

Answers With Rationales for Thinking Exercises

Exemplar 14A. Delirium (Mental Health Nursing: Older Adult)

Thinking Exercise 14A-1

Answers

A, D, F, G

Rationales

Older adults are often at high risk for acute confusion (delirium) when they experience physical stress, such as surgery and new-onset health problems; and emotional stress, such as relocating from their home to an acute care setting (Choices A, D, and F). The client had surgery for a lower GI bleed, and she may be anemic as a result (Choice G). There is no indication that she has infection, fluid overload, or substance use disorder, but if she did have any of these problems, they would likely contribute to developing or worsening delirium.

Cognitive Skill

Analyze Cues

References

Halter, 2018, pp. 431–432; Ignatavicius et al., 2018, pp. 17, 38

Thinking Exercise 14A-2

Answers

- Hypertension controlled by hydrochlorothiazide and diet
- Two falls at home without major injury in the past 6 months
- Diabetes mellitus type 2 controlled by diet and metformin

Rationales

The client is receiving thiazide-type diuretic therapy for hypertension, which can cause hyponatremia (decreased serum sodium). Signs and symptoms of hyponatremia include weakness, dizziness, and acute confusion. The client has already fallen at home, most likely related to this electrolyte imbalance or orthostatic hypotension, another adverse effect of diuretic therapy. The nurse would also be concerned about her history of diabetes mellitus (DM) because the client had surgery, which can cause her blood glucose to increase. DM makes the client more susceptible to slower wound healing and infection.

Cognitive Skill

Recognize Cues

References

Ignatavicius et al., 2018, pp. 173–174, 725–726, 1303–1304

Thinking Exercise 14A-3

Answers

Nursing Action	Indicated	Contraindicated	Non-Essential
Request that the surgeon change the client's analgesic medication to a nonopioid drug.	X		
Be sure that environmental orientation cues are available, such as a large clock, in the client's room.	X		
Place the client on fall precautions.	X		
Continue to monitor serum sodium levels.	X		
Monitor pulse and blood pressure every 1 to 2 hours.	X		
Request a prescription for an antipsychotic medication.		X	
Reorient the client frequently.	X		
Request that a family member or friend stay with the client at night.	X		
Prepare to administer a blood or blood product transfusion.			X
Ask family to bring in familiar or favorite items that may help reorient or distract client from pulling out IV.	X		

Rationales

The client has delirium (acute confusion), which is usually reversible if the cause is removed or resolved. Opioid analgesic medications often cause delirium, especially in older adults. Therefore the nurse would request a change in the client's drug therapy for pain management. The main approach to managing delirium is to reorient the client and to provide environmental cues like large clocks to help with reorientation. The client is in a strange environment and might benefit from being with family members or friends and having some familiar or favorite items with her during her hospital stay. Antipsychotic medications are contraindicated for delirium unless the client has ongoing psychotic behaviors such as delusions and hallucinations. The nurse would continue to monitor the client's serum sodium levels because they have markedly decreased to below the normal range. Hyponatremia can contribute to acute confusion. The client's blood pressure has also decreased in a few hours and needs to be monitored more frequently. There is no indication that the client is anemic at this time, and therefore a blood or blood product transfusion is not necessary.

Cognitive Skill

Generate Solutions

References

Halter, 2018, pp. 431–432; Ignatavicius et al., 2018, pp. 17, 38

Thinking Exercise 14A-4

Answers

The client is experiencing a visual hallucination most likely due to delirium. Her acute confusion is most likely the result of urinary tract infection, anemia, or electrolyte imbalance. The nurse would request a complete blood cell count, basic metabolic panel, and urine culture, and carefully monitor the client's vital signs and voiding patterns.

Rationales

The client's increase in acute confusion may be due to postoperative complications, such as urinary tract infection (UTI) because she had a urinary catheter, postoperative anemia, or electrolyte imbalance due to medication or vomiting. The nurse would requests laboratory tests to verify if any of these complications are present, and assess the client carefully for changes in vital signs or voiding patterns. If the client has a UTI, she would likely have frequent urination in small amounts.

Cognitive Skill

Prioritize Hypotheses

References

Ignatavicius et al., 2018, pp. 173–174, 1354–1357

Thinking Exercise 14A-5

Answers

Assessment Finding	Effective	Ineffective	Unrelated
Alert and oriented × 3	X		
Has not had additional hallucinations	X		
Had a small stool this morning			X
Understands discharge instructions	X		
Has minimal surgical pain			X
No episodes of screaming or crying out for the past 3 days	X		
Has short-term memory loss at times		X	

Rationales

The client has no indications of delirium but continues to have short-term memory loss at times. This change will most likely improve as the client continues her recovery from surgery. Having a stool and minimal pain are not related to the client's delirium.

Cognitive Skill

Evaluate Outcomes

References

Halter, 2018, pp. 431–432; Ignatavicius et al., 2018, pp. 17, 38

Exemplar 14B. Alzheimer's Disease (Mental Health Nursing: Middle-Age Adult)

Thinking Exercise 14B-1

Answers

- Participated in football and ice hockey in high school and college
- Mother resides in a nursing home due to chronic heart failure, chronic kidney disease, and late-stage Alzheimer's disease
- Fell off a ladder last year and suffered a mild concussion
- Recently has had "problems with finding the right words at times"

Rationales

Although the client is under 65 years of age, he is at risk for Alzheimer's disease (AD) or other dementia because of his participation in very physical sports and a head injury from a fall. He is also at high risk because he has an immediate family member who has dementia. The nurse would be concerned that he is experiencing problems finding the words that he wants when communicating. This is a typical finding associated with AD.

Cognitive Skill

Recognize Cues

Reference

Halter, 2018, pp. 436–437

Thinking Exercise 14B-2

Answers

A, B, C, F, H

Rationales

Alzheimer's disease (AD) is a chronic, irreversible disease that progresses in three well-identified stages over many years (Choices A and B). During these stages, the client will need emotional support from friends and family (Choice C). While the client is lucid, he should plan advance directives with his family (Choice F). The best approach to manage early AD is to keep as physically and mentally active as possible (Choice H). Eventually the disease will cause impaired mobility and inability to perform ADLs.

Cognitive Skill

Take Action

Reference

Halter, 2018, pp. 437–444

Thinking Exercise 14B-3

Answers

Medication	Dose, Route, Frequency	Drug Class	Indication
Donepezil	10 mg orally once at bedtime	Cholinesterase inhibitor	Alzheimer's disease
Enalapril	5 mg orally once each day	Angiotensin-converting enzyme inhibitor	**Hypertension**
Furosemide	20 mg orally once in the morning	**High-ceiling (loop) diuretic**	Hypertension
Pantoprazole	**40 mg orally once each day**	Proton pump inhibitor	Gastroesophageal reflux disease (GERD)
Ibuprofen	200 mg orally 3-4 times each day	NSAID	Chronic low back pain and headaches

Cognitive Skill

Analyze Cues

References

Burchum & Rosenthal, 2019, pp. 201–203, 462–464, 486, 489, 859–860, 966

Thinking Exercise 14B-4

Answers

A, C, D, F, G, H, I

Rationales

Communicating with a client who has Alzheimer's disease or any other type of dementia can be very challenging. Many clients become frustrated, confrontational, and agitated when they have problems understanding what is being said or are cognitively overstimulated. Therefore distraction; decreased stimulation; use of short, simple language; and limiting choices that the client has to make help decrease these negative emotions (Choices A, C, D, and H). Fatigue or fear of the unfamiliar can exacerbate these emotions. Providing rest periods, a structure, and a consistent daily routine can decrease anxiety and provide comfort (Choices F and G). Reorienting clients who have moderate or severe AD is usually not effective because their reality is not the same as for those without dementia. Instead, validating the client's feelings is more comforting and reassuring (Choice I).

Cognitive Skill

Take Action

References

Halter, 2018, pp. 437–444; Ignatavicius et al., 2018, pp. 863–865

Thinking Exercise 14B-5

Answers

A, B, D, E, F, G

Rationales

The client's wife needs to practice self-care interventions to better help cope with her caregiving responsibilities. Humor, taking one day at a time, relaxing, having short respite periods, and being realistic in client expectations can help the caregiver cope with stress and prevent burnout (Choices A, B, D, E, and G). More information about caregiver coping and stress prevention is available from the Alzheimer's Association. This organization can also provide contact information about support groups that are available for family and friend caregivers (Choice F).

Cognitive Skill

Generate Solutions

Reference

Ignatavicius et al., 2018, pp. 866–867

CHAPTER 15 **Mood and Affect:** *Depression*

Answers With Rationales for Thinking Exercises

Exemplar 15. Depression (Mental Health Nursing: Adolescent)

Thinking Exercise 15-1

Answers

A, B, C, D, E, G, H, I, J

Rationales

Adolescents who have major depressive disorder (clinical depression) often rebel and cope with their sadness by substance use and/or increased sexual activity (Choices A, D, and G). Clients of all ages with depression often express that nothing they do gives them joy or pleasure (Choice I). Most clients who are depressed also verbalize that they have minimal energy, decreased appetite, insomnia, memory loss, and problems concentrating or focusing (Choices B, E, H, and J). Some clients become so severely depressed that they have suicidal ideation or attempt suicide (Choice C).

Cognitive Skill

Analyze Cues

Reference

Halter, 2018, pp. 245–253

Thinking Exercise 15-2

Answers

- Client's mother has a history of anorexia nervosa and major depressive disorder
- Client's height = 5 ft, 8 in (172.7 cm)
- Client's weight = 102 lb (46.3 kg)
- Small parallel linear scars on both upper thighs
- Dry flaky skin on most of her body
- Hair dry and brittle

Rationales

Clinical depression and eating disorders tend to have a genetic link and are more likely to occur in anyone if an immediate family member has these problems. The nurse would be concerned about the client's weight because she is underweight for her height. Her dry skin and brittle hair indicate that she is consuming inadequate nutrients. The small parallel linear scars indicate that the client is likely engaging in cutting behaviors, a type of nonsuicidal self-injury.

Cognitive Skill

Recognize Cues

References

Halter, 2018, pp. 245–253, 486–487

Thinking Exercise 15-3

Answers

Fluoxetine is a selective serotonin reuptake inhibitor that can be effective for treating both depression and eating disorders. The nurse teaches the client and her parents that this drug can cause common side effects including weight gain, nervousness, and sexual dysfunction. In addition, the nurse teaches them that this class of drugs makes clients at increased risk for suicide and the client must be monitored closely. A rare and life-threatening adverse effect of fluoxetine is serotonin syndrome, which can cause increased vital sign values, GI distress, seizures, and possibly apnea (death). Teach the client and family to call 911 if these signs and symptoms occur.

Cognitive Skill

Prioritize Hypotheses

Reference

Burchum & Rosenthal, 2019, pp. 355–359

Thinking Exercise 15-4

Answers

A, B, C, D, E, F

Rationales

All of the questions except Choice G are important for the therapist to ask the client who is depressed to ensure that the client is not in danger of potentially harming herself. Some clients threaten suicide, but having a plan on how to carry out the suicide would be the most serious concern to the therapist or nurse.

Cognitive Skill

Analyze Cues

Reference

Halter, 2018, pp. 478–480

Thinking Exercise 15-5

Answers

A, B, C, D, F

Rationales

All of the questions except Choice E are important for the therapist to ask the client who engages in nonsuicidal self-injury behaviors such as cutting. It is not important to determine how the client makes the cuts because the device has to be sharp enough to break the skin. Most "cutters" are female, and many engage in cutting behaviors as part of a group of girls.

Cognitive Skill

Take Action

Reference

Halter, 2018, pp. 486–487

Thinking Exercise 15-6

Answers

Assessment Finding	Effective	Ineffective	Unrelated
Continues to engage in cutting behaviors at times		X	
Adheres to the treatment plan each week	X		
Gained 10 lb (2.3 kg) in 2 months	X		
Has dinner with the family most nights	X		
Grades in school improving	X		
Acne worsened during the past month			X
Joined the tennis team at school	X		

Rationales

The client's signs and symptoms have improved since beginning and adhering to treatment for major depressive disorder and mild bulimia nervosa. She has gained weight, has begun to participate in school and family activities, and improved her grades. The client's acne has gotten worse, but this change is not related to her mental health problems. She is continuing the cutting behaviors at times, so interventions so far have not stopped her self-injury.

Cognitive Skill

Evaluate Outcomes

Reference

Halter, 2018, pp. 341–346

CHAPTER 16 Stress and Coping: *Generalized Anxiety Disorder*

Answers With Rationales for Thinking Exercises

Exemplar 16. Generalized Anxiety Disorder (Mental Health Nursing: Young Adult)

Thinking Exercise 16-1

Answers

- History of depression as a teenager but currently not being treated for this problem
- States that she has been extremely worried most days for the past 7 to 8 months about many day-to-day things and reports having difficulty controlling the worry
- Married for 1½ years and is starting out her practice as a clinical psychologist
- Husband lost his job 6 months ago due to his company's closure; remains unemployed
- Has student loans from graduate school and is having problems making payments
- Wants to get pregnant someday but feels too stressed to think about it now
- Is having problems sleeping—either getting to sleep or staying asleep
- Has been taking melatonin to help her sleep but is finding it only slightly effective
- Reports always feeling tired and having problems concentrating at work

Rationales

The nurse recognizes that the client has experienced increased stress for over 6 months that is causing sleep disturbances and excessive worry. Finances as a newly married woman have been the major source of her worries. Her history of depression is important because she may experience acute depression as a result of her stress level and inability to cope.

Cognitive Skill

Recognize Cues

Reference

Halter, 2018, pp. 277–278

Thinking Exercise 16-2

Answers

The nurse teaches the client that nonpharmacologic interventions for managing GAD include cognitive behavioral therapy, biofeedback, and relaxation techniques. If the client needs drug therapy to treat her mental health problem, the first-line drug classes used are selective serotonin reuptake inhibitors and serotonin-norepinephrine reuptake inhibitors. Buspirone is another preferred drug for GAD. Unlike other anxiolytics, this drug is not a central nervous system depressant, has no abuse potential, and can be used on a long-term basis.

Cognitive Skill

Prioritize Hypotheses

Reference

Burchum & Rosenthal, 2019, pp. 399–401

Thinking Exercise 16-3

Answers

Potential Health Teaching	Appropriate Health Teaching
"Your drug dosage will likely be increased based on how well this dosage reduces your anxiety."	X
"Take the drug in the morning on an empty stomach to decrease the risk of nausea."	
"If you begin thinking about harming yourself, let your primary health care provider know immediately."	X
"This drug may decrease your appetite, so monitor your weight."	X
"This drug can make you sleepy."	X
"Follow up with your primary health care provider to check your blood pressure, which may increase."	X

Rationales

Venlafaxine is a serotonin-norepinephrine reuptake inhibitor that is approved for use in clients with depression or generalized anxiety disorder. The most common side effect is nausea, and therefore the nurse would not recommend that the drug be taken in the morning on an empty stomach. Instead, the client should take the drug at night and possibly with food. The drug can decrease appetite, cause sleepiness, and increase diastolic blood pressure. Therefore teaching about these side effects is important. Venlafaxine can increase the risk of suicide in both adolescents and young adults.

Cognitive Skill

Take Action

References

Burchum & Rosenthal, 2019, pp. 361, 400

Thinking Exercise 16-4

Answers

A, C, D, E, H

Rationales

The client is taking several medications that can cause dizziness. When these drugs are taken together, the risk for dizziness and lightheadedness increases, and these effects should be reported (Choice A). The nurse teaches the client to avoid over-the-counter cough and cold medications that contain dextromethorphan and supplements such as St. John's wort because when combined with an SSRI and/or SNRI, the client may experience serotonin syndrome, a potentially life-threatening toxic effect (Choices C and D). Triptans can also contribute to the risk of serotonin syndrome. Signs and symptoms of this syndrome include increased body temperature, dilated pupils, delirium, diarrhea with abdominal pain, increased reflexes, tremors or muscle spasms, tachycardia, and profuse sweating. The client should seek medical attention if serotonin syndrome occurs (Choice E). The client should also check her blood pressure regularly because venlafaxine can cause increased blood pressure, but not an increased pulse (Choice H).

Cognitive Skill

Take Action

References

Halter, 2018, pp. 258–261; Burchum & Rosenthal, 2019, pp. 320–324, 359–364

Thinking Exercise 16-5

Answers

Assessment Finding	Effective	Ineffective	Unrelated
Unintentional weight loss of 10 lb (4.5 kg) in the past 6 weeks		X	
Sleeping pattern improving	X		
Feels less worried most of the time	X		
Participates in yoga class 3 to 4 days a week	X		
No longer eating red meat in her diet			X
Husband starting new job next week			X
Has decided to try to get pregnant starting next month	X		
Was able to pay her student loan payment last month			X

Rationales

The client is currently engaging in relaxation techniques (yoga), is sleeping better, and is feeling less worried. She feels less stressed now because she and her husband are considering trying to start a family. However, the client has unexpectedly lost weight, which may be the result of drug therapy. The primary health care provider may need to change the client's medication during this office visit. Although her life situation has improved, those factors are not the result of nursing interventions to decrease her anxiety.

Cognitive Skill

Evaluate Outcomes

Reference

Halter, 2018, pp. 277–278

CHAPTER 17 **Reproduction:** *Uterine Leiomyoma/Hysterectomy*

Answers With Rationales for Thinking Exercises

Exemplar 17. Uterine Leiomyoma/Hysterectomy (Medical-Surgical Nursing: Middle-Age Adult)

Thinking Exercise 17-1

Answers

A, C, D, E

Rationales

Uterine fibroids are often large and cause a feeling of pelvic pressure and abdominal bloating (Choices A and D). Some women also have changes in urinary or bowel elimination patterns, including urinary incontinence or retention or constipation (Choice C). Diarrhea is not a common assessment finding. Because the client has heavy vaginal bleeding that often occurs in women who have uterine fibroids, she may be anemic (Choice E).

Cognitive Skill

Recognize Cues

Reference

Ignatavicius et al., 2018, pp. 1459–1460

Thinking Exercise 17-2

Answers

Medication	Dose, Route, Frequency	Drug Class	Indication
Levothyroxine	50 mcg orally once daily 30-60 min before breakfast	Thyroid replacement drug	Hypothyroidism
Dabigatran	150 mg orally twice daily	Direct thrombin inhibitor	**Atrial fibrillation**
Citalopram	40 mg orally once daily	**Selective serotonin reuptake inhibitor**	Depression
Lisinopril	**10 mg orally once daily**	Angiotensin-converting enzyme inhibitor	Hypertension
Simvastatin	40 mg orally once daily	HMG-CoA reductase inhibitor	Hypercholesterolemia

Cognitive Skill

Analyze Cues

References

Burchum & Rosenthal, 2019, pp. 355, 357, 359–361, 486, 489, 579–580, 583, 616–618, 715–717

Thinking Exercise 17-3

Answers

B, C, E, F, G, H, I

Rationales

The nurse teaches the client about actions that will help prevent potential postoperative complications, including venous thromboembolism, atelectasis, paralytic ileus, dehydration, and bleeding. Using an incentive spirometer and deep breathing every 1 to 2 hours can help prevent pulmonary complications such as atelectasis (Choices B and H). Ambulating early after surgery and using sequential compression devices can help prevent venous thromboembolism (Choices C and E). The nurse reminds the client to drink plenty of fluids so that the IV can be removed and the client can resume her usual diet (Choices F and I). The nurse also tells the client that her blood count (CBC) will be monitored in case she is experiencing internal bleeding. For some clients, the hemoglobin and hematocrit decrease (anemia) due to blood loss during surgery (Choice G).

Cognitive Skill

Take Action

References

Ignatavicius et al., 2018, pp. 1461–1463; also see Chapter 16

Thinking Exercise 17-4

Answers

The nurse teaches the client to monitor for potential postoperative complications such as venous thromboembolism, infection, and internal abdominal bleeding. Signs and symptoms of these complications include elevated temperature, reddened swollen calf, and severe abdominal pain and swelling.

Rationales

Clients who have open traditional abdominal surgery under general anesthesia are at risk for numerous postoperative complications. One of the most important nursing actions is to teach clients to monitor for signs and symptoms of these complications at home and to immediately report relevant signs and symptoms to their primary health care provider for early management. If not treated early or effectively, the client may be at risk for life-threatening problems, such as hypovolemic shock, pulmonary embolus, and sepsis.

Cognitive Skill

Prioritize Hypotheses

References

Ignatavicius et al., 2018, pp. 1461–1463, also see Chapter 16

Thinking Exercise 17-5

Answers

Assessment Finding	Effective	Ineffective	Unrelated
Incision healed without infection	X		
Urinary incontinence		X	
Normal body temperature	X		
No vaginal bleeding	X		
Reports having periods of flatus			X
Reports occasional constipation			X

Rationales

At 6 weeks after surgery, the client's incision should be healed and she should not have a fever or other signs of infection. The client would also be expected to not have any more vaginal bleeding as she did as a result of the fibroids before surgery. Urinary incontinence is not a common complication of hysterectomy. It is possible that the trauma of surgery could have caused her incontinence, and it will need to be further evaluated. Having occasional constipation is unrelated to the surgery and could be due to her decreased activity during her postoperative recovery. Flatus is often common in clients who have bowel elimination problems, such as constipation or diarrhea.

Cognitive Skill

Evaluate Outcomes

References

Ignatavicius et al., 2018, pp. 1461–1463, also see Chapter 16

CHAPTER 18 Reproduction: *Childbearing Family*

Answers With Rationales for Thinking Exercises

Exemplar 18A. Uncomplicated Prenatal Woman

Thinking Exercise 18A-1

Answers

The client's gravida is 4 and her parity is 3. The number of term deliveries is 1, the number of preterm deliveries is 2, the number of aborted deliveries is 0, and the number of living children is 3. The client's estimated date of delivery is September 19, 2020.

Rationales

An obstetric history is often abbreviated as GTPAL. Gravida (G) is the number of times that a woman has been pregnant, regardless of the duration of the pregnancy or the number of fetuses. The client was pregnant in 2012, 2013, and 2014 and is currently pregnant, for four total pregnancies. To calculate parity (P), the pregnancy must reach 20 weeks' gestation, and this client delivered after 20 weeks for her previous three pregnancies. Preterm pregnancy is a pregnancy that extends from 20 to 36⁶⁄₇ weeks' gestation at delivery. Term (T) pregnancies are divided into early term, full term, and late term, but the time period generally extends from 37 to 41⁶⁄₇ weeks' gestation at delivery. Pregnancies that end prior to 20 weeks' gestation, either spontaneously or electively, are referred to as abortions (A). The (L) in the obstetric history stands for "living children" and is based on the current number of living children. The estimated date of delivery is based on Naegele's rule, which is calculated from the first date of the last menstrual period (LMP) by subtracting 3 months (12 −3 = 9) and adding 7 (12 + 7 = 19) days. This calculation means that the client's estimated due date is 9/19/2020.

Cognitive Skill

Analyze Cues

References

Lowdermilk et al., 2020, pp. 58, 264, 270–284, 486, 824–837

Thinking Exercise 18A-2

Answers

A, B, C, F, H

Rationales

The initial assessment for the pregnant client includes urine, cervical, and blood samples to evaluate the mother's health, as well as to promote early identification of infectious or metabolic conditions that might negatively affect the fetus and pregnancy. Laboratory tests include blood type, baseline hemoglobin and hematocrit, platelets, rubella status, renal function, urinalysis, cultures for *Neisseria gonorrhea,* chlamydia, and syphilis, and HIV status (Choices B, C, F, H). Nutrition and weight gain are addressed at every visit, but in the first trimester the focus is on minimizing the effects of pregnancy-related nausea and vomiting and determining the optimal weight gain for the pregnant woman (Choice A).

Cognitive Skill

Take Action

Reference

Lowdermilk et al., 2020, pp. 269–290

Thinking Exercise 18A-3

Answers

Assessment Finding	Expected	Requires Nursing Follow-Up
Temperature = 98.6°F (37°C)	X	
Respiratory rate = 14 breaths/min	X	
Heart rate = 76 beats/min	X	
Blood pressure = 132/ 78 mm Hg		X
Timing of initial visit (9 weeks)	X	
Previous term delivery(s)	X	
Previous preterm delivery(s)		X

Continued

Assessment Finding	Expected	Requires Nursing Follow-Up
Estimated date of delivery (EDD)	X	
Height: 66 in (167.64 cm)	X	
Daily sertraline		X
Acetaminophen as needed for pain	X	
Naproxen sodium as needed for pain		X

Rationales

Results for temperature, heart rate, respiratory rate, obstetric history, and current medications are all appropriate and expected. The blood pressure is borderline high; this should be followed up on to see if it is chronic or acute and should be treated accordingly. All NSAID medications are contraindicated throughout the pregnancy owing to interference with neural tube development and risk of bleeding. Sertraline is contraindicated in the third trimester, so the client needs to be transitioned to a replacement medication, or an alternative therapy should be discussed. Understanding the impetus and outcome of the preterm delivery is always important in order to identify any potential implications for the current pregnancy. History of a preterm delivery is one of the biggest risk factors for preterm delivery with the current pregnancy.

Cognitive Skill

Recognize Cues

References

Lowdermilk et al., 2020, pp. 249–260, 274–276, 283–288; Burchum & Rosenthal, 2019, pp. 359–360, 860, 864–866

Thinking Exercise 18A-4

Answers

During the client's first trimester, routine primary health care provider visits will be every 4 weeks. The primary health care provider will order an ultrasound to check for fetal anatomy that could indicate fetal anomalies. The client can expect to hear the heartbeat during the second trimester and feel fetal movements after 16 weeks. A noninvasive way to monitor the growth of the fetus is by measuring the fundal height and is done at every visit after 20 weeks' gestation but may have a 2-week margin of error.

Cognitive Skill

Analyze Cues

Rationales

Although routine prenatal visits can be individualized based on the client's health and needs, they generally are not more frequent than every 4 weeks in the first trimester and increase in frequency as the pregnancy develops. Ultrasound during pregnancy is used to assess for multiple fetuses, fetal measurements, weeks of gestation, and biparietal diameter (BPD) to evaluate potential complications. It also gives the mother a more accurate expected date of delivery (EDD). Fundal heights are generally consistent with gestation from 18 to 30 weeks and are thus used as a noninvasive means of evaluating fetal development.

Cognitive Skill

Analyze Cues

Reference

Lowdermilk et al., 2020, pp. 269–290

Thinking Exercise 18A-5

Answers

Diagnostic Test	Indication for Performing	Nursing Implications
Fetal nonstress test	Used to evaluate the viability of the fetus and the placenta's ability to perfuse the fetus	Place client on external fetal monitor and instruct her to push the button every time the fetus moves.
Alpha-fetoprotein	**Screening marker used to identify increased risk for birth defects**	Perform test after 10 weeks' gestation and include gestation with serum sample.
Fetal biophysical profile	Used to identify if a fetus is in distress and assesses fetal heart rate reactivity, breathing and body movements, muscle tone, and amniotic fluid volume	**The overall score will dictate if and when the test has to be repeated.**
Chorionic villus sampling	Genetic testing that can be done at 8–12 wk for pregnancies associated with high risk for genetic defects	Potential complications include spontaneous or accidental abortion.
Amniocentesis	**Used to measure fetal maturity, fetal distress, and risk for respiratory distress syndrome**	Test is contraindicated in clients with abruptio placentae and may cause amniotic fluid emboli.
Glucose tolerance test	Can be used to evaluate clients with hypoglycemia	**Instruct the client to fast for 12 hours prior to the test.**

Cognitive Skill

Generate Solutions

References

Lowdermilk et. al., 2020, pp. 273–277, 565–576; Pagana & Pagana, 2018, pp. 48–49, 234–235, 509–510, 569–570, 824–825, 1034–1036

Thinking Exercise 18A-6

Answers

Assessment Finding	Effective	Ineffective	Unrelated
Temperature = 98.6°F (37°C)	X		
Blood pressure = 142/88 mm Hg		X	
Client reports six fetal kicks every hour	X		
Group B streptococci (+)			X
1-hour glucose tolerance test results = 133 mg/dL (10 mmol/L)	X		
Client reports having car seat, clothes, diapers, and bassinet	X		
Client plans to breast-feed	X		
Urinalysis results = 3+ protein, negative for bacteria		X	
Client denies completing childbirth preparation class			X

Rationales

The nurse evaluates the client's physiologic status and psychological adaptation to the pregnancy. Having elevated blood pressure, especially late in pregnancy, is concerning for possible complications. Kick counts or fetal movement is also very important to monitor, as decreased fetal movement is often a precursor to spontaneous abortion. Although no research has been done to determine the optimal number of kicks or movements, generally four or more times in an hour is an acceptable number to indicate a healthy fetus. Although the pregnant mother has tested positive for group B streptococcus (GBS), it is unrelated to whether or not nursing actions up to this point have been effective, because we cannot prevent GBS infections. However, during childbirth, the client will need to be adequately treated as prophylaxis for the newborn. Although perinatal classes and education are important, they are not required.

Cognitive Skill

Evaluate Outcomes

References

Lowdermilk et al., 2020, pp. 264–288, 567; Pagana & Pagana, 2018, p. 234

Exemplar 18B. Complicated Prenatal Woman

Thinking Exercise 18B-1

Answers

Assessment Finding	Expected	Requires Nursing Follow-Up
Temperature = 98°F (36.7°C)	X	
Heart rate = 100 beats/min	X	
Respiratory rate = 22 breaths/min	X	
Blood pressure = 168/98 mm Hg		X
Headache rated at 8/10 on a 0 to 10 pain scale		X
Constant epigastric pain		X
Hemoglobin = 11 g/dL (110 g/L)	X	
Platelets = 128,000/mm³ (128 × 10⁹/L)		X
Urine protein = 2+		X
Urine ketones = 1+		X
Clonus = negative	X	
DTRs = 2+ in lower and upper extremities	X	
Breath sounds = clear in all fields	X	
Visual disturbances		X
Client reports that primary health care provider is "watching my blood pressure"		X

Rationales

Any possible positive assessment that might lead the provider to suspect preeclampsia requires follow-up, including high blood pressure, severe headache, urine protein, and visual disturbances. The client's platelet count is also low and requires follow-up by the nurse.

Cognitive Skill

Recognize Cues

Reference

Lowdermilk et al., 2020, pp. 586–594

Thinking Exercise 18B-2

Answers

A, C, E

Rationales

Expectant management includes the use of antihypertensive medication to maintain a BP less than 160/110 mm Hg (Choice A). Prescription blood pressure parameters will allow the interprofessional health care team to have the same desired outcomes (Choice C). Comparing the client's prenatal and current blood pressure will assist the team in knowing how elevated the client's blood pressure is from "normal" (Choice E). Placing a pregnant client on her back after 20 weeks' gestation can result in vena cava syndrome and is never recommended. Blood pressure should remain consistent throughout pregnancy.

Cognitive Skill

Take Action

Reference

Lowdermilk et al., 2020, pp. 592–594

Thinking Exercise 18B-3

Answers

A, F

Rationales

Magnesium sulfate is the drug of choice for preventing and treating seizure activity for the client and neurologic protection for the fetus (Choice A). Weekly nonstress tests will monitor both the client and the fetus for worsening symptoms (Choice F).

Cognitive Skill

Take Action

References

Lowdermilk et al., 2020, pp. 578, 587–590; Burchum & Rosenthal, 2019, pp. 474–475

Thinking Exercise 18B-4

Answers

- Blood type
- Current blood pressure
- Previous deliveries
- Rubella status

Rationales

The mother's blood type is Rh negative, so she will need to receive an injection of RhoGAM if compatibility is an issue, depending on the father's blood type. Blood pressure is elevated and the client should be assessed for preeclampsia. Previous obstetric history includes two preterm deliveries and only two living children, but her para is 3. She will need to have an MMR immunization after delivery for her rubella status.

Cognitive Skill

Recognize Cues

References

Lowdermilk et al., 2020, pp. 283, 412, 433, 583–584, 684, 784–785

Thinking Exercise 18B-5

Answers

Nurse's Response	Therapeutic	Nontherapeutic
"Spontaneous abortions are for the best and you are lucky it happened early."		X
"You can always have other children."		X
"We will be monitoring your bleeding for your safety."	X	
"Fluid replacement and nutrition are important for your physical healing."	X	
"Talking to someone you trust is vital for your mental healing."		X
"Who can I call to be with you during this time?"	X	

Rationales

Fluid replacement and nutrition are important for healing, and monitoring bleeding is the most important concern. Emotional support is also important, but talking to a trusted person is not absolutely vital.

Cognitive Skill

Generate Solutions

Reference

Lowdermilk et al., 2020, pp. 600–601

Exemplar 18C. Uncomplicated Intrapartum Care

Thinking Exercise 18C-1

Answers

The first stage of labor lasts from the time dilation begins to the time when the cervix is fully dilated. The second stage of labor lasts from the time of full cervical dilation to the birth of the infant. The third stage of labor lasts from the infant's birth to the expulsion of the placenta. The fourth stage of labor begins with the delivery of the placenta and includes at least the first 2 hours after birth.

Cognitive Skill

Take Action

Reference

Lowdermilk et al., 2020, pp. 228–230

Thinking Exercise 18C-2

Answers

Health Teaching	Indicated	Non-Essential
Contractions every 5 minutes for at least an hour with a pattern of increasing regularity, frequency, duration, and intensity	X	
Awakening less than twice per night with the need to urinate		X
Any gush or trickle of fluid from the vagina	X	
Vaginal bleeding	X	
"Nesting" or feeling the need to clean		X
Feeling the baby move more than usual		X
Decreased fetal movement	X	
Any feeling that something is wrong.	X	

Rationales

Awakening once nightly to urinate, nesting, and feeling the baby move often are all normal occurrences in late pregnancy. The other changes indicate that the client is likely going into labor or having a complication, such as placenta previa or fetal distress. Therefore the client needs to return to the hospital to keep both herself and the fetus healthy.

Cognitive Skill

Prioritize Hypotheses

References

Lowdermilk et al., 2020, pp. 273, 327

Thinking Exercise 18C-3

Answers

C, D, G

Rationales

Contractions are measured with 1 minute being represented by the dark bold line. The contraction pattern is represented in minutes. A contraction pattern that is every minute would display a contraction starting at each and every dark bold line (or comparable) (Choice C). The fetus's oxygenation has very little, if anything, to do with variability. Moderate variability is displayed, and that is considered good (as opposed to absent or marked) (Choice D). There are no decelerations on the strip displayed. Strength of contractions, when using an external monitor, cannot be visualized on the fetal monitor strip. When using an external monitor, only the health care professional's touch can assess strength. An average fetal heart rate is 110 to 160, and this monitor strip shows a baseline of 120 (Choice G).

Cognitive Skill

Analyze Cues

Reference

Lowdermilk et al., 2020, pp. 358–359

Thinking Exercise 18C-4

Answers

B, C, F, H

Rationales

An average fetal heart rate is 110 to 160 beats/min, and this strip shows a baseline within that range at 145 (Choice H). Accelerations are defined as an increase in fetal heart rate of 15 beats for 15 seconds, and this strip displays data that meet that definition. Accelerations are a positive fetal sign (Choices B and C). There are no decelerations on the strip displayed (Choice F). The variability of this fetus is not marked, and variability does not change based on the stage of labor. Different types of decelerations indicate different things. Not all decelerations prove fetal compromise. For example, some decelerations show head compression, and others show decreased oxygenation.

Cognitive Skill

Analyze Cues

References

Lowdermilk et al., 2020, pp. 358, 364–369

Thinking Exercise 18C-5

Answers

B, E, F

Rationales

When using an external monitor, only the health care professional's touch can assess strength. Contractions are measured with 1 minute being represented by the dark bold line. Contraction pattern is represented in minutes (2 to 3 minutes) (Choice B). Duration of contractions is measured from the start of a contraction to the end of that same contraction. Duration is represented in seconds, with each small box representing 10 seconds (50 to 70 seconds) (Choice F). Resting tone is the time between each contraction. Adequate resting tone is at least 1 minute between each contraction (Choice E). False labor can be diagnosed only with a vaginal exam that reveals no cervical change. False versus true labor is not assessed using a fetal monitor strip. Marked contraction pattern is not a definition for a contraction pattern. With pushing efforts, a strip may show a "spikey" top to the contractions, but coughing or sneezing can create the same effect.

Cognitive Skill

Prioritize Hypotheses

References

Lowdermilk et al., 2016, pp. 358, 364–369

Exemplar 18D. Complicated Intrapartum Care

Thinking Exercise 18D-1

Answers

Nursing Action	Anticipated	Contraindicated	Non-Essential
Apply pressure to fetal presenting part and off of the cord.	X		
Apply oxygen to client at 10 L per mask.	X		
Encourage client's support person to remain calm.			X
Attempt to replace cord back into the client's uterus.		X	
Remove pressure from the client's cervix after 60 seconds.		X	
Remain with client until delivery of the infant.	X		

Rationales

Applying pressure to the fetal presenting part and off of the cord enables as much oxygen as possible to reach the fetus via the umbilical cord. Providing extra oxygen to the client will increase oxygen availability to the fetus. Encouraging all support persons to remain calm is important but not essential. Replacing the cord is never indicated and always contraindicated because of the risk of harm to the mother and fetus. Pressure should never be applied to a client's cervix. The nurse would never leave the client in an emergency situation.

Cognitive Skill

Generate Solutions

Reference

Lowdermilk et al., 2020, pp. 716–717

Thinking Exercise 18D-2

Answers

Nursing Action	Potential Intrapartum Complication	Appropriate Nursing Action for Each Intrapartum Complication
1 Apply pressure to fetal presenting part and off of the cord.	Prolapsed cord	1 Apply pressure to fetal presenting part and off of the cord. 2 Apply oxygen to client at 10 L per mask. 8 Remain with client until delivery of the infant.
2 Apply oxygen to client at 10 L per mask.	Abruptio placentae	2 Apply oxygen to client at 10 L per mask. 8 Remain with client until delivery of the infant.
3 Encourage client's support person to leave the room.	Eclampsia seizure	2 Apply oxygen to client at 10 L per mask. 3 Encourage client's support person to leave the room. 4 Compare the client's prenatal and current blood pressure values. 9 Titrate or administer magnesium sulfate.
4 Compare the client's prenatal and current blood pressure values.	Chorioamnionitis	10 Administer ampicillin.

Continued

Nursing Action	Potential Intrapartum Complication	Appropriate Nursing Action for Each Intrapartum Complication
5 Monitor blood glucose levels hourly.		
6 Attempt to replace cord back into the client's uterus.		
7 Remove pressure off the client's cervix after 60 seconds.		
8 Remain with client until delivery of the infant.		
9 Titrate or administer magnesium sulfate.		
10 Administer ampicillin.		

Rationales

Nursing actions for intrapartum complications are to achieve optimal outcome for both mother and baby. Oxygenation and circulatory status are the top concerns for which actions should be taken.

Cognitive Skill

Take Action

References

Lowdermilk et al., 2020, pp. 594, 607, 691, 716

Thinking Exercise 18D-3

Answers

A, B, G

Rationales

Assessing the O_2 saturation will indicate the oxygen concentration that is being transferred from the lungs to the extremities (Choice A). Anytime a client is feeling short of breath, oxygen application will decrease anxiety and increase oxygenation (Choice B). Having support persons leave the room is not indicated at this time and could possibly increase the client's anxiety. Having the client's head lower than her uterus will not increase oxygenation and could increase shortness of breath. Comparing blood pressure values and assessing fluid membrane status do not indicate oxygenation issues. The nurse always remains with the client during any complication or emergency (Choice G).

Cognitive Skill

Take Action

References

Lowdermilk et al., 2020, pp. 716–717, 728–730

Thinking Exercise 18D-4

Answers

- 103 lb (46.8 kg), 110 lb (50 kg)
- 12/2016 SAB 12 weeks
- 11/2017 Vaginal delivery 30 weeks

- 12/2018 SAB at 16 weeks
- Diagnosed 11/2018 with incompetent cervix
- Twin pregnancy
- Vaginal spotting after cerclage placement at 14 weeks
- Hispanic descent
- Smokes approximately 1 pack per day (PPD)
- Employed as a Certified Nursing Assistant, working night shift, 12 hours, full-time in a long-term care facility

Rationales

The nurse recognizes that a low prepregnancy weight of the mother, previous preterm deliveries, the need to have a cerclage to tighten the cervix, and vaginal bleeding during the second trimester are all high-risk factors for preterm labor. This risk is increased when the pregnant woman smokes, has twin gestation, and works in a job that requires strenuous or extended activity involving standing, walking, and lifting. Spontaneous preterm labor is also commonly found in nonwhite women, which includes Hispanic descent.

Cognitive Skill

Recognize Cues

References

Lowdermilk et al., 2020, pp. 300, 684

Thinking Exercise 18D-5

Answers

B, C, E

Rationales

Betamethasone is given intramuscularly in two doses and 24 hours apart (Choice E). Indications include acceleration of fetal lung maturity to reduce the incidence and severity of respiratory distress syndrome (Choices B and C). Greatest benefits accrue if at least 24 hours elapse between the initial dose and birth of the preterm infant.

Cognitive Skill

Take Action

References

Lowdermilk et al., 2020, p. 683; Burchum & Rosenthal, 2019, pp. 873–875

Exemplar 18E. Uncomplicated Postpartum Care

Thinking Exercise 18E-1

Answers

First, the nurse will ask the client to empty her **bladder** to prevent **uterus** displacement. Next, the nurse will assist the client to a **supine** position with her knees flexed. Then, the nurse will apply clean gloves and lower the perineal pads to observe lochia as the **fundus** is palpated. To **support** and anchor the lower uterine segment, the nurse's nondominant hand is placed above the woman's symphysis pubis. Finally, palpation begins at the **umbilicus,** and the nurse gently palpates until the **fundus** is located.

Rationales

This is the evidence-based procedure for doing a postpartum fundal assessment.

Cognitive Skill

Take Action

References

Lowdermilk et al., 2020, pp. 424–425, 428

Thinking Exercise 18E-2

Answers

A, C, E

Rationales

Grand multiparity is defined as five or more births (Choice A). Overdistention of the uterus is caused by a large infant (Choice C). These factors and an operative delivery (Choice E) place the client at a higher risk of hemorrhage.

Cognitive Skill

Analyze Cues

References

Lowdermilk et al., 2020. pp. 428, 565

Thinking Exercise 18E-3

Answers

Assessment Findings	Expected	Requires Nursing Follow-Up
Temperature = 98.6°F (37°C)	X	
Blood type is A negative		X
Hepatitis B status is negative	X	
Blood pressure = 132/78 mm Hg	X	
Had a total of four prenatal visits		X
Had one previous term delivery	X	
Rubella status is nonimmune		X
Uses ibuprofen and oxycodone regularly for pain		X
No colostrum noted with hand expression		X
No running water available at her home		X

Rationales

A negative blood type needs follow-up to determine if RhoGAM is needed for Rh incompatibility. Inadequate prenatal care requires follow-up to determine if follow-up care is available for this client and why prenatal care is so important. Rubella status needs follow-up to make sure that the client receives a rubella booster immunization. Oxycodone is an opioid and follow-up is needed to educate on general opioid use and also with breast-feeding. The client has no colostrum by this time and a breast-feeding consultation is needed. Client should have running water for cleanliness, and a resources follow-up is needed.

Cognitive Skill

Recognize Cues

Reference

Lowdermilk et al., 2020, pp. 425–428

Thinking Exercise 18E-4

Answers

- Continues to rate her pain at 5/10 (on a 0 to 10 pain scale) with medication administration
- Having trouble sleeping
- Has first baby in family
- Babysat once for a neighbor's 6-year-old
- Father of the baby not involved
- Infant boy has many characteristics of father of the baby
- Cesarean birth

Rationales

The nurse is concerned about the client's poor pain control and insomnia while caring for a newborn. In addition, the client has no infant-caring experience. Her baby looks like the father, but he is not involved, which may increase the mother's resentment of the baby and affect bonding. A surgical birth can inhibit adaptation because of the lengthier recovery.

Cognitive Skill

Recognize Cues

Reference

Lowdermilk et al., 2016, pp. 442–445

Thinking Exercise 18E-5

Answers

Assessment Finding	Effective	Ineffective	Unrelated
Temperature = 98.2°F (36.8°C)	X		
Pain = 2 (on a 0 to 10 pain scale)	X		
Lochia = serosa, moderate amount		X	
Nipples are tender with blisters		X	
No clots noted in past 24 hours	X		
Fundus is firm and 2 fingerbreadths below the umbilicus	X		
1+ pitting edema in lower extremities bilaterally		X	
Client denies difficulty urinating	X		
Family present at bedside	X		
Blood glucose = 96 mg/dL (5.3 mmol/L)			X

Rationales

Blood glucose is not related to usual postpartum care. Having mild pain, a normal temperature, no clots, fundus firm at 2 fingerbreadths, no difficulty urinating, and family present at discharge are all expected and indicate that her care has been effective. Lochia should not still be moderate, and the client should not have tissue breakdown on her nipples or pitting edema. These issues may require follow-up.

Cognitive Skill

Evaluate Cues

Reference

Lowdermilk et al., 2020, pp. 436–438

Exemplar 18F. Complicated Postpartum Care

Thinking Exercise 18F-1

Answers

A, B, E, G

Rationales

Notifying the primary health care provider of an increased blood pressure, especially when the client is on medication to decrease blood pressure, is crucial (Choice A). Therefore administering an antihypertensive medication is a priority (Choice B). A magnesium level will guide the magnesium infusion rate. It is always essential to stay with a client in an emergency situation (Choices E and G). Positioning with the client's head elevated will not affect eclampsia.

Cognitive Skill

Take Action

Reference

Lowdermilk et al., 2020, pp. 593–594

Thinking Exercise 18F-2

Answers

- Gravida 6 para 5 (G6P5)
- 9-lb (4082-g) baby
- Precipitous birth within 30 minutes of arrival at hospital
- Large clots expelled with recent fundal check
- Feeling light-headed and dizzy when getting up to go to the bathroom

Rationales

Risk factors and causes of postpartum hemorrhage include uterine atony caused by an overdistended uterus (large fetus and high parity), precipitous birth, and symptoms of excessive blood loss (large clots and feeling light-headed and dizzy).

Cognitive Skill

Recognize Cues

Reference

Lowdermilk et al., 2020, p. 721

Thinking Exercise 18F-3

Answers

A, B, C, G

Rationales

Protocols are primary health care provider or agency order sets that allow nurses to administer medications to clients experiencing complications within certain parameters. There are no contraindications to administering oxytocin to a client having a postpartum hemorrhage (Choice A). Assessing the fundus in a bleeding postpartum client is always the first intervention to determine firmness of the uterus; therefore assess where the bleeding could be originating from (Choice B). Administering misoprostol rectally is appropriate and avoids the dilution of medication that administering it vaginally with bleeding could cause (Choice C). Methylergonovine and dinoprostone are contraindicated in clients who have hypertension. The nurse notifies the primary health care provider when a postpartum client has a hemorrhage (Choice G).

Cognitive Skill

Take Action

Reference

Lowdermilk et al., 2016, pp. 723–725

Thinking Exercise 18F-4

Answers

A, D, E

Rationales

The correct choices are all symptoms of postpartum affective mood disorders (Choices A, D, and E). The remaining choices are all expected postpartum reactions and symptoms.

Cognitive Skill

Take Action

Reference

Lowdermilk et al., 2020, p. 434

Thinking Exercise 18F-5

Answers

Assessment Finding	Effective	Ineffective	Unrelated
Heart rate = 82 beats/min	X		
Blood pressure = 112/67 mm Hg	X		
Reports feeling light-headed and dizzy when getting up to go to the bathroom		X	
Hemoglobin = 9.7 g/dL (97 g/L)		X	
Incision is clean, dry, slightly pink with staples intact	X		
Pain = 4 (on a 0 to 10 pain scale) after ibuprofen for pain relief		X	
Reports breast-feeding is going well; newborn is gaining weight			X
Verbalizes that she will take iron supplements with orange juice until next appointment with primary health care provider	X		

Rationales

Symptoms of dizziness and low hemoglobin should be addressed prior to discharge because the client should not continue to be symptomatic with a low hemoglobin to be considered ready for discharge. Pain should be lower than a 4 on a 0 to 10 pain scale with medication administration and needs to be followed up.

Cognitive Skill

Evaluate Outcomes

References

Lowdermilk et al., 2016, pp. 427–428, 727

Exemplar 18G. Uncomplicated Newborn Care

Thinking Exercise 18G-1

Answers

A, B, D, E, G

Rationales

Assessing the newborn for any respiratory or cardiac complications is the priority for the nurse; this includes assessing for hypoxia (Choices B and D). However, giving routine oxygen is no longer recommended, so the newborn must be cyanotic or in respiratory distress to receive oxygen. Protecting the newborn from various infections is part of the initial treatment of a newborn; this includes giving hepatitis B vaccine (Choice A). Vitamin K is given shortly after birth to protect the newborn from hemorrhage because the gut is sterile and the newborn is not able to synthesize vitamin K for clotting purposes at birth (Choice E). Maintaining a stable body temperature of the newborn, promoting bonding time with the mother, and breast-feeding success can be accomplished by placing the newborn in skin-to-skin contact with the mother (Choice G). This is often referred to as kangaroo care. Completing a hearing test and an oximetry test to identify congenital cardiac heart defects are also recommended procedures in the newborn time period, but these can wait until after the transitional period.

Cognitive Skill

Take Action

References

Hockenberry & Wilson, 2019, pp. 196–235; Lowdermilk, et al., 2020, pp. 461–465, 486–506, 515–522

Thinking Exercise 18G-2

Answers

Assessment Finding	Expected	Common Variation	Unexpected
Heart rate = 134 beats/min	X		
Pale mucous membranes			X
Bluish tint of fingers and toes		X	
Jittery activity			X
Fontanels are soft with edema of soft scalp tissue		X	

Assessment Finding	Expected	Common Variation	Unexpected
Cries without tears	X		
Positive red reflex	X		
Large dark bluish areas of pigmentation on lower back		X	
Small white bumps along the midline of the hard palate		X	

Rationales

The normal newborn's heart rate fluctuates between 120 and 140 beats/min, accelerating when crying and decreasing when asleep, so a heart rate of 134 is considered a normal finding. A newborn's tear ducts do not function at birth, and a normal response to the ophthalmic examination is for the newborn to have a positive red reflex. These are all normal and expected findings. Common variations seen in newborns include Epstein pearls and changes in pigmentation as seen in stork bites, birth marks, and Mongolian spots. Other common variations include acrocyanosis for up to 24 hours after birth and molding or caputs, which are associated with soft-tissue swelling. Unexpected findings that the nurse should follow up on urgently include pallor of the mucous membranes, which is suggestive of central cyanosis. Jitteriness of the newborn is often associated with blood glucose instability and requires follow-up.

Cognitive Skill

Analyze Cues

References

Hockenberry & Wilson, 2019, pp. 205–209; Lowdermilk, et al., 2020, pp. 461–480, 510–511

Thinking Exercise 18G-3

Answers

To accurately assess the newborn, the nurse will count heart rate and respirations for 60 seconds, measure the weight of the baby without clothes or diaper at the same time of day daily, and monitor the feeding patterns of the newborn daily. These feeding patterns are then compared with expected intake to identify potential growth difficulties.

Rationales

To accurately assess the newborn, the nurse will count heart rate and respirations for 60 seconds because of the natural fluctuations in a newborn's heart rate and breathing. The best way to obtain accurate weights of the baby is without clothes or diapers, and at the same time of day every day with the same scale. Daily weights are critical for the evaluation of whether or not feeding in the newborn is adequate and demonstrates that the newborn is growing appropriately.

Cognitive Skill

Take Action

References

Hockenberry & Wilson, 2019, pp. 199, 204–209, 227; Lowdermilk, et al., 2020, pp. 462–463, 506, 533–536, 544–546

Thinking Exercise 18G-4

Answers

Screening	Indicated	Contraindicated	Non-Essential
Type and screen blood		X	
Metabolic panel	X		
Bilirubin	X		
Car seat screening			X
Pulse oximetry	X		
Urinalysis		X	
Hearing	X		
Finger prints			X
Blood glucose	X		

Rationales

To type and screen the newborn is not only non-essential due to the mother having A+ blood, it is contraindicated because it would be an unnecessary expense and invasive procedure. A urinalysis is also not needed in the absence of symptoms. However, testing the baby's blood glucose would be indicated because the infant is large for gestational age. Hearing screens, pulse oximetry, and metabolic newborn screening tests are routine standard care for newborns. Having fingerprints done is usually appreciated by the parents and family, but not necessary for the newborn's well-being. A newborn weighing over 2500 g does not qualify to have a car seat screening performed. This newborn has at least two risk factors for having elevated bilirubin: premature and precipitous delivery.

Cognitive Skill

Generate Solutions

References

Hockenberry & Wilson, 2019, pp. 233–234; Lowdermilk et al., 2020, pp. 3, 33–40, 487–514, 524–526; Pagana & Pagana, 2018, p. 109

Thinking Exercise 18G-5

Answers

Assessment Finding	Effective	Ineffective	Unrelated
Temperature = 99.1°F (37.2°C)	X		
Heart rate = 144 beats/min	X		
Respirations = 54 breaths/min	X		
Oxygen saturation = 99% (on room air)	X		
Bilirubin = 14 mg/dL (205 mcmol/L)		X	
Birth weight = 9 lb 13 oz (4.46 kg) Current weight = 9 lb 6 oz (4.29 kg)	X		

Assessment Finding	Effective	Ineffective	Unrelated
Baby has minimal periods of wakefulness		X	
Breast-feeding every 2.5–3 hours		X	
Urine output = 4 wet diapers in 12 hours	X		
Bowel movement = dark green, thick, and large amount	X		
Baby has had photographs taken			X
Security safety bands are intact			X

Rationales

The newborn's vital signs are all within usual newborn parameters. Areas of concern include the fact that the baby has minimal periods of wakefulness and elevated bilirubin for age. The newborn appears to be feeding adequately to promote urine and bowel elimination, even though there has been a slight weight loss, commonly seen in newborns. Having photographs taken is unrelated to evaluating the newborn's status and readiness for discharge, and the security safety bands are kept intact until discharge.

Cognitive Skill

Evaluate Outcomes

References

Lowdermilk et al., 2020, pp. 484, 506–530, 544–546; Hockenberry & Wilson, 2019, pp. 256–259; Pagana & Pagana, 2018, pp. 108–109

CHAPTER 19 Perfusion: *Complex Health Problems*

Answers With Rationales for Thinking Exercises

Exemplar 19A. Myocardial Infarction (Medical-Surgical Nursing: Middle-Age Adult)

Thinking Exercise 19A-1

Answers

Nursing Action	Indicated	Contraindicated	Non-Essential
Apply supplemental oxygen.	X		
Assess pain intensity level.	X		
Conduct a head-to-toe assessment.			X
Obtain an electrocardiogram (ECG).	X		
Obtain a comprehensive metabolic profile (CMP).	X		
Obtain a chest x-ray.	X		
Insert an indwelling urinary catheter.		X	

Rationales

The client has the hallmark signs of myocardial infarction for an older woman, which is causing cardiac tissue ischemia. Assessing pain further determines the source of the client's reports of chest pain, back pain, and shortness of breath. Applying supplemental oxygen aids the body in providing oxygen to the cardiac tissues. An ECG consists of images of the electrical pattern of the heart's electrical conduction and can give insight to areas of cardiac ischemia. A head-to-toe assessment is non-essential to the other three actions, which are focused on assessing the client's potentially fatal condition. Blood draws for laboratory tests are needed in this case to determine electrolyte levels for conduction and cardiac stress markers. A chest x-ray is prescribed to rule out pericarditis and other pulmonary causes for the client's signs and symptoms. At this time, the client's urinary output can be monitored with noninvasive means, and an indwelling urinary catheter would be a source of possible infection.

Cognitive Skill

Generate Solutions

Reference

Ignatavicius et al., 2018, pp. 769–779

Thinking Exercise 19A-2

Answers

- Troponin T
- Creatine kinase MB (CKMB)
- Serum magnesium

Rationales

Troponin and CKMB are cardiac enzymes that become elevated in clients with myocardial infarction and resulting cardiac ischemia. CKMB is initially slower to respond and takes less time to resolve in response to cardiac distress than troponin. Both should be examined in order to gain insight about the length of time the heart has been in distress. Magnesium is needed for correct heart contractility. No other blood levels are outside of critical limits.

Cognitive Skill

Recognize Cues

References

Pagana & Pagana, 2018, pp. 167, 315, 451; Pagana et al., 2019, pp. 201–204, 367–369, 531–534

Thinking Exercise 19A-3

Answers

Nursing Action	Potential Postprocedure Complication	Appropriate Nursing Action for Prevention of Postprocedure Complication
1 Assess the neurovascular status of the right hand.	Acute kidney injury	**7** Monitor urine output.
2 Maintain continuous cardiac telemetry monitoring.	Dysrhythmia	**2** Maintain continuous cardiac telemetry monitoring.
3 Increase the intravenous fluid rate of infusion.	Hypotension	**3** Increase the intravenous fluid rate of infusion.

Nursing Action	Potential Postprocedure Complication	Appropriate Nursing Action for Prevention of Postprocedure Complication
4 Monitor level of consciousness and vital signs.	Stroke	4 Monitor level of consciousness and vital signs.
5 Maintain sequential or pneumatic compression devices.	Procedure site hematoma	1 Assess the neurovascular status of the right hand.
6 Monitor oxygen saturation.		
7 Monitor urine output.		

Rationales

Cardiac catheterization is an invasive procedure with many potential complications. Acute kidney injury (AKI) can occur due to the use of contrast dye during the procedure and decreased cardiac output. The nurse monitors for AKI by assessing for decreased urinary output. Dysrhythmia from cardiac tissue damage is best monitored continuously through telemetry. Severe hypotension can be life threatening. Therefore the best nursing action to take if the client's blood pressure begins to decrease is to increase the rate of intravenous fluid infusion, which increases blood volume. Cardiac catheterization can result in a stroke caused by emboli being released into the arterial system. The nurse frequently assesses the client's level of consciousness during vital sign checks to monitor for neurologic changes that are associated with the development of a stroke. Surgical site hematoma from the arterial puncture to access the coronary vessels can be monitored by assessing the neurovascular status of the accessed limb and observing for swelling, warmth, and pain at the insertion site.

Cognitive Skill

Take Action

Reference

Ignatavicius et al., 2018, pp. 657–659

Thinking Exercise 19A-4

Answers

Medication	Purpose	Common Side/Adverse Effect
Aspirin	Prevent platelet aggregation	Black tarry stools or bleeding gums
Atorvastatin	Reduce the risk of recurrent MI	Unexplained muscle pain, cramping, or tenderness
Carvedilol	Decrease the force of cardiac contraction	Increased shortness of breath
Clopidogrel	Prevent platelet aggregation	Black tarry stools or bleeding gums
Lisinopril	Prevent the development of heart failure	Swelling of the tongue and throat

Rationales

Both aspirin and clopidogrel are given to reduce platelet aggregation and clot formation. Because of this action, they can cause GI bleeding, often manifesting with black tarry stools and bleeding gums. Beta-adrenergic blockers like carvedilol decrease the heart rate and the force of cardiac contraction, causing improved perfusion of the cardiac muscle between beats. However, beta-adrenergic blockers can cause bronchospasm, resulting in shortness of breath, especially in people with asthma. Lisinopril is an angiotensin-converting enzyme inhibitor that prevents ventricular remodeling and reduces the likelihood of heart failure. A major side effect of ACE inhibitors is angioedema, which causes the tongue, throat, and glottis to swell. Atorvastatin lowers low-density lipoprotein (LDL) levels, which helps to prevent atherosclerotic plaques from forming and creating another blocked blood vessel. Statin drugs have been shown to cause muscle injury, which manifests most commonly as cramping, pain, and tenderness.

Cognitive Skill

Analyze Cues

References

Ignatavicius et al., 2018, p. 776; Burchum & Rosenthal, 2019, pp. 485–489, 521, 578–583

Thinking Exercise 19A-5

Answers

B, D, E, F, H

Rationales

Modifiable risk factors for coronary artery disease (CAD) include smoking; high-fat, high-sodium diet; high serum cholesterol; decreased physical activity; diabetes mellitus; hypertension; and obesity. Clients should be advised to quit tobacco use, not decrease it. Lowering sodium consumption has been shown to lower the risk of CAD. Clients should be advised to eat foods that lower their low-density lipoprotein (LDL) levels (Choice B). Exercise periods should occur three to four times per week, for approximately 40 minutes (Choice D). Walking for 30 minutes a day also increases activity and cardiac function. Managing hemoglobin A_{1c} is a key component of managing diabetes mellitus (Choice E). Regularly monitoring blood pressure levels and seeking treatment for high blood pressure are key to CAD management and prevention (Choice F). Obese clients need to talk with their primary health care provider about starting a weight reduction program (Choice H).

Cognitive Skill

Take Action

Reference

Ignatavicius et al., 2018, p. 771

Exemplar 19B. Atrial Fibrillation/Stroke (Medical-Surgical Nursing: Older Adult)

Thinking Exercise 19B-1

Answers

A 75-year-old male client is diagnosed with new-onset atrial fibrillation. The nurse would administer diltiazem IV push to convert this dysrhythmia to normal sinus rhythm. However, this drug puts the client at risk for immediate hypotension and bradycardia, and therefore it should be injected over 2 to 3 minutes.

Rationales

Diltiazem is a calcium channel blocker commonly used to treat cardiac dysrhythmias including atrial fibrillation and atrial flutter. To reverse sudden cases of atrial fibrillation, the client receives the medication in intravenous form. During and immediately after IV administration, the nurse observes the client for bradycardia and hypotension. Because of the possibility for these adverse effects, the drug must be administered over 2 to 3 minutes.

Cognitive Skill

Prioritize Hypotheses

References

Ignatavicius et al., 2018, pp. 679–682; Burchum & Rosenthal, 2019, pp. 503–504

Thinking Exercise 19B-2

Answers

A 75-year-old male client is diagnosed with new-onset atrial fibrillation. The nurse understands that atrial fibrillation puts the client at increased risk for embolus formation and heart failure. In addition to medication administration, vital sign checks, and focused cardiac assessments, the nurse implements telemetry and prepares for possible cardioversion.

Rationales

Because atrial fibrillation decreases the emptying of the atria, it is very possible for emboli to form and be dispersed throughout the cardiovascular system, resulting in pulmonary embolism, stroke, and/or venous thromboembolism. The disruption in electrical conduction puts the client at risk for heart failure. Clients with atrial fibrillation wear telemetry devices to continually monitor the conduction pattern. If medical interventions are not successful, the primary health care provider may decide to use cardioversion to shock the heart back into normal sinus rhythm.

Cognitive Skill

Prioritize Hypotheses

References

Ignatavicius et al., 2018, pp. 679–682; Burchum & Rosenthal, 2019, pp. 503–504

Thinking Exercise 19B-3

Answers

A, B, F, H

Rationales

Clients with atrial fibrillation are placed on an anticoagulant or antiplatelet therapy to prevent formation of emboli. Therefore the nurse teaches the client about Bleeding Precautions (Choice A). Clients should reposition slowly to avoid falls and possible bleeding events (Choice B). Clients with atrial fibrillation are at increased risk for stroke for two reasons: (1) thromboemboli that develop in the atria, which never quite empty, and (2) bleeding in the brain from anticoagulant therapy. Stroke education is very important for the client and family (Choice F). There is a risk of skin burns from external cardiac conversion, in which a defibrillator is synched with the heart and then a shock is delivered to regain atrial sinus rhythm. Skin care and any burns should be covered (Choice H).

Cognitive Skill

Take Action

References

Ignatavicius et al., 2018 pp. 681–683; Burchum & Rosenthal, 2019, pp. 612–616

Thinking Exercise 19B-4

Answers

A, B, C, D, E, F

Rationales

Choices A through F are modifiable risk factors for developing a stroke, meaning that the client can make lifestyle decisions to decrease stroke risk. History of stroke and hypertension are nonmodifiable risk factors for developing a stroke because they cannot be altered.

Cognitive Skill

Take Action

Reference

Ignatavicius et al., 2018, p. 930

Thinking Exercise 19B-5

Answers

- Heart rate
- Respirations
- Blood pressure
- Oxygen saturation
- Pain (headache)
- Glasgow Coma Scale score
- Pupil size and response
- Orientation
- Hand grasp
- Foot strength

Rationales

The client is exhibiting signs of stroke. Strokes affect a variety of areas in the body as a response to low oxygen levels in the brain. Blood pressure and heart rate increase to try and increase blood flow. Pain, impaired cognition, cranial nerve involvement (pupillary changes), and motor changes occur due to a lack of cerebral tissue perfusion.

Cognitive Skill

Recognize Cues

Reference

Ignatavicius et al., 2018, pp. 930–935

Thinking Exercise 19B-6

Answers

Nursing Action	Indicated	Contraindicated	Non-Essential
Apply supplemental oxygen.	X		
Call Imaging for stat CT and MRI.	X		
Perform the National Institutes of Health Stroke Scale Neurologic Exam.	X		
Obtain a comprehensive metabolic panel (CMP).			X
Provide a low-stimulation room.			X

Nursing Action	Indicated	Contraindicated	Non-Essential
Keep the head of the client's bed (HOB) at less than 20 degrees.		X	
Initiate IV access.	X		

Rationales

Applying supplemental oxygen will increase the amount of blood oxygen available to the affected area of the brain. Stroke is only confirmed through diagnostic imaging testing. Performing the National Institutes of Health Stroke Scale Neurologic Exam yields information about where the stroke is located and the areas of the brain that are not being perfused. There is no need for a CMP because strokes cannot be diagnosed using laboratory testing. The client who is having a stroke does not need a low-stimulation room. Keeping the head of the bed at less than 20 degrees increases work of breathing and intracranial pressure, which can worsen the effects of the stroke. The client will need to have IV access for medications and/or other interventions.

Cognitive Skill

Generate Solutions

Reference

Ignatavicius et al., 2018, pp. 935–938

Exemplar 19C. Hypovolemic Shock (Medical-Surgical Nursing: Older Adult)

Thinking Exercise 19C-1

Answers

Nursing Action	Indicated	Contraindicated	Non-Essential
Administer a normal saline 1000-mL bolus.	X		
Administer oxygen via nasal cannula (NC).	X		
Draw type and screen for possible blood transfusion.	X		
Ambulate the client to the toilet.		X	
Position the head of the bed at 45–60 degrees.		X	
Frequently check client mental status and level of consciousness (LOC).	X		
Educate the client about incentive spirometry.			X

Rationales

The client is experiencing hypovolemic shock, even though there is no external signs of bleeding. Care for clients in this condition focuses on returning the client's intravascular volume to normal levels and preventing complications. Therefore increasing the vascular volume with a normal saline bolus, administering supplemental oxygen to maximize circulating oxygen levels, drawing a type and screen for possible blood transfusion, and conducting a mental status assessment are necessary actions. Ambulating the client to the bathroom is contraindicated because having the client stand will shift intravascular volume away from major organs and possibly cause organ failure. Raising the head of the bed 45 to 60 degrees is contraindicated. Instead, the bed should be placed flat or at no greater than 30 degrees, and the feet and knees may need to be elevated to help perfuse the client's major organs. At this time, educating the client about incentive spirometry is not essential.

Cognitive Skill

Generate Solutions

Reference

Ignatavicius et al., 2018, pp. 758–760

Thinking Exercise 19C-2

Answers

Medication	Dose, Route, Frequency	Drug Class	Indication
Aspirin	**81 mg orally once daily**	Antiplatelet agent	Primary prevention of myocardial infarction and ischemic stroke
Metformin	850 mg orally twice a day	Biguanide	Diabetes mellitus to lower blood glucose
Metoprolol/ hydrochlorothiazide	100 mg/50 mg orally once daily	Beta-adrenergic blocker/ diuretic	**Hypertension**
Naproxen sodium	250 mg orally PRN twice a day	**NSAID**	Osteoarthritic pain
Rivaroxaban	10 mg orally once daily	Thrombin inhibitor	**Prevention of embolic events**

Cognitive Skill

Analyze Cues

References

Burchum & Rosenthal, 2019, pp. 516–517, 619–620, 621–622, 692–695, 858

Thinking Exercise 19C-3

Answers

F, G

Rationales

NSAIDS such as naproxen sodium decrease platelet aggregation, and an alternate chronic pain management drug should be used (Choice F). Rivaroxaban is used to prevent emboli and therefore should be withheld at this time (Choice G).

Cognitive Skill

Take Action

References

Burchum & Rosenthal, 2016, pp. 619–620, 621–622, 692–695, 858

Thinking Exercise 19C-4

Answers

- Prothrombin time
- International normalized ratio (INR)
- Blood urea nitrogen
- Creatinine
- Lactate

Rationales

The prothrombin time and INR both indicate that the client has slower clotting, most likely influenced by antiplatelet medications, NSAIDs, or both. The BUN and creatinine levels indicate kidney involvement caused by hypovolemia and lack of oxygen needed to properly perfuse the nephrons. High lactate levels indicate that the cells of the body are using anaerobic metabolism to function due to a lack of oxygen.

Cognitive Skill

Recognize Cues

References

Pagana & Pagana, 2018, pp. 171, 292, 391–394, 453; Pagana et al., 2019, pp. 205–208, 343-344, 446–449, 534–537

Thinking Exercise 19C-5

Answers

- Blood pressure
- Respirations
- Oxygen saturation
- Temperature
- Glasgow Coma Scale
- Orientation
- Lung sounds
- Pulses - Pedal

Rationales

The client is exhibiting signs of transfusion-related circulatory overload (TACO). Hypertension and the bounding pedal pulses are related to the increase in circulatory volume. Gas exchange is not effective because the lungs are taking on the extra volume and not able to move oxygen into the system or carbon dioxide out of the system. This lack of exchange manifests as increased work of breathing, increased oxygen demands, increased temperature, crackles in the lungs, decreased orientation, and decreased Glasgow Coma Scale scores. Clients with TACO will also be restless and exhibit distended jugular veins.

Cognitive Skill

Recognize Cues

Reference

Ignatavicius et al., 2018, p. 835

Thinking Exercise 19C-6

Answers

A, B, C, E

Rationales

Clients who are at risk for bleeding should use a soft-bristle toothbrush and avoid flossing to prevent gum bleeding (Choice A). Aspirin and other NSAIDs should be avoided because they decrease the ability of the platelets to aggregate (clump) (Choice B). The nurse would also teach the client to avoid contact sports and any activities in which bumping, scraping, or other injury may occur (Choice C). If the client experiences a bump, she should immediately apply ice to constrict blood vessels and prevent bruising or a hematoma. A rectal suppository will not be needed if the client eats high-fiber foods, has adequate fluids, and exercises on a regular basis (Choice E).

Cognitive Skill

Take Action

Reference

Ignatavicius et al., 2018, p. 827

CHAPTER 20 Mobility: *Spinal Cord Injury*

Answers With Rationales for Thinking Exercises

Exemplar 20. Spinal Cord Injury (Pediatric Nursing: Adolescent)

Thinking Exercise 20-1

Answers

A, B, E, G

Rationales

Priority interventions for the client with a spinal cord injury focus on the ABCs, or airway, breathing, and circulation. Therefore managing the ventilator and maintaining a patent airway is the first priority (Choice B). Using the log-roll method for turning and maintaining a cervical collar are essential interventions to prevent secondary injury to the spinal cord that could worsen the level of paralysis for the client (Choice A). Monitoring for respiratory failure and progression of the paralysis by performing frequent neurologic checks is especially important during the first few days following the injury (Choice E). Obtaining additional details about the accident, treating the scalp abrasion, and maintaining a neutral temperature are not priorities at this time until the client is stabilized (Choices C, F, and H). IV fluids are recommended in the acute phase of injury to prevent hypovolemia and potential shock (Choice G). The client's assessment findings do not indicate that he has a urinary tract infection. Therefore antibiotics are not indicated at this time (Choice D).

Cognitive Skill

Take Action

References

Ignatavicius et al., 2018, pp. 853, 896–897, 910–911; Hockenberry et al., 2019, pp. 1327–1335

Thinking Exercise 20-2

Answers

The nurse recognizes that clients with spinal cord injury suffer both physiologically and psychologically. The priority desired outcomes of treatment for this client are to stabilize the injury and prevent secondary damage to his spinal cord. Additional client outcomes include establishing a bowel and bladder regimen. Other outcomes include maintaining the greatest amount of mobility as possible, monitoring the client's adaptation to his paralysis, and preventing pressure injury.

Rationales

Spinal cord injury (SCI) is a physical trauma that affects the client's self-image and feeling of self-worth due to dependence on other people to perform ADLs, basic body functions, and ambulation. The major desired outcome for clients who have an SCI is to prevent further cord injury by stabilizing the vertebral column. The client will likely have a spastic bowel and bladder and therefore lose voluntary control until a bowel and bladder regimen is established. The nurse and interprofessional team would collaborate to help the client optimize his mobility skills and prevent pressure injury below the level of spinal cord injury.

Cognitive Skill

Prioritize Hypotheses

References

Ignatavicius et al., 2018, pp. 98–99, 895–902; Hockenberry et al., 2019, pp. 1335–1337

Thinking Exercise 20-3

Answers

Nursing actions	Anticipated	Contraindicated	Non-Essential
Monitor vital signs per facility standard.	X		
Encourage coughing and deep breathing exercises.	X		
Administer analgesic as prescribed.	X		
Reposition the client every 4 hours.		X	
Apply sequential compression devices.	X		
Keep NPO until the client voids and reports no nausea.		X	
Obtain a prescription for echocardiogram.			X
Consult clergy or social worker for family support.	X		
Collaborate with respiratory therapy to maintain oxygenation as needed.	X		
Complete a dietary assessment.			X
Obtain a prescription for an indwelling urinary catheter.		X	
Monitor the client's level of sensory perception every 4 hours.	X		
Collaborate with physical therapy to promote independence.	X		

Rationales

Monitoring for secondary injury or complications such as respiratory distress, pneumonia, skin breakdown, and the effects of immobility is part of nursing care for the client with a spinal cord injury. Interventions include encouraging deep breathing, providing DVT prophylaxis such as sequential compression devices, monitoring vital signs, assessing sensory perception for improvement or worsening, and collaborating with interprofessional services to provide support and promote client independence. Managing acute pain is important to prevent chronic pain later. Although repositioning is also part of routine care, this must be done more frequently than every 4 hours. Rather, repositioning should be done every 1 to 2 hours. Determining whether or not to keep the adolescent NPO is primarily based on the sedation status postoperatively and not on the ability to void or the presence of nausea. Non-essential actions for this client include dietary assessment (which is more important later in the treatment) and obtaining an echocardiogram without any cardiac symptoms. Bowel and bladder routines are important to establish as soon as possible to avoid more invasive interventions such as use of an indwelling urinary catheter.

Cognitive Skill

Generate Solutions

References

Ignatavicius et al., 2018, pp. 98, 895–902, 910–911; Hockenberry et al., 2019, pp. 1331–1335

Thinking Exercise 20-4

Answers

A, D, E, F, G, H

Rationales

Assessing the client's adaptation or response to his paralysis is ongoing. Therapeutic responses are open ended and allow the adolescent to explore his feelings and verbalize them, which in turn helps him to cope with the spinal cord injury (Choices E, F, and H). The nurse's goal is to provide hope, reaffirm the client's abilities, facilitate the grieving process for the adolescent and family, and focus on the client's future (Choice D). Questions that can be answered with a "yes" or "no" are generally not therapeutic. Encouraging engagement with peers and referring to support groups are very appropriate actions to support both the adolescent and the family (Choices A and G).

Cognitive Skill

Take Action

References

Ignatavicius et al., 2018, pp. 896–897, 910; Hockenberry et al., 2019, pp. 81–87, 595–602

Thinking Exercise 20-5

Answers

Nursing Action	Potential Spinal Cord Injury Complication	Appropriate Nursing Action for Complication
1 Remove restrictive clothing and check for urinary distention.	Pneumonia	**2** Perform cough assist as needed.
2 Perform cough assist as needed.	Urinary tract infection	**5** Facilitate frequent bladder emptying.

Nursing Action	Potential Spinal Cord Injury Complication	Appropriate Nursing Action for Complication
3 Administer beta-blocking agent per agency protocol.	Autonomic dysreflexia	**1** Remove restrictive clothing and check for urinary distention.
4 Teach the client to do wheelchair push-ups hourly.	Joint contractures	**7** Perform frequent range-of-motion exercises.
5 Facilitate frequent bladder emptying.	Pressure injuries	**4** Teach the client to do wheelchair push-ups hourly.
6 Administer a daily rectal suppository.		
7 Perform frequent range-of-motion exercises.		
8 Apply cervical traction.		

Rationales

Due to the inability of clients who have quadriplegia to cough effectively, the nurse needs to perform a "cough assist" to prevent atelectasis and pooling of secretions, which could lead to pneumonia. Urinary tract infections occur at an increased rate for clients who have spinal cord injuries due to the inability to empty the bladder completely and development of bacteriuria. Autonomic dysreflexia is a life-threatening medical emergency that must be recognized and treated without delay. This response by the body is often triggered by infection, bladder overdistention, constriction of the thorax, restrictive clothing, and room temperature fluctuations. Immobility of extremities can lead to joint contractures, which may be prevented by performing frequent range-of-motion exercises. Decreased sensory perception and immobility are leading causes for pressure injuries in clients with spinal cord injury. Treatment includes routine and frequent repositioning—for example, performing frequent push-ups in a wheelchair to relieve pressure on the buttocks.

Cognitive Skill

Take Action

References

Ignatavicius et al., 2018, pp. 895–903, 911; Hockenberry et al., 2019, pp. 1331–1335

Thinking Exercise 20-6

Answers

Assessment Finding	Effective	Ineffective	Unrelated
Temperature = 98.5°F (36.9°C)	X		
Heart rate = 68 beats/min and regular	X		
Respiratory rate = 16 breaths/min	X		
Blood pressure = 114/58 mm Hg	X		
Oxygen saturation = 88% (on room air)		X	
Glasgow Coma Scale score = 15	X		
Level of sensory and function impairment has not progressed	X		

Continued

Assessment Finding	Effective	Ineffective	Unrelated
Client is able to assist physical therapy with transfers and exercises	X		
Adolescent cries easily and expresses a lack of hope		X	
Nonblanching redness noted on sacrum		X	
Pain score = 0/10 on a 0 to 10 pain intensity scale			X
Lung sounds are clear bilaterally	X		
Client reports daily bowel movement is soft and brown	X		

Rationales

The primary goals of rehabilitation include maximizing the client's potential for mobility and independent living, which means that the client must be able to physically and emotionally tolerate a wide range of intensive therapies. The client's vital signs have stabilized, but the client continues to have some level of respiratory distress as evidenced by low oxygen saturation even with clear lung sounds. Other assessment findings that indicate that interventions were ineffective is that the client is tearful and likely has not adapted to the spinal cord injury. In addition, the client has a stage 1 pressure injury, a common complication of immobility. Pain is not a common problem for most clients with a spinal cord injury owing to loss of peripheral sensation. Daily bowel movements indicate that the bowel regimen is successful.

Cognitive Skill

Evaluate Outcomes

References

Ignatavicius et al., 2018, pp. 87–101, 452; Hockenberry et al., 2019, pp. 1331–1337

CHAPTER 21 Cognition: *Traumatic Brain Injury*

Answers With Rationales for Thinking Exercises

Exemplar 21. Traumatic Brain Injury (Medical-Surgical Nursing: Older Adult and Young Adult)

Thinking Exercise 21-1

Answers

- Glasgow Coma Scale score
- PERRLA
- Level of consciousness
- Orientation

Rationales

The client needs follow-up for the Glasgow Coma Scale (GCS) score, PERRLA (because of decreasing GCS score), level of consciousness (LOC), and orientation. According to the client information provided, the GCS score is 13 (Eye opening, 3; Motor response, 6; Verbal response, 4) and the LOC is lethargic (drowsy but easily awakened). These are all signs of neurologic impairment, and follow-up is needed to determine the cause.

Cognitive Skill

Recognize Cues

Reference

Ignatavicius et al., 2018, pp. 846–850

Thinking Exercise 21-2

Answers

Nursing Action	Indicated	Contraindicated	Non-Essential
Apply supplemental oxygen.	X		
Conduct a head-to-toe assessment.	X		
Obtain an electrocardiogram (ECG).			X
Obtain a comprehensive metabolic profile (CMP).			X
Obtain a chest x-ray.			X
Insert an indwelling urinary catheter.		X	
Assess pain intensity and quality.	X		

Rationales

The client has a low oxygen saturation rate, so supplemental oxygen therapy is required. A head-to-toe assessment is indicated to determine changes in the client's perfusion. Currently there is no need for an ECG or chest x-ray. Although laboratory analysis of a blood draw may be useful in this situation, a CMP is not indicated. Mental status changes are not an indication for inserting a urinary catheter, which would expose the client to an increased risk of urinary tract infection. Pain should be assessed, especially headache, which can indicate increasing intracranial pressure.

Cognitive Skill

Generate Solutions

Reference

Ignatavicius et al., 2018, pp. 941–948

Thinking Exercise 21-3

Answers

A, B, D, F, H

Rationales

The client may have a subdural hematoma, as indicated by the changes in orientation, level of consciousness, and vital signs. These changes indicate possible Cushing triad: bradycardia, widened pulse pressure, and hypertension. A head CT scan can help diagnose cranial perfusion health problems (Choice A). The nurse gives a 500-mL bolus of saline to increase circulating volume, helping the diastolic blood pressure (Choice B). A CBC is not indicated because the anoxia to the brain causes increased hemoglobin and hematocrit (Choice C). The National Institutes of Health Stroke Scale assesses motor, sensory, language, and muscular function to help find the area of the brain that is injured (Choice D). There is not enough information to administer alteplase (rtPA); if the client is experiencing a hemorrhagic stroke, alteplase will worsen the bleeding (Choice E). The client should have a blood glucose test because hypoglycemia can mimic cerebral anoxia (Choice F). At this time, there is no indication for intubation (Choice G). Pupillary size and responses can indicate increased intracranial pressure. Dilated, unequal, and ovoid pupils are all signs of brain herniation, a life-threatening complication (Choice H).

Cognitive Skill

Take Action

Reference

Ignatavicius et al., 2018, pp. 941–948

Thinking Exercise 21-4

Answers

Nursing Action	Potential Complication	Appropriate Nursing Action for Potential Complication
1 Apply and maintain sequential or pneumatic compression stockings or devices.	Increased carbon dioxide	**2** Apply continuous capnography.
2 Apply continuous capnography.	Hypothermia	**3** Apply warm blankets.
3 Apply warm blankets.	Increased ICP and decreased gas exchange	**4** Elevate the head of the client's bed to more than 30 degrees.
4 Elevate the head of the client's bed to more than 30 degrees.	Increased brain swelling and damage	**6** Perform mental status checks every hour.
5 Insert an indwelling urinary catheter.	Venous thromboembolism (VTE)	**1** Apply and maintain sequential or pneumatic compression stockings or devices.
6 Perform mental status checks every hour.		
7 Monitor vital signs every 15 minutes.		

Rationales

Applying continuous capnography allows the nurse to monitor the amount of carbon dioxide (CO_2) being exhaled. Too much CO_2 in the brain's blood supply causes cerebral dilation and increased ICP. Too little CO_2 in the blood supply causes cerebral vasoconstriction and ischemia. Applying warm blankets gently increases the client's temperature and allows for oxygenation of the peripheral tissues through circulation. Elevating the head of the bed decreases intracranial pressure through gravitational pull on cerebrospinal fluid, increases oxygenation by decreasing the work of the lungs, and increases comfort by decreasing abdominal pressure and work of breathing. Hourly mental status checks allow the nurse to monitor increased swelling and damage. Because the client is intubated and unable to move freely, venous thromboembolism prevention needs to be initiated and maintained.

Cognitive Skill

Take Action

Reference

Ignatavicius et al., 2018, pp. 941–948

Thinking Exercise 21-5

Answers

A, B, C, D, E, F, G, H

Rationales

Most clients with moderate-to-severe brain injuries have long-term physical, cognitive, and emotional deficits. Because of their brain injury, they often have emotional lability, temper outbursts, and memory problems as they adjust to what they are able to accomplish (Choices A and C). Clients with this level of brain injury will need constant supervision to ensure their safety, and may never be able to care for themselves independently (Choice B). Because of these needs, primary caregivers may experience significant role strain and need respite care to keep themselves healthy. The family of the client may feel anger toward the client for all of the changes that need to be made. Local support groups can help families adjust to their new responsibilities and be a worthwhile resource for the family (Choices D, E, and F). Any client who has suffered a brain injury is at an increased risk for seizures. Therefore the nurse needs to teach caregivers what to do in case of a seizure (Choice G). Clients who have a structured environment usually have less emotional and behavioral problems (Choice H).

Cognitive Skill

Take Action

Reference

Ignatavicius et al., 2018, pp. 949–950

Thinking Exercise 21-6

Answers

	Indicated	Non-Essential
Screened for medical conditions	X	
Comatose as determined by a primary health care provider, diagnostic testing, and history	X	
Normal or near normal core body temperature	X	
Normal systolic blood pressure (>100 mm Hg)	X	
Neurologic examination by a neurologist or intensivist	X	
Donation coordinated by a local organ-procurement organization	X	

Rationales

All of these considerations are required for a client to be a successful organ donor. Being comatose, as determined through more than one source of information, and neurologic testing are required to ensure brain death. The medical condition screening, temperature, and blood pressure requirements are necessary to ensure that the procured tissues from the donor will be viable in the recipient. Organ donation is coordinated by local organ-procurement organizations.

Cognitive Skill

Generate Solutions

Reference

Ignatavicius et al., 2018, pp. 947–948

CHAPTER 22 Infection: *Sepsis*

Answers With Rationales for Thinking Exercises

Exemplar 22. Sepsis (Medical-Surgical Nursing: Older Adult)

Thinking Exercise 22-1

Answers

Nursing Action	Indicated	Contraindicated	Non-Essential
Administer a normal saline 1000-mL bolus.	X		
Administer oxygen via nasal cannula.	X		
Draw a comprehensive metabolic profile (CMP).	X		
Obtain a sputum sample.	X		
Position the head of the bed at 30 to 60 degrees.			X
Prepare for central line insertion.	X		
Notify the imaging department of the need for emergent head CT.			X

Rationales

The client's vital signs indicate she is volume deficient, so administering a bolus is an appropriate intervention. If the vitals do not change after the bolus, the client may be experiencing sepsis and system-wide inflammation processes. Administering oxygen is an important intervention because the client is at the borderline, if not below, desirable oxygen saturation rates. A CMP is indicated to look at the anion gap, an indicator of blood pH. The nurse obtains a sputum sample to determine if pneumonia is present. The head of the client's bed can be at any position the client feels is comfortable and is therefore non-essential until the primary health care provider is ready to insert the central line. The client will most likely need multiple sites for IV access and may need to have vasopressors administered to improve her vital signs. Therefore, preparing for a central line is indicated. At this time, there is no indication for a head CT scan.

Cognitive Skill

Generate Solutions

Reference

Ignatavicius et al., 2018, pp. 761–766

Thinking Exercise 22-2

Answers

- Heart rate
- Respirations
- Blood pressure
- Oxygen saturation

- Orientation
- Capillary refill
- Edema

Rationales

The client is demonstrating worsening of cardiac output, further decrease in mentation, and third spacing of fluids. This is likely due to systemic inflammation from sepsis and a depletion of blood volume.

Cognitive Skill

Recognize Cues

Reference

Ignatavicius et al., 2018, pp. 761–766

Thinking Exercise 22-3

Answers

- White blood cell count
- Neutrophils
- Serum lactate

Rationales

These laboratory findings are consistent with sepsis. White blood cell and neutrophil counts decrease in sepsis because these cells are fighting the systemic infection. This process uses extra oxygen, causing cellular anaerobic metabolism. As a result, the serum lactate rises. The nurse would carefully monitor the culture results so that the antibiotic regimen being used for the client can be switched from broad-spectrum antibiotics to microbial-specific ones as indicated by the culture and sensitivity results.

Cognitive Skill

Recognize Cues

References

Ignatavicius et al., 2018, pp. 761–766; Pagana & Pagana, 2018, pp. 120–123, 171, 251–253, 292–293, 315–316, 362–364, 368–369, 453–454, 467–473, 896; Pagana et al., 2019, pp. 152–154, 205, 299–302, 367–369, 416–418, 420–423, 534–536, 549–554, 737–738, 791–793, 991–1005, 1007–1009

Thinking Exercise 22-4

Answers

When making recommendations, the nurse would be sure to include ceftriaxone and IV normal saline (NS). The client weighs 70 kg; therefore the nurse estimates the client needs at least an additional 1100 mL of fluid volume resuscitation to support circulation. In addition, vasopressors are suggested in order to maintain a mean arterial pressure (MAP) of 65.

Rationales

Until culture studies reveal the microorganism causing the sepsis, broad-spectrum antibiotics with gram-negative activity such as ceftriaxone are recommended. Isotonic normal saline is the IV fluid of choice for fluid volume resuscitation. Because the client weighs 70 kg, she should receive 2100 mL total of IV fluid and 1000 has already been infused. Therefore the client needs 1100 mL more of IV fluid. The ideal mean arterial pressure (MAP) in clients experiencing sepsis is at least 65, and vasopressors are titrated in order to achieve this value. If the MAP is above 65, the vasopressor is stopped and not restarted unless the MAP is below 65.

Cognitive Skill

Take Action

References

Burchum & Rosenthal, 2019, pp. 1019–1021; Ignatavicius et al., 2018, pp. 761–766

Thinking Exercise 22-5

Answers

A, B, C, D, E, F, G

Rationales

Clients with elevated serum lactate have the level rechecked after 6 hours from the initial draw (Choice A). Because the client has a low blood pressure (90/50 mm Hg) and a mean arterial pressure (MAP) below 65, the client needs vital sign monitoring every 15 minutes, and vasopressors should be started (Choices B and C). Once the drugs are started, the nurse would need to continue monitoring vital signs every 15 minutes to determine the effectiveness of drug therapy and determine when the medication should be stopped. Vasopressors are not used if the MAP is greater than 65. Vasopressor drugs can damage the peripheral tissues and vessels, so they are best administered through a central line (Choice D). This line also allows central venous pressure measurements, if desired. An indwelling urinary catheter allows the nurse to monitor hourly output from the kidneys to help determine fluid volume status (Choice E). Clients with sepsis often have a low cardiac output from a lack of blood volume, so frequent cardiac and skin assessments can help assess fluid volume status. Blood vessels are very dilated in sepsis, causing third spacing of the infused IV fluids and edema. The nurse would also assess the skin for pallor, temperature, mottling, petechiae, and ecchymoses, which are signs of worsening perfusion and septic shock (Choices F and G).

Cognitive Skill

Take Action

Reference

Ignatavicius et al., 2018, pp. 761–766

CHAPTER 23 Gas Exchange: *Chest Trauma*

Answers With Rationales for Thinking Exercises

Exemplar 23. Chest Trauma (Medical-Surgical Nursing: Middle-Age Adult)

Thinking Exercise 23-1

Answers

- Unable to answer questions or follow commands
- Bilateral chest bruising
- Abdominal bruising
- Heart rate = 110 beats/min
- Blood pressure = 96/65 mm Hg
- Oxygen saturation = 92% (on manual bag/valve and 100% Fio_2)

Rationales

Chest and abdominal bruising indicates trauma to these areas and a potential for internal bleeding. Tachycardia indicates pain or possible blood loss. The nurse would need to monitor heart rate and blood pressure (which is low) to determine if further action is needed. The inability to follow commands and answer questions and 92% oxygenation on manual bag-valve and 100% Fio_2 are important because these findings are consistent with the client's need for mechanical ventilation to have adequate oxygenation.

Cognitive Skill

Recognize Cues

References

Ignatavicius et al., 2018, pp. 129–131, 628–639

Thinking Exercise 23-2

Answers

Nursing Action	Emergent	Contraindicated	Non-Emergent
Administer 2 units of blood.		X	
Contact respiratory therapy department for a mechanical ventilator.	X		
Draw a comprehensive metabolic profile (CMP).			X
Get a chest x-ray to confirm endotracheal tube placement.	X		
Raise the head of the bed to 30 degrees.	X		
Prepare for central line insertion.			X
Notify imaging department about need for emergent head and neck CT.	X		

Rationales

The client is intubated and is not alert enough for extubating, so a mechanical ventilator is needed to maintain breathing. A chest x-ray is used to confirm the endotracheal tube is at the most effective position in the trachea. Positioning the head of bed to 30 degrees helps with breathing efforts and prevents aspiration of gastric contents. Clients with probable head and neck trauma have CTs to rule out injury before the cervical collar can be removed. At this time, the client is not demonstrating a need for blood and there is a chance for transfusion reaction. IV fluids would be a more appropriate choice to help with the slight volume deficiency. A complete metabolic profile will most likely be completed, but these lab values are not an immediate need. Although a central line may be inserted later, there is no immediate indication for this type of access.

Cognitive Skill

Generate Solutions

References

Ignatavicius et al., 2018, pp. 129–131, 628–639

Thinking Exercise 23-3

Answers

Nursing Action	Potential Complication	Appropriate Nursing Action for Each Potential Complication
1 Apply continuous oximetry.	Acute pain	**11** Titrate sedation per facility policy and administer analgesic.
2 Assess mucous membranes.	Impaired oxygenation	**1** Apply continuous oximetry.
3 Administer prophylactic IV antibiotic therapy.	Hypovolemia	**5** Take vital signs every hour.
4 Insert an oral-gastric tube.	Infection	**9** Perform oral care every 2 hours.
5 Take vital signs every hour.	Impaired tissue integrity	**10** Reposition the client every 2 hours.
6 Ensure continuous cardiac monitoring.	Aspiration	**4** Insert an oral-gastric tube.
7 Monitor intake and output.		
8 Monitor for low-grade fever.		
9 Perform oral care every 2 hours.		
10 Reposition the client every 2 hours.		
11 Titrate sedation per facility policy and administer analgesic.		

Rationales

Because the client is on a mechanical ventilator, sedation and analgesics are the most appropriate interventions to promote client comfort. When a client is artificially ventilated, the oxygenation status should be continually monitored to ensure the appropriate settings are being used. Taking vital signs every hour is the best way listed to evaluate whether the client has adequate blood volume. Performing oral care every 2 hours prevents microbial growth and ventilator-associated pneumonia (VAP), a potentially fatal hospital-acquired infection. The client is unable to turn herself and avoid pressure injury, so the nurse must ensure repositioning at least every 2 hours. It is very common for intubated clients to vomit. Inserting an oral-gastric tub prevents aspiration of gastric contents through suction if needed.

Cognitive Skill

Take Action

Reference

Ignatavicius et al., 2018, pp. 628–639

Thinking Exercise 23-4

Answers

The first thing the nurse would check is the client to determine the cause of the alarm. Then the nurse would check the monitors. The nurse determines the alarms are due to low client oxygenation, hypertension, tachycardia, and high peak inspiratory pressure (PIP). Consequently, the nurse suctions the client, which results in no clinical change. The nurse then double-checks the current ventilator settings against previous documentation and notes that there have been no changes to the previous settings. The nurse notifies the primary health care provider and gives an SBAR report. The provider prescribes a repeat bedside chest x-ray. After reviewing the results of the bedside test, the nurse prepares for bedside chest tube insertion to relieve hemothorax in the lower left chest.

Rationales

The nurse would always check the client first to determine the severity of the situation and to ensure that the monitoring leads are attached correctly. Next, the monitors are checked for data to help guide decisions. The most common cause of a PIP alarm is mucus and secretions in the endotracheal tube, which can occlude the airway, causing tachycardia and low oxygenation. A repeat chest x-ray helps to diagnose the cause for the client presentation. Common signs of hemothorax include tachycardia, poor oxygenation, hypertension, and anxiety. Chest tubes for hemothorax are inserted low in the thoracic cavity to alleviate fluid accumulation.

Cognitive Skill

Take Action

Reference

Ignatavicius et al., 2018, pp. 628–639

Thinking Exercise 23-5

Answer

E

Rationales

If the chest tube disconnects from the chest tube drainage system, the chest tube becomes a conduit for microbes to enter the pleural space. Placing the open end of the tube in sterile water prevents microbes from using the tube as a means to enter the pleural space (Choice E). The chest tube dressing should be sterile and tight against the chest to prevent leaks rather than clean and loose (Choice A). The drainage system should be placed below the level of chest tube insertion and the chest tubes should not be "stripped" (Choices C and D). Gentle rather than vigorous bubbling should be present in the water-seal chamber. Excessive bubbling indicates a possible leak in the system (Choice G). Drainage is measured hourly during the first 24 hours after chest tube insertion and then measured according to facility policy (Choice F). The nursing staff would get the client out of bed and encourage deep breathing to prevent respiratory distress or infection (Choice B).

Cognitive Skill

Take Action

Reference

Ignatavicius et al., 2018, p. 592

CHAPTER 24 Elimination: *Complex Health Problems*

Answers With Rationales for Thinking Exercises

Exemplar 24A. Chronic Kidney Disease (Medical-Surgical Nursing: Middle-Age Adult)

Thinking Exercise 24A-1

Answers

- Glycosylated hemoglobin (A1c)
- Blood urea nitrogen (BUN)

- Serum creatinine
- Serum calcium
- Serum phosphate
- Glomerular filtration rate (GFR)

Rationales

The client has had high blood glucose over the past year as evidenced by the average A1c. The client's polyuria is most likely associated with worsening kidney function, as evidenced by a decreased GFR, increased BUN and creatinine, decreased calcium, and increased serum phosphate. High blood sugars damage the nephrons and can worsen kidney failure. Calcium and phosphate have an inverse relationship. In chronic kidney disease, serum phosphate tends to increase because the kidneys have difficulty removing excess phosphorus (phosphate) owing to its molecular size. When phosphate increases, serum calcium decreases, which puts the client at risk for cardiac dysrhythmias.

Cognitive Skill

Recognize Cues

References

Ignatavicius et al., 2018, pp. 1395–1399; Pagana & Pagana, 2018, pp. 120–122, 174–175, 238–240, 351–353, 453–456; Pagana et al., 2019, pp. 152–154, 205–209, 281–283, 403–405

Thinking Exercise 24A-2

Answers

The nurse understands that chronic kidney disease (CKD) management requires changes in **nutrition** and **prescribed medications** to slow or prevent progression of the disease. These changes are designed to lower **blood pressure**, balance **electrolytes**, and maintain appropriate **fluid volume**. If these changes are not successfully made, the client's CKD status can change to stage 5 and result in the need for kidney replacement therapies such as dialysis and/or transplant.

Rationales

For client safety, nurses teach clients to make needed changes in nutrition and take prescribed drugs appropriately. These actions help to lower blood pressure and maintain adequate fluid status. These changes also aid the kidneys in electrolyte balance. If changes are not made by the client, the kidneys will eventually fail, which is categorized as stage 5, and the client will need renal replacement therapy.

Cognitive Skill

Analyze Cues

Reference

Ignatavicius et al., 2018, p. 1339

Thinking Exercise 24A-3

Answers

A, B, C, D, E, F, H

Rationales

Clients in stage 2 or 3 chronic kidney disease (CKD) begin getting education on dialysis methods so that they can make an informed decision about care before they reach end-stage kidney disease (ESKD). If the client chooses hemodialysis, an arteriovenous (AV) fistula is placed and needs time to heal before it can be used as a viable dialysis port (Choice A). If the client chooses peritoneal dialysis, a catheter is placed in the abdomen, which can be used within a few days after placement (Choice B). Clients need education about electrolyte imbalance signs and symptoms because they are not able to excrete excess electrolytes and may experience dysrhythmias or mental status changes due to the excesses (Choice C). Clients who have later stages of CKD have decreased serum calcium, which can cause atherosclerosis and cardiac dysrhythmias—major contributors to myocardial infarction (Choice D). In CKD stage 3 and higher, proteins in the blood build up easily, hyperlipidemia results from fat metabolism changes, and excess phosphates are not excreted. Dietary restrictions are needed to minimize these pathophysiologic changes (Choice E). Participation in 30 to 60 minutes a day of moderately intense exercise and limiting alcohol can help slow progression of CKD to total kidney failure (Choices F and H).

Cognitive Skill

Take Action

Reference

Ignatavicius et al., 2018, pp. 1399–1402

Thinking Exercise 24A-4

Answers

Nursing Action	Indicated	Contraindicated	Non-Essential
Administer oral medications during the dialysis treatment according to the client's home schedule.		X	
Perform a clean dressing change to the access site.		X	
Perform frequent assessments of mental status.	X		
Provide a low-stimulation environment during the dialysis treatment.			X
Use the dialysis catheter for IV fluids after dialysis is completed.		X	
Weigh the client before and after dialysis.	X		

Rationales

Because the nurse is accessing the circulatory system and moving fluid outside of the body to normalize the client's blood volume, 15-minute vital sign and mental status checks are needed to ensure the client has enough fluid volume in the body to function. Administering oral medications according to the client's home schedule is not effective because the dialysis unit also removes medications. Hemodialysis catheters are central lines and need sterile dressings rather than clean ones. A low-stimulation environment is not essential to the success of the client receiving hemodialysis. Using the dialysis catheter for IV fluids after the session concludes is not safe because the catheter is designed for blood inflow and outflow. Weighing the client before and after dialysis is necessary to determine the fluid volume removed from the client during the procedure.

Cognitive Skill

Take Action

Reference

Ignatavicius et al., 2018, pp. 1411–1414

Thinking Exercise 24A-5

Answers

Nursing Action	Potential Dialysis Complication	Appropriate Nursing Action for Dialysis Complication
1 Monitor the client's finger stick blood glucose.	Abdominal pain	**7** Warm the dialysate before infusion.
2 Monitor the client's vital signs frequently.	Catheter site infection	**6** Monitor for warmth and redness at catheter site.
3 Monitor the client's level of consciousness.	Hyperglycemia	**1** Monitor the client's finger stick blood glucose.
4 Apply a mask to both the nurse and client during dialysis catheter access and use.	Peritonitis	**4** Apply a mask to both the nurse and client during dialysis catheter access and use.
5 Monitor the color and clarity of the effluent.	Perforated bowel	**5** Monitor the color and clarity of the effluent.
6 Monitor for warmth and redness at catheter site.		
7 Warm the dialysate before infusion.		

Rationales

Cold or room-temperature dialysate can cause abdominal pain and cramping. Warming the dialysate using an appropriate warmer *(not a microwave)* can ease this pain. Exit site infection is the most frequent complication of peritoneal dialysis catheter insertion. Because the infection can easily travel into the client's system and cause sepsis, the site should be monitored for warmth and redness frequently. Glucose is a major ingredient in dialysate and can cross the peritoneal membrane and increase blood glucose levels. Therefore blood sugars must be checked in order to make sure the dialysate's glucose is not crossing into the client's system. A perforated bowel will leak stool into the peritoneal cavity, which will cause the effluent to be dark and cloudy, rather than nearly clear and colorless. Sterile technique, including masking the nurse and client during catheter access, helps to prevent peritonitis, which can be fatal.

Cognitive Skill

Generate Solutions

Reference

Ignatavicius et al., 2018, pp. 1417–1421

Exemplar 24B. Intestinal Obstruction (Medical-Surgical Nursing: Young Adult, Older Adult)

Thinking Exercise 24B-1

Answers

During the client interview, the nurse asks the client about whether she has had nausea and abdominal pain. The client states that those symptoms "come and go." During the focused physical examination, the nurse inspects the abdomen for distention. Then the nurse auscultates the abdomen and expects that bowel sounds may be absent distal to the obstruction. The nurse anticipates a prescription for a CT scan to aid the primary health care provider in diagnosis. In addition to acute pain, if an intestinal obstruction is confirmed, the client is at risk for dehydration.

Rationales

Commonly reported symptoms associated with intestinal obstruction include nausea, vomiting, abdominal pain, and/or cramping. The abdomen becomes distended and there may be masses seen on inspection. Bowel sounds that are distal to the obstruction are hypoactive or absent. Soft-tissue imaging, such as CT, MRI, or abdominal ultrasound, helps confirm the presence of an intestinal obstruction. If left untreated, the client will develop dehydration and electrolyte imbalances and possibly will die from an intestinal blockage.

Cognitive Skill

Analyze Cues

Reference

Ignatavicius et al., 2018, pp. 1121–1123

Thinking Exercise 24B-2

Answers

Nursing Action	Potential Postoperative Complication	Appropriate Nursing Action for Postoperative Complication
1 Assess the incision site for dehiscence and drainage.	Acute kidney injury	**7** Monitor the client's urine output.
2 Ensure continuous cardiac telemetry monitoring.	Electrolyte imbalance	**2** Ensure continuous cardiac telemetry monitoring.
3 Increase the intravenous fluid rate of infusion.	Respiratory depression	**4** Monitor the client's level of consciousness and vital signs.
4 Monitor the client's level of consciousness and vital signs.	Hypotension	**3** Increase the intravenous fluid rate of infusion.
5 Maintain sequential or pneumatic compression devices.	Venous thromboembolism	**5** Maintain sequential or pneumatic compression devices.
6 Monitor the client's oxygen saturation levels.		
7 Monitor the client's urine output.		
8 Recheck the client's blood glucose.		

Rationales

Because of possible reduced fluid intake before and during surgery, the client is at risk for acute kidney injury due to dehydration. Monitoring urine output evaluates kidney function through urine production. Cardiac telemetry monitors for dysrhythmias caused by electrolyte imbalances. New-onset confusion can be an early sign of respiratory depression and manifests before oxygenation monitoring detects low blood oxygen. The best action for the nurse to take when the client is hypotensive is to increase the rate of intravenous fluid infusion. Maintaining sequential or pneumatic compression devices helps prevent venous stasis and venous thromboembolism in postoperative clients.

Cognitive Skill

Generate Solutions

Reference

Ignatavicius et al., 2018, pp. 272–275

Thinking Exercise 24B-3

Answers

A, B, C, D, E, F, G, H

Rationales

All of these statements support healthy bowel elimination. Raw fruits and vegetables, as well as fiber supplements, add bulk to the stool, making it easier to pass. Water is needed to pass stool. Dehydration can cause the stool to become too hard and dry to pass. Laxatives can decrease abdominal muscle tone and should be used only sparingly. Activating the abdominal muscles through core strengthening aids peristalsis. Prune juice stimulates peristalsis. Diarrhea and oozing stool can be signs of a forming impaction. Using a toilet or bedside commode puts the body in a position that makes passing stool easier than on a bedpan.

Cognitive Skill

Evaluate Outcomes

Reference

Ignatavicius et al., 2018, p. 1126

Thinking Exercise 24B-4

Answers

Assessment Finding	Effective	Ineffective	Unrelated
Staples missing and visible pink tissue at surgical site		X	
Reports mild pain at the incision site	X		
Voiding using a urinal			X
Capillary refill is less than 3 sec	X		
Bilateral +1 pitting edema in ankles and feet	X		

Rationales

Missing staples and pink tissue are signs of wound dehiscence. The surgical site should have all staples accounted for and approximated. Mild pain at the incision site is an expected finding. Using a urinal to void is unrelated to the surgical case. Capillary refill of less than 3 seconds indicates adequate perfusion. Edema in the lower extremities is an expected finding, considering intravenous fluids given in the operating room and postoperative bedrest.

Cognitive Skill

Evaluate Outcomes

Reference

Ignatavicius et al., 2018, pp. 275–278

Thinking Exercise 24B-5

Answers

B

Rationales

Nasogastric (NG) tubes are placed to relieve pressure on the intestines and rest the bowels (Choice B). Abdominal CTs or ultrasounds are used to confirm intestinal obstructions, rather than plain x-rays (Choice A). Many clients with obstructions respond well to nonsurgical management of their conditions, especially nonmechanical causes for the obstruction (Choice C). Walking is an excellent way to promote bowel motility, and therefore bedrest is contraindicated (Choice D). Most clients with intestinal obstruction do not have lengthy hospital stays unless complications arise (Choice E). Clients with NG tubes are NPO with no food or liquids in order to rest the intestines (Choices F and G). Diarrhea can be a sign of partial intestinal obstruction, and the body is using intestinal motility in an attempt to move whatever is causing the obstruction (Choice H).

Cognitive Skill

Take Action

Reference

Ignatavicius et al., 2018, pp. 1123–1125

CHAPTER 25 Metabolism: *Complex Health Problems*

Answers With Rationales for Thinking Exercises

Exemplar 25A. Diabetic Ketoacidosis (Pediatric Nursing: Adolescent)

Thinking Exercise 25A-1

Answers

- History of diabetes mellitus type 1
- Blood glucose = 330 mg/dL (18.3 mmol/L)
- Lethargic
- Heart rate = 120 beats/min
- Blood pressure = 88/42 mm Hg
- Deep rapid respirations
- Breath smells of rotting fruit

Rationales

The client's mother indicates that the client has diabetes mellitus type 1 and a blood glucose level of 330 mg/dL (18.3 mmol/L), and he has been physically active for 3 days. These statements, in addition to the client's lethargy, alert the nurse to assess for complications of hyperglycemia. Deep rapid respirations, called Kussmaul respirations, are a compensation mechanism that assists the body to exhale additional carbon dioxide to correct acidosis. Without adequate insulin the body is unable to use glucose for energy and begins using stored fat. The breakdown of fat for energy produces ketone bodies. The client's acidic or fruity breath is a sign that the client is metabolizing fat instead of glucose. Although the client is lethargic, his ability to follow simple commands is a positive sign. The client's blood pressure and heart rate indicate that the client is dehydrated.

Cognitive Skill

Recognize Cues

References

Ignatavicius et al., 2018, pp. 1282–1283, 1311–1314; Pagana et al., 2019, pp. 269–271

Thinking Exercise 25A-2

Answers

Based on the assessment findings and laboratory results, the nurse suspects that the client is experiencing **diabetic ketoacidosis** because his **serum glucose** is very high and his other laboratory results indicate that he has **metabolic acidosis**. The nurse anticipates that the client will need **IV fluid replacement** and **IV regular insulin** as soon as possible to manage his diabetic complication.

Rationales

Diabetic ketoacidosis is a complication that occurs in clients who have diabetes mellitus type 1 and is characterized by uncontrolled hyperglycemia, metabolic acidosis, and increased production of ketones. The client's deep and rapid respirations are consistent with a client who is experiencing metabolic acidosis. Hyperglycemia causes dehydration and therefore the client needs IV fluid replacement and IV regular insulin because it is a fast-acting type of insulin needed to reduce the current blood glucose level.

Cognitive Skill

Prioritize Hypotheses

References

Ignatavicius et al., 2018, pp. 1282–1283, 1311–1314

Thinking Exercise 25A-3

Answers

Nursing Action	Indicated	Contraindicated	Non-Essential
Initiate potassium replacement per hospital protocol.	X		
Check the client's blood glucose level hourly.	X		
Administer 4 units regular insulin subcutaneously.		X	
Help the client drink 120 mL of fruit juice.		X	
Insert an indwelling urinary catheter to closely monitor output.			X
Monitor the client for postural (orthostatic) hypotension.	X		
Check the client's vital signs every 15 minutes.	X		

Rationales

To determine the effectiveness of the treatment plan, the nurse monitors the client's fluid, electrolytes, and blood glucose levels. Checking the client's vital signs every 15 minutes and monitoring for postural hypotension assists the nurse in determining fluid replacement needs. If the client's blood pressure does not respond to the fluids, the nurse will need to contact the primary health care provider and recommend additional fluid replacement therapy. Checking the client's blood glucose level hourly is essential when administering intravenous insulin. Blood glucose levels usually correct more quickly than the metabolic acidosis, but insulin therapy must continue so that the client's body continues to use glucose for energy instead of stored fat. To prevent hypoglycemia, the nurse will contact the primary health care provider when the client's blood glucose levels reach 250 mg/dL (13.8 mmol/L) and recommend changing the intravenous fluids to 5% dextrose in 0.45% saline. Hypokalemia occurs with insulin therapy, correction of acidosis, and increase in fluid volume. The nurse initiates potassium replacement per protocol to eliminate complications associated with hypokalemia. Insulin therapy is administered intravenously to lower blood glucose levels and maintain glucose metabolism while correcting acidosis. Insulin would not be administered subcutaneously. The client is experiencing hyperglycemia. The administration of fruit juice is treatment for hypoglycemia and would be contraindicated. The nurse must monitor the client's urine output hourly, but a urinary catheter is not needed because the client is able to use a urinal.

Cognitive Skill

Generate Solutions

Reference

Ignatavicius et al., 2018, pp. 1311–1314

Thinking Exercise 25A-4

Answers

Assessment Finding	Effective	Ineffective	Unrelated
Blood glucose = 198 mg/dL (11 mmol/L)	X		
Yellow nasal drainage present			X
Arterial pH = 7.33		X	
Serum creatinine = 1.1 mg/dL (97 mcmol/L)	X		
Bowel sounds hypoactive × 4		X	
Urine ketones = negative	X		

Rationales

The collaborative management for the client is focused on correcting fluid and electrolyte imbalances and blood glucose levels while helping the body to adjust the pH level back to normal. A blood glucose level of 198 mg/dL (11 mmol/L) and serum creatinine level of 1.1 mg/dL demonstrate that insulin infusion and fluid replacement therapy have been effective without causing hypoglycemia, a common complication of diabetic ketoacidosis treatment. Negative urinary ketones, a normal laboratory finding, indicate that the body is no longer breaking down stored fat for energy. With a pH level at 7.33, the client's metabolic acidosis has not yet resolved and further intervention may be required. The client's hypoactive bowel sounds are most likely a manifestation of hypokalemia, a common complication of fluid resuscitation. The nurse must follow up on this assessment finding to prevent cardiac dysrhythmias and paralytic ileus. Nasal drainage is not related to diabetic ketoacidosis or to the treatment plan.

Cognitive Skill

Evaluate Outcomes

Reference

Ignatavicius et al., 2018, pp. 1313–1316

Thinking Exercise 25A-5

Answers

A, C, E, F, G

Rationales

Common precipitating factors for diabetic ketoacidosis include infection, physical or mental stressors, and inadequate insulin dosing. Intensive exercise, as this diabetic client most likely experienced at baseball camp, increases metabolic needs, and glucose cannot be used to meet metabolic needs without appropriate doses of insulin. Precipitating factors for this client include exercising 6 hours each day (Choice E) and not administering prescribed insulin appropriately (Choices C and F). The client would need both long-acting and short-acting insulin to meet his metabolic needs during the baseball camp. Taking his long-acting insulin each morning as prescribed is not a contributing factor. Administering his insulin doses into scar tissue, which slows absorption, and not taking short-acting insulin with meals, which eliminates the body's ability to use any of the food just eaten for energy, are both factors that contribute to hyperglycemia, ketogenesis (conversion of fats into acids), and diabetic ketoacidosis. Eating large meals, including 16 slices of pizza (Choice A), also causes hyperglycemia, especially when insulin is not administered. Hyperglycemia disturbs fluid and electrolyte imbalances. Excessive glucose excreted in the urine results in osmotic diuresis, manifesting as polyuria (Choice G), and contributes to dehydration, a key characteristic of diabetic ketoacidosis.

Cognitive Skill

Analyze Cues

References

Ignatavicius et al., 2018, pp. 1282–1283, 1294–1296, 1299–1301, 1304–1307, 1311–1313

Thinking Exercise 25A-6

Answers

Client's Response	Effective	Ineffective	Unrelated
"I will check my blood sugar levels every 4 hours when exercising and playing baseball."	X		
"I will hold my long-acting insulin doses when I choose not to take my short-acting insulin doses."		X	
"When exercising I will drink only water and not sugar-filled sports drinks."		X	
"I will wear protective sports equipment during baseball games and practice."			X
"I will rotate injection sites because scar tissue slows the absorption of insulin administered."	X		
"I will contact my mother if my blood sugar level is ever more than 250 mg/dL (13.8 mmol/L)."	X		

Rationales

When clients who have diabetes mellitus are experiencing stress from exercise, illness, or some other source, blood glucose monitoring should occur every 4 to 6 hours to identify and treat hyperglycemia effectively. The nurse teaches the client to contact the primary health care provider if blood glucose levels rise above 250 mg/dL (13.8 mmol/L). A adolescent would be taught to contact his mother if his blood glucose levels are elevated so that she can intervene and contact the primary health care provider. Prescribed insulin doses including long-acting and short-acting insulins should not be held. Long-acting insulin maintains a basal level, and short-acting insulin adjusts for food consumed. Insulin injection sites must be rotated, allowing each injection site to heal completely before the site is used again. Exercising increases fluid and electrolyte losses. The nurse also teaches the client to drink sports drinks when exercising strenuously to replace electrolytes, but the client must assess blood glucose levels and administer additional insulin as necessary for the body to metabolize the drink for energy. Wearing protective sports equipment is essential to the client's safety but is not related to the management of diabetes mellitus, nor to prevention of diabetic ketoacidosis episodes.

Cognitive Skill

Evaluate Outcomes

References

Ignatavicius et al., 2018, pp. 1294–1295, 1300–1301, 1314; Pagana et al., 2019, pp. 269–271

Exemplar 25B. Cirrhosis (Medical-Surgical Nursing: Older Adult)

Thinking Exercise 25B-1

Answers

- Mucous membranes are pale and yellow
- Capillary refill = 4 seconds
- Bowel sounds = hypoactive $\times$ 4
- Abdomen is distended and firm
- Petechiae on lower arms and legs
- Client reports severe pruritus

Rationales

The client has a suspected GI bleed and anemia and is at risk for hypovolemic shock, which has resulted in a capillary refill time greater than 3 seconds and pale mucous membranes. The nurse must also look for signs of advancing liver failure, which is evidenced by yellow mucous membranes, hypoactive bowel sounds, a firm and distended abdomen, petechiae on the skin, and reports of pruritus.

Cognitive Skill

Recognize Cues

Reference

Ignatavicius et al., 2018, pp. 1170–1178

Thinking Exercise 25B-2

Answers

Nursing Action	Indicated	Contraindicated	Non-Essential
Obtain consent for the transfusion.	X		
Bathe the client with warm soapy water.		X	
Draw type and screen for blood transfusion.	X		
Ambulate the client to the toilet.		X	

Continued

Nursing Action	Indicated	Contraindicated	Non-Essential
Position the client's head of the bed at between 45 and 60 degrees.			X
Frequently check client vital signs.	X		
Educate the client about incentive spirometry.			X

Rationales

Blood transfusion requires that a consent form be signed and a type and screen be drawn before the transfusion can begin. During the transfusion, the nurse would check the client's vital signs frequently to evaluate for transfusion reactions—either anaphylaxis or fluid volume overload. Using warm soapy water to bathe the client can exacerbate his pruritus; cool water and minimal or no soap should be used. Ambulating the client to the toilet is contraindicated because of his anemia; using a bedside commode is a safer option for toileting. The head of the bed can be positioned for client comfort. The client has not displayed signs of pneumonia, so incentive spirometry education is non-essential at this time.

Cognitive Skill

Generate Solutions

Reference

Ignatavicius et al., 2018, pp. 832–835

Thinking Exercise 25B-3

Answers

Nursing Action	Potential Complication	Appropriate Nursing Action for Complication
1 Monitor oxygen saturation.	Impaired comfort	**3** Administer IV morphine.
2 Assess mucous membranes for jaundice.	Paracentesis insertion site infection	**7** Monitor for a low-grade fever and check insertion site.
3 Administer IV morphine.	Hypervolemia	**6** Monitor intake and output.
4 Monitor level of consciousness.	Electrolyte imbalance	**5** Maintain continuous cardiac monitoring.
5 Maintain continuous cardiac monitoring.	Hepatic encephalopathy	**4** Monitor level of consciousness.
6 Monitor intake and output.		
7 Monitor for a low-grade fever and check needle insertion site.		

Rationales

Clients with liver failure have pain before and after paracentesis, and opioids are effective in helping to manage that pain. The paracentesis site should be checked for warmth, redness, and drainage. It is common for the site to have clear drainage immediately after paracentesis, but purulence can indicate peritonitis, which can lead to a low-grade fever. Clients with ascites should have intake, output, and daily weight monitoring to determine appropriate blood volume status. Changes in level of consciousness can be from shunting of portal venous blood or increased serum ammonia levels and indicate further liver failure. Continuous cardiac monitoring, in addition to blood studies, can show changes such as dehydration, serum potassium, and serum sodium.

Cognitive Skill

Take Action

Reference

Ignatavicius et al., 2018, pp. 1170–1178

Thinking Exercise 25B-4

Answers

A, B, C, D, E, F, G, H

Rationales

Clients who receive a liver transplant must be free from cardiac and pulmonary disease or infection to be considered good candidates for transplant (Choices A and B). Once a transplant occurs, the client will be on antirejection medication for the rest of his life, so medical adherence is vital to the success of the procedure (Choice C). Liver tissue can come from a living or deceased donor, since only part of the organ (usually one lobe) is used (Choice D). Even with proper management, the client's body may reject the new liver (Choice E). Fever and right upper quadrant pain are hallmark signs of liver rejection (Choice G). Antirejection medications suppress the immune response, which increases the client's risk for developing cancer (Choice F). Keeping up with vaccination schedules is also important because of the client's suppressed immune system (Choice H).

Cognitive Skill

Take Action

Reference

Ignatavicius et al., 2018, pp. 1187–1189

Thinking Exercise 25B-5

Answers

Assessment Finding	Effective	Ineffective	Unrelated
Is oriented to person, place, and time	X		
Reports mild abdominal pain	X		
Voided 150 mL in 8 hr using a urinal		X	
Capillary refill is less than 3 sec	X		
Oxygen saturation is 95% on room air.	X		
Bilateral +1 pitting edema in ankles and feet		X	

Rationales

The goal of care in this phase for the client is to keep as much physiologic stability as possible. Being oriented to person, place, and time indicates no worsening of brain function. Liver failure can cause a great amount of abdominal pain due to pressure from ascites, so mild pain is considered effective. Capillary refill of less than 3 seconds indicates good perfusion. An oxygen saturation of 95% on room air means there is adequate oxygen exchange in the lungs. Voiding less than 240 mL in 8 hours is cause for concern (less than 30 mL/hr) and indicates that the kidneys have been affected. Either the client is dehydrated or his nephrons have been damaged so badly by circulating bilirubin that they are decreasing their ability to make urine. Bilateral pitting edema in the ankles and feet indicates that there is a circulatory issue causing fluid to leak from the blood vessels and pool in the tissues.

Cognitive Skill

Evaluate Outcomes

Reference

Ignatavicius et al., 2018, pp. 1170–1178

Exemplar 25C. Acute Pancreatitis (Medical-Surgical Nursing: Middle-Age Adult)

Thinking Exercise 25C-1

Answers

A, B, D, E, G

Rationales

The client's initial appearance and report alerts the nurse to acute pancreatitis or an exacerbation of chronic pancreatitis. At this time, the nurse would not attempt to complete a health history nor a CAGE assessment, as the client's pain level must be addressed before he will be able to answer questions appropriately. The nurse would complete a full pain assessment including location, severity, onset, duration, contributing factors, and relieving factors (Choice G). In addition, the nurse would assess for other manifestations of pancreatitis including abdominal rigidity and gray-blue discoloration caused by pancreatic enzyme leakage into cutaneous tissue from the peritoneal cavity (Choices B and E). Complications of pancreatitis would also be assessed. Shock is a life-threatening complication of pancreatitis that would be monitored by assessing vital signs frequently (Choice A). Respiratory complications may also occur with pancreatitis, including hypoxia, atelectasis, pneumonia, and pleural effusions. Auscultating lung fields and assessing for signs of dyspnea are essential for early identification of these respiratory complications (Choice D).

Cognitive Skill

Analyze Cues

Reference

Ignatavicius et al., 2018, pp. 1197–1200

Thinking Exercise 25C-2

Answers

Nursing Action	Indicated	Contraindicated	Non-Essential
Provide the client with a low-fat diet.		X	
Help the client into a side-lying position with knees flexed.	X		
Teach the client to use an incentive spirometer.			X
Monitor vital signs every 15 minutes.	X		
Provide pain relief by pushing the client's PCA button.		X	

Nursing Action	Indicated	Contraindicated	Non-Essential
Assess glucose management with a hemoglobin A1c level.			X
Provide an emesis basin and measure amount vomited.		X	
Assist the client in performing frequent oral care.	X		

Rationales

This client is at risk for shock from pancreatic hemorrhage, fluid volume shifts, and/or toxic effects of abdominal sepsis from enzyme damage. The nurse monitors the client's vital signs frequently to identify changes in hemodynamic status early. During the acute phase of pancreatitis, the client would be kept NPO to rest the pancreas and reduce pancreatic enzyme secretion. Providing the client with a diet at this time would be contraindicated, especially since the client is vomiting bile. Instead of providing an emesis basin for the client's vomiting, the nurse would obtain an order for a nasogastric tube to decompress and empty the stomach. Because the client is NPO, the nurse or assistive personnel would assist the client in performing frequent oral hygiene to keep mucous membranes moist and free of inflammation or crusts. Clients with pancreatitis may experience intermittent hyperglycemia owing to a release of glucagon and decreased release of insulin, but this is an acute issue. Acute hyperglycemia is best assessed by serum blood glucose levels and not hemoglobin A1c levels. The client is at risk for respiratory complications, but a client in acute pain from pancreatitis is not ready to learn about or use an incentive spirometer.

Cognitive Skill

Generate Solutions

Reference

Ignatavicius et al., 2018, pp. 1198–1201

Thinking Exercise 25C-3

Answers

Assessment Finding	Effective	Ineffective	Unrelated
Blood pressure = 125/63 mm Hg	X		
Bilateral crackles present on auscultation		X	
Alert and oriented, denies anxiety	X		
Positive Chvostek sign		X	
Reports a personal history of alcoholism			X
Bowel sounds active × 4			X
Abdominal pain rated 3/10 on a 0 to 10 pain intensity scale	X		

Rationales

Management of acute pancreatitis is focused on decreasing pain and preventing complications. The client currently rates his abdominal pain at 3/10, which indicates that treatment is working to decrease his pain, which was previously rated at 10/10. The client's blood pressure and mental status indicate fluid resuscitation has been effective in stabilizing hemodynamic status. The nurse may want to know if the client has a history of alcoholism, but this information does not assist in determining if implemented interventions were effective. The client's mental status indicates that he is not currently experiencing any alcohol withdrawal symptoms. Bilateral crackles present on auscultation indicate a respiratory complication and must be monitored closely to prevent respiratory failure. A positive Chvostek sign relates to hypocalcemia, another complication of pancreatitis. Calcium replacement therapy is needed to prevent additional issues. Paralytic ileus is another complication of pancreatitis, but bowel sounds are not a good assessment of peristalsis. This information does not provide the nurse with necessary data to determine whether treatment is effective. Passage of flatus or a bowel movement is a reliable indicator of peristalsis and should be used to determine intervention effectiveness.

Cognitive Skill

Evaluate Outcomes

Reference

Ignatavicius et al., 2018, pp. 1198–1201

Thinking Exercise 25C-4

Answers

Nursing Action	Potential Complication	Appropriate Nursing Action for Each Complication
1 Weigh the client daily and report a significant increase from the previous day.	Hyperglycemia	**3** Assess finger stick blood sugars every 4 hours.
2 Have a second nurse check the prescription and solution prior to administration.	Fluid overload	**1** Weigh the client daily and report a significant increase from the previous day.
3 Assess finger stick blood sugars every 4 hours.	Infection	**6** Assess the IV site daily and change the dressing per agency policy.
4 Change the IV tubing every 3 days.	Hypoglycemia	**7** Infuse 10% dextrose in water if TPN solution is temporarily unavailable.
5 Adjust the infusion rate to ensure the entire TPN bag infuses within 24 hours.		
6 Assess the IV site daily and change the dressing per agency policy.		
7 Infuse 10% dextrose in water if TPN solution is temporarily unavailable.		

Rationales

Total parenteral nutrition (TPN) solutions contain high concentrations of dextrose and proteins. The high sugar content puts the client at risk for hyperglycemia, and insulin may be added to the solution by the pharmacist to help prevent this complication. With or without insulin in the solution, the nurse would obtain finger stick blood sugars every 4 hours, document results to trend glucose levels, and administer additional insulin if necessary to prevent hyperglycemia. Vascular fluids may shift because of the high concentration of the TPN solution; therefore the nurse must monitor the client's weight and intake and output. A significant increase in weight from one day to the next indicates fluid overload and must be reported to prevent respiratory complications. TPN is only infused through a central IV catheter.

Central IV catheters, in general, place the client at risk for infection, but infusing a high-glucose solution through the catheter increases the client's risk. When administering TPN, the nurse must assess the IV site daily, change the IV tubing every day when spiking a new infusion bag, and change the dressing per facility protocol. In nondiabetic clients, the pancreas produces increased amounts of insulin to metabolize the dextrose-concentrated TPN solution. If the infusion is stopped abruptly, the high levels of insulin without any glucose will cause a hypoglycemic event. Therefore the nurse infuses a 10% or 20% dextrose solution if TPN is temporarily unavailable. The nurse would have a second nurse check the prescription and solution prior to administering to ensure client safety, although this action does not directly prevent or identify any of the potential complications listed.

Cognitive Skill

Take Action

References

Ignatavicius et al., 2018, pp. 1201–1203, 1224

Thinking Exercise 25C-5

Answers

The nurse teaches the client to eat small, frequent meals that contain high-**protein**, moderate-**carbohydrate**, and low-**fat** foods. GI stimulants such as **caffeine** and **spices** should be avoided. The client is taught to abstain from drinking alcohol because if alcohol is consumed, acute **pain** will return and further **autodigestion** of the pancreas may lead to chronic pancreatitis. In addition to nutritional teaching, the nurse teaches the client to contact the primary health care provider with symptoms of biliary tract disease including **jaundice**, **clay-colored stools**, and/or **dark urine**.

Rationales

The nurse would collaborate with a registered dietitian nutritionist to teach the client about long-term dietary management. The client would be taught to eat bland, low-fat, high-protein, and moderate-carbohydrate meals. Food high in protein and moderate in carbohydrates assist in the healing process, and food high in fat is avoided because it causes the pancreas to secrete more digestive enzymes. The nurse would teach the client to avoid foods that make symptoms worse, such as caffeinated beverages, spicy foods, and alcohol. Ingestion of alcohol increases the client's risk for recurring acute pancreatitis episodes, manifesting with acute pain, and possible progression to chronic pancreatitis. Pancreatitis results in autodigestion and fibrosis of the pancreas. The nurse would teach the client to be alert for the signs and symptoms of biliary tract disease or cholecystitis, including jaundice, clay-colored stools, and dark urine. Gallstones can cause an episode of acute pancreatitis.

Cognitive Skill

Take Action

References

Ignatavicius et al., 2018, pp. 1193–1194, 1197, 1201–1204

CHAPTER 26 Tissue Integrity: *Burns*

Answers With Rationales for Thinking Exercises

Exemplar 26. Burns (Medical-Surgical Nursing: Young Adult)

Thinking Exercise 26-1

Answers

Nursing Action	Indicated	Contraindicated	Non-Essential
Obtain a 12-lead ECG.			X
Initiate an IV line.	X		
Administer oxygen therapy.			X
Remove eschar to prevent infection.			X
Manage the client's pain with analgesia.	X		
Administer tetanus toxoid for prophylaxis.	X		
Help the client take a shower.		X	

Rationales

Clients who have superficial and superficial partial thickness burns have pain and are at risk for tetanus. These burns do not create eschar. Starting an IV line allows access for IV analgesia and fluids as the client may require, and administering preventive tetanus toxoid is important for tetanus prevention. At this time, it appears that the client does not have any airway or breathing issues. Therefore oxygen is not needed. An ECG is also not indicated at this time. To prevent infection, the client should not take a shower until healing occurs.

Cognitive Skill

Generate Solutions

Reference

Ignatavicius et al., 2018, pp. 482–497

Thinking Exercise 26-2

Answers

Using the Rule of Nines, the nurse calculates that the client has burns on an estimated 10% of her body. The client is at risk for developing infection and edema as a result of her burns. The nurse applies a wound dressing after giving the client a(n) analgesic.

Rationales

The total anterior and posterior of a person's arm represent 9% (4.5% for each side) of the body. However, this client's hands are not affected and they each account for 1%. The client has bilateral anterior arm burns (3.5% for each arm for a total of 7%), and burns on about half of her posterior arms

(½ of 7% is 3.5%). Adding 7% plus 3.5% provides an estimate of about 10% to 10.5%. The client's burns are not deep, but the skin, which usually protects a person from infection, has been disrupted. Therefore she is at high risk for a local wound infection. Skin and underlying tissue damage also places the client at risk for edema around the wounds. In addition to skin damage, the burns damaged peripheral nerves, causing moderate to severe pain. Therefore the client requires analgesic medication to promote comfort.

Cognitive Skill

Analyze Cues

Reference

Ignatavicius et al., 2018, pp. 482–497

Thinking Exercise 26-3

Answers

A, B, C, D, E, F, G, H, I

Rationales

The client is at risk for airway obstruction or breathing issues due to possible smoke inhalation. Therefore Choices B, C, E, G, and I are important interventions to manage this potential problem. The client's airways were likely burned from smoke inhalation. The other choices (A, D, F, and H) are appropriate interventions for any client who has sustained recent burns.

Cognitive Skill

Take Action

Reference

Ignatavicius et al., 2018, pp. 482–497

Thinking Exercise 26-4

Answers

C, D

Rationales

The client is now in the acute phase of burn injury in which he is at high risk for sepsis and respiratory infections, such as pneumonia (Choices C and D). Most of the other choices are more common in the first phase of burn injury, which is the resuscitation phase. In the current phase, the client would be expected to lose weight rather than gain it. Posttraumatic stress disorder often manifests later in the rehabilitation phase of burn injury.

Cognitive Skill

Analyze Cues

Reference

Ignatavicius et al., 2018, pp. 497–504

Thinking Exercise 26-5

Answers

> **Nurses' Notes**
>
> 9/18/20 7 a.m. (0700) Client states that his pain is often a 4-5/10 on a 0 to 10 pain intensity scale. PT in this a.m. to begin exercises to prevent joint contractures. States he always feels hungry, especially after working with the therapist. Has lost 10 pounds since admission 3 days ago even though he is on a high-calorie diet. Serum albumin and prealbumin this a.m. continue to be below normal limits. _____ K.S. Atkins, RN

Rationales

The client's pain is not under control and requires attention to increase client comfort. At this time he is in the acute phase of burn injury and has increased body metabolism, causing weight loss. It is clear that his metabolic needs are not being met, and the nurse would collaborate with the registered dietitian nutritionist to change his plan of care to achieve the desired outcome of preventing the client from losing more weight.

Cognitive Skill

Recognize Cues

Reference

Ignatavicius et al., 2018, pp. 497–450

CHAPTER 27 Stress and Coping: *Substance Use Disorder*

Answers With Rationales for Thinking Exercises

Exemplar 27. Substance Use Disorder (Pediatric Nursing/Mental Health Nursing: Adolescent)

Thinking Exercise 27-1

Answers

- Client is "doubled over" in pain, but also unable to walk without swaying and bumping into the wall
- Client talks with slurred words, has difficulty focusing, and falls asleep repeatedly during assessment
- History of attention deficit hyperactivity disorder (ADHD) and asthma
- Home medications: amphetamine/dextroamphetamine daily
- Father's occupation is nurse
- Reports casual social acquaintances
- "Struggles" in school per parents
- Rates severe abdominal pain as "15" on a 0 to 10 pain scale; slightly worse in left lower quadrant
- Respiratory rate = 12 breaths/min
- Amylase = 250 units/L
- Lipase = 260 units/L
- ALT = 40 units/L
- Alkaline phosphatase = 360 units/L
- Blood alcohol level = 236 mg/dL or 51.2 mmol/L
- Oriented to self, but somnolent
- Distended abdomen with hypoactive bowel sounds and tender to palpation
- Mildly diaphoretic, otherwise skin intact

Rationales

The adolescent appears to be under the influence of drugs and alcohol based on his mental state and difficulty with speaking and ambulation. Health history results that have significantly increased association with substance use include taking amphetamines daily for ADHD, having minimal social relationships, and having difficulty learning. Difficulty learning can be a contributing causative factor to substance use or may be the result of substance use. The serum laboratory results and distended, painful abdomen are suggestive of some level of liver or pancreas injury as a result of alcoholism. The client's clinical manifestations also support complications related to alcoholism. A respiratory rate of 10 breaths/min suggests respiratory depression, which can lead to some level of more serious respiratory distress.

Cognitive Skill

Recognize Cues

References

Halter, 2018, pp. 408–422; Pagana & Pagana, 2018, pp. 36, 43–44, 55, 206–207, 302, 412–413; Hockenberry & Wilson, 2019, pp. 543, 581–583

Thinking Exercise 27-2

Answers

B, D, E, F

Rationales

It is very important to ask how, what, and when questions to elicit a thorough history and understanding of the client's substance use disorder. Asking questions in a matter-of-fact tone and being nonjudgmental helps the client feel more comfortable and answer truthfully (Choices B, D, E, and F). Listening to the client's responses is a significant component of the assessment. Questions that begin with "Why" are not therapeutic, as they are perceived as being judgmental.

Cognitive Skill

Take Action

References

Halter, 2018, pp. 408, 422–423; Hockenberry & Wilson, 2019, pp. 530–540

Thinking Exercise 27-3

Answers

A, B, C, D, E, F

Rationales

The desired outcomes for the client are to facilitate a safe detoxification without injury and participate in therapeutic interventions that include referral for treatment (Choice A). The nurse will want to be sure to include parents and family members because they also need therapy to help process this experience and understand their loved one (Choices D and F). Therapeutic outcomes for the client include helping the client to increase his problem-solving skills, identifying community resources that support remaining drug free, and decreasing his projection or rationalization behaviors (Choice C). Although relapse is a very common complication following detoxification, all clients should be attempting to abstain for some period of time (Choice B). After the client returns to the community, he should not miss school (Choice E).

Cognitive Skill

Generate Solutions

References

Halter, 2018, pp. 423–427; Hockenberry & Wilson, 2019, pp. 532, 543, 581–582

Thinking Exercise 27-4

Answers

Clinical Manifestations of Drug Withdrawal	Drug	Expected Clinical Manifestations From Drug Withdrawal
1 Client reports insomnia, or sleep disturbances.	Sedative-hypnotics	**3, 9, 11**
2 Client experiences dulled thinking and lethargy.	Cocaine	**1, 2, 5, 8**
3 Client reports hallucinations.	Heroin	**1, 4, 5, 6, 10**
4 Client reports muscle aches or bone pain.	Oxycodone	**1, 4, 10**
5 Client demonstrates restlessness or depression.	Phencyclidine (PCP)	**5, 8**
6 Client reports cold flashes and goose bumps.	Flunitrazepam	**3, 4, 5, 7, 9**
7 Client demonstrates extreme anxiety and irritability.		
8 Client reports vivid unpleasant dreams, and/or increased appetite.		
9 Client exhibits seizure activity or delirium.		
10 Client reports nausea or vomiting or stomach cramping.		
11 Client demonstrates elevated pulse, hyperthermia, and blood pressure.		

Cognitive Skill

Analyze Cues

References

Halter, 2018, pp. 414–425; Hockenberry & Wilson, 2019, pp. 580–581

Thinking Exercise 27-5

Answers

Nursing Action	Indicated	Contraindicated	Non-Essential
Monitor the client's respiratory rate every 4 hours.	X		
Complete the Clinical Institute Withdrawal From Alcohol (CIWA-Ar) scale every 4 hours and as needed.	X		
Encourage the client to use denial as a coping mechanism.		X	
Complete a search of the client's personal belongings.	X		
Schedule time for an initial family therapy session.	X		
Administer naloxone			X
Recognize that substance use disorder is a disease influenced by genetic factors.	X		

Nursing Action	Indicated	Contraindicated	Non-Essential
Arrange and encourage client counseling.	X		
Redirect client when he projects anger.	X		
Provide an empathetic, warm, and nonjudgmental environment.	X		
Require that the client participate in group activities.		X	
Administer acetaminophen as needed for headaches.		X	

Rationales

Monitoring the client for withdrawal symptoms; especially respiratory distress or failure, is the priority for the nurse to maintain client safety during the acute phase of withdrawal, or about the first 72 hours. It is also important for the nurse to maintain a therapeutic and comfortable environment so that the client feels safe and improves his response to treatment. Counseling for both the client and the family is essential. By referring to the addiction as a disease, the nurse helps the client feel less guilt and improves self-esteem. Naloxone is an opioid antagonist and therefore non-essential because the client did not test positive for opioids. Acetaminophen is contraindicated because the drug can cause liver toxicity and the client already has a compromised liver function, most likely as a result of the client's alcohol dependence. Allowing the client to continue to rationalize or deny responsibility or accountability for his treatment is nontherapeutic and therefore contraindicated.

Cognitive Skill

Generate Solutions

References

Halter, 2018, pp. 408–427; Hockenberry & Wilson, 2019, pp. 578–583

Thinking Exercise 27-6

Answers

Assessment Finding	Effective	Ineffective	Unrelated
The client reports that he cannot stay sober without help.	X		
The client shares that his parents' "nagging" makes him want to drink.		X	
The client actively engages in and attends self-help groups.	X		
The client plans to look for a new group of friends.	X		
The client is able to express feelings of sadness.	X		
The client reports satisfaction with body image.			X
The client denies experiencing flashbacks or hallucinations.			X
The client expresses hopelessness that he will be able to stay sober.		X	
The client sings and dances in the unit hallway.			X

Rationales

Substance use rehabilitation programs are based on three fundamental concepts: (1) People are powerless over their addiction and therefore they cannot remain substance free without help; (2) although people are not responsible for their disease, they are responsible for their recovery; and (3) clinical findings that support the effectiveness of detoxification treatment include the client's ability to take responsibility for treatment, without blaming others. Evidence that the client has completed the withdrawal phase without injury also supports that outcomes are being met. For successful rehabilitation, the client should not have feelings of hopelessness.

Cognitive Skill

Evaluate Outcomes

References

Halter, 2018, pp. 416–428; Hockenberry & Wilson, 2019, pp. 532, 543, 580–582

CHAPTER 28 Management of Care: *Complex Health Problems*

Answers With Rationales for Thinking Exercises

Exemplar 28. Complex Health Problems (Medical-Surgical Nursing: Middle-Age and Older Adult)

Thinking Exercise 28-1

Answers

After report from the previous shift, the nurse most likely would assess Client # 4 as the priority because this client is at risk for blood transfusion reaction. The second client that the nurse would assess is Client # 1 because this client is at risk for embolic stroke.

Rationales

Client #4 is currently receiving a unit of packed red blood cells and may experience a life-threatening reaction such as respiratory distress, or other complications such as elevated temperature or urticaria (hives). Client #1 is also at risk for embolic stroke, which is a common and potentially life-threatening complication resulting from new-onset atrial fibrillation.

Cognitive Skill

Prioritize Hypotheses

Thinking Exercise 28-2

Answer

E

Rationales

All of the clients except for Client #5 have very complex and unstable physical health problems, and several have additional major mental health problems. Client #5 has a history of many health problems but she is ready for discharge (Choice E). Therefore she is more stable and has more predictable outcomes when compared with the other four clients, which is within the scope of practice of the LPN/LVN.

Cognitive Skill

Take Action

Thinking Exercise 28-3

Answers

Nursing Actions	Assigned Client	Appropriate Nursing Action for Assigned Client
1 Administer prescribed antibiotic therapy.	Client #1	**2** Assess client's neurologic status frequently.
2 Assess client's neurologic status frequently.	Client #2	**6** Monitor for new-onset cardiac dysrhythmias.
3 Review medications for home care follow-up.	Client #3	**4** Assess for orthostatic hypotension.
4 Assess for orthostatic hypotension.	Client #4	**5** Monitor hemoglobin and hematocrit values.
5 Monitor hemoglobin and hematocrit values.	Client #5	**3** Review medications for home care follow-up.
6 Monitor for new-onset cardiac dysrhythmias.		
7 Consult with physical and occupational therapy providers.		

Rationales

Client #1 has new-onset atrial fibrillation and is at risk for stroke. Therefore the nurse would monitor the client carefully for changes in neurologic status to determine the presence of an embolic stroke. Client #2 has severe hypokalemia for which he is receiving IV potassium supplements. Potassium is essential for muscle functioning including the myocardium. Therefore a low potassium level can cause a cardiac dysrhythmia. Clients who have Parkinson disease are also often at risk for orthostatic hypotension. However, he requires total care and is likely immobile, preventing him from being out of bed and changing to a standing position in which orthostatic (postural) hypotension typically occurs. Because he is ADL dependent, a referral for rehabilitation is not appropriate. Client #3 has severe dehydration, which often causes hypotension, especially when the client changes position from lying or sitting to standing. Client #4 has GI bleeding and is receiving a blood transfusion to increase her hemoglobin and hematocrit, which requires monitoring. Client #5 is preparing for discharge, and the nurse would perform medication reconciliation to ensure she will take the drugs that are needed to continue her management at home. Antibiotic therapy is not appropriate to manage viral pneumonia.

Cognitive Skill

Take Action

Thinking Exercise 28-4

Answers

A, B, D, G

Rationales

It is not within the scope of practice for assistive personnel to provide client education or perform client assessments. However, they may take and document vital signs and oxygen saturation if taught how to do those procedures (Choice A). They may record and document the client's intake and urinary output (Choice B). Assistive personnel also provide personal client care, including bathing and turning clients to prevent skin breakdown (Choices D and G).

Cognitive Skill

Take Action

Thinking Exercise 28-5

Answers

A, B, C, E, F, G

Rationales

All of these activities are within the scope of practice for the LPN/LVN if he or she is taught how to perform them, with the exception of Choice D. The comprehensive health assessment is performed only by the RN; the LPN/LVN may perform a focused assessment as needed, depending on the client's condition.

Cognitive Skill

Take Action

CHAPTER 29 Pharmacology in Management of Common Health Problems

Answers With Rationales for Thinking Exercises

Exemplar 29A. Drugs That Affect Nutrition and Elimination (Medical-Surgical Nursing: Older Adult; Pediatric Nursing)

Thinking Exercise 29A-1

Answers

A, B, E, F, G, H

Rationales

The nurse would teach the client the need to take all medication doses because two of the drugs are antibiotics to treat the infection (Choice A). However, many antibiotics can cause GI distress, especially nausea and diarrhea, which can cause dehydration in a client over 65 years of age (Choice B). Pantoprazole is a proton pump inhibitor that can cause magnesium and bone loss. Therefore the client should have a baseline serum magnesium and bone density scan for comparison after the drug regimen is discontinued (Choices E and F). Pantoprazole also decreases gastric pH, which can predispose older adults to pneumonia (Choice G). Alcohol can cause a severe interaction with metronidazole, including possible vomiting, severe headache, and seizures. The nurse would teach the importance of avoiding alcohol while the client is taking this drug (Choice H).

Cognitive Skill

Take Action

References

Burchum & Rosenthal, 2019, pp. 956–966, 1099

Thinking Exercise 29A-2

Answers

The child weighs 57 lb today; therefore the nurse calculates his prescribed dose of polyethylene glycol to be 21 g once daily. The nurse teaches the mother to give the child a(n) full glass of water with each dose of docusate sodium and report adverse effects of his new drug therapy, including excessive diarrhea, increased abdominal bloating, and flatulence.

Rationales

The child weighs 57 lb, which converts to 25.9 kg (57/2.2 = 25.9). The amount of polyethylene glycol that he is supposed to take is 0.8 g/kg of body weight; 25.9 kg × 0.8 = 20.72 g of medication, which is rounded to 21 g. Water helps to decrease constipation and promote bowel elimination. Adverse effects of taking both a stool softener and laxative include excessive diarrhea, abdominal bloating and cramping, and excess flatulence (gas).

Cognitive Skill

Take Action

Reference

Burchum & Rosenthal, 2019, pp. 973–978

Thinking Exercise 29A-3

Answers

Assessment Finding	Effective	Ineffective	Unrelated
Serum potassium = 3.2 mEq/L (3.2 mmol/L)		X	
Serum sodium = 136 mEq/L (136 mmol/L)	X		
Increased sexual desire and erection	X		
No chest pain or dyspnea	X		
Blood pressure = 118/66 mm Hg	X		
Frequent tearing eyes and sneezing when outdoors			X
1+ to 2+ edema in both ankles		X	

Rationales

All of the assessment findings are within normal limits except for the client's serum potassium (which is low) and his peripheral edema at 1+ to 2+ in both ankles. Therefore these abnormal findings indicate that the treatment plan, including drug therapy, is not as effective as it needs to be. The client's report of frequent tearing eyes and sneezing when outdoors suggests that the client has allergies, which are not related to his primary health problem of heart failure.

Cognitive Skill

Evaluate Outcomes

Reference

Burchum & Rosenthal, 2019, pp. 464–465

Thinking Exercise 29A-4

Answers

Nursing Action	Anticipated	Contraindicated	Non-Essential
Draw a comprehensive metabolic panel (CMP).			X
Carefully monitor the client's intake and output.	X		
Initiate oxygen therapy.	X		
Continue to carefully monitor daily weights.	X		
Prepare to administer IV push furosemide stat.	X		
Keep the client in a supine flat position.		X	
Monitor the client's vital signs frequently.	X		

Rationales

The client has a history of heart failure, has peripheral edema and new-onset shortness of breath, and gained 4 lb (1.82 kg) of body fluid in 2 days. All of these findings indicate worsening heart failure (affecting left and right sides of the heart) requiring actions such as carefully monitoring intake and output, starting oxygen therapy, and monitoring daily weights. The nurse would anticipate that the primary health care provider would prescribe IV push furosemide, a fast-acting loop diuretic, to decrease body fluid volume. The client should be placed in a semi-Fowler or Fowler (sitting) position to ease the client's breathing. It is not essential to draw a CMP at this time.

Cognitive Skill

Generate Solutions

Reference

Burchum & Rosenthal, 2019, pp. 462–464

Thinking Exercise 29A-5

Answers

For safe medication administration, the nurse will administer the IV push furosemide over 1 to 2 minutes. Within an hour of administration, the client would be expected to void a large amount. If needed, IV push furosemide may be repeated in 1 to 2 hours.

Rationales

IV furosemide is given slowly when given via IV push. As a fast-acting loop diuretic, the client would be expected to void to get rid of excessive fluid volume. If the client does not respond as expected, the drug may be safely repeated in 1 to 2 hours.

Cognitive Skill

Evaluate Outcomes

Reference

Burchum & Rosenthal, 2019, pp. 462–464

Exemplar 29B. Drugs That Affect Clotting (Medical-Surgical Nursing: Middle-Age and Older Adult)

Thinking Exercise 29B-1

Answers

B, D, E, F

Rationales

Sodium heparin is a fast-acting anticoagulant that acts in the bloodstream to prevent further clotting. Therefore it can affect the aPTT, platelet count, and complete blood cell count (Choices B, D, and F). In addition, the anti-factor Xa heparin assay is monitored when clients are receiving this medication to evaluate the drug level (Choice E). INR and PT are monitored in clients receiving warfarin.

Cognitive Skill

Recognize Cues

References

Burchum & Rosenthal, 2019, pp. 607–611, 629–630

Thinking Exercise 29B-2

Answers

During IV heparin administration, the nurse would monitor the client for possible adverse drug effects, especially bleeding or hemorrhage. To monitor for this complication, the nurse would assess for common signs of blood loss, including decreased blood pressure and increased pulse. Other indications of bleeding include hematuria, red or black stools, ecchymosis, and decreased level of consciousness.

Rationales

Blood loss causes hypovolemia or dehydration. In this state, the pressure of blood against the arterial vessel walls is lessened, resulting in a decreased blood pressure. To compensate for less intravascular fluid volume (blood), the heart beats more quickly to circulate blood throughout the body to perfuse major organs and the periphery. The nurse monitors for signs of overt bleeding, including blood in the urine and/or stool. In addition, a decrease in level of consciousness may indicate bleeding in the cerebrum of the brain.

Cognitive Skill

Prioritize Hypotheses

Reference

Burchum & Rosenthal, 2019, pp. 607–611

Thinking Exercise 29B-3

Answers

A, B, C, D, E, F, G, H

Rationales

Warfarin is administered orally and is a slower-acting anticoagulant that works directly in the liver to decrease clotting. However, because it is an anticoagulant, the client is at risk for bleeding and should follow Bleeding Precautions. These precautions include avoiding any sharp objects (such as hard toothbrushes or razors) (Choices E and F) and monitoring for any unusual bleeding or bruising, which should be reported immediately to the primary health care provider after stopping the drug (Choices C and G). The nurse teaches the client to avoid any drug, including over-the-counter drugs, that can cause bleeding and to follow up with laboratory testing to monitor coagulation study levels (Choices B and D). The client needs to avoid pregnancy because the drug is toxic for a fetus and can interact with many other drugs (Choice A). Even her dentist needs to know that she is on warfarin in case there is a need for oral surgery or tooth extraction (Choice H). The client should not change her diet while on warfarin.

Cognitive Skill

Take Action

References

Burchum & Rosenthal, 2019, pp. 612–616, 630–631

Thinking Exercise 29B-4

Answers

Health Teaching	Essential	Unrelated
"Report any unexpected bleeding to your primary health care provider."	X	
"Continue taking your newly prescribed medications until your prescriber tells you not to do so."	X	
"Drink a glass of water after each dose of your new drugs."		X
"Eat foods high in Vitamin K and calcium to help prevent clotting."		X
"Avoid taking other medications that can cause bleeding, such as nonsteroidal anti-inflammatory drugs like ibuprofen."	X	
"Follow up with the prescribed laboratory testing needed to monitor your clotting values."		X

Rationales

Both aspirin and clopidogrel are antiplatelet drugs rather than anticoagulants. Antiplatelet drugs do not affect coagulation studies, and follow-up laboratory testing is not needed. However, the client is at risk for bleeding. The nurse teaches the client to report any unusual or unexpected bleeding to her primary health care provider, but to continue taking the drugs unless the provider discontinues them. Stopping these drugs quickly can result in clot formation that could lead to a myocardial infarction or other clotting event. Drinking a certain amount of water or changing one's diet is not necessary when the client is taking antiplatelet drugs.

Cognitive Skill

Generate Solutions

References

Burchum & Rosenthal, 2019, pp. 622–624, 631–632

Exemplar 29C. Drugs That Affect Perfusion (Medical-Surgical Nursing: Middle-Age and Older Adult)

Thinking Exercise 29C-1

Answers

A, B, D, G, H

Rationales

Losartan is an angiotensin II receptor blocker (ARB) that helps protect kidney function, especially for clients who have diabetes mellitus (Choice A). As with other antihypertensive drugs, the client should monitor his blood pressure frequently at home and change positions slowly because of potential orthostatic (postural) hypotension (Choices B and H). The nurse teaches the client that this drug can cause angioedema, although rare, which manifests with swelling and tightness in the lips, mouth, and throat. If these changes occur, the client or client's family needs to call 911 (Choice D). Clients on any antihypertensive drug should be sure to keep all follow-up appointments with their primary health care provider (Choice G).

Cognitive Skill

Take Action

Reference

Burchum & Rosenthal, 2019, pp. 489–491

Thinking Exercise 29C-2

Answers

In view of the client's blood pressure pattern and the peak action of amlodipine, the nurse would recommend that the client take his amlodipine in early morning. He should also avoid drinking grapefruit juice because it interferes with the drug's metabolism in the intestines.

Rationales

Amlodipine is a calcium channel blocker that has a peak onset of 6 to 12 hours. The client's blood pressure increases in the late afternoon, so if the drug is taken early in the day, it will be working at its peak action to keep his blood pressure within normal range. Many drugs, including amlodipine, are affected by grapefruit juice, which can interfere with drug metabolism.

Cognitive Skill

Take Action

Reference

Burchum & Rosenthal, 2019, pp. 497–499

Thinking Exercise 29C-3

Answers

B, C, E, F, G

Rationales

Verapamil is a calcium channel blocker commonly used for angina pectoris to suppress impulse conduction through the AV node of the heart. Therefore, the nurse reminds the client to call 911 if there are other episodes of angina (Choice G). Verapamil should not be taken with beta blockers or digoxin because these drugs also decrease AV conduction, and AV heart block could result (Choice B). The nurse teaches the client to monitor his pulse and blood pressure because the drug can lower these vital signs (Choice E) and to follow up with primary health care provider appointments (Choice F). Many drugs, including verapamil, are affected by grapefruit juice, which can interfere with drug metabolism (Choice C).

Cognitive Skill

Take Action

Reference

Burchum & Rosenthal, 2019, pp. 497–501

Thinking Exercise 29C-4

Answers

- Reports new dry "hacking" cough that occurs almost every day
- Has replaced sodium-based salt with potassium-based salt in his diet

Rationales

Lisinopril is an angiotensin-converting enzyme (ACE) inhibitor. Drugs in this class can cause a dry cough that is very annoying to clients who take them. If clients experience a cough, they are usually placed on a different type of drug. ACE inhibitors can also cause hyperkalemia. Taking potassium-based salt can increase serum potassium, making the client more likely to develop hyperkalemia, which can cause cardiac dysrhythmias.

Cognitive Skill

Recognize Cues

Reference

Burchum & Rosenthal, 2019, pp. 485–489

Thinking Exercise 29C-5

Answers

The nurse performs a focused cardiovascular assessment because the client is at risk for dysrhythmias and hypokalemia because she takes both digoxin and HCTZ. In addition, the client is at risk for drug toxicity, which can be prevented by monitoring the client's digoxin and potassium levels.

Rationales

The client taking both digoxin and a thiazide diuretic is at risk for decreased potassium levels, which can cause dysrhythmias. Therefore the health care team monitors the client's digoxin level for toxicity and potassium levels to ensure that they are within the normal range.

Cognitive Skill

Analyze Cues

References

Burchum & Rosenthal, 2019, pp. 464–465, 536–541

Exemplar 29D. Drugs That Promote Comfort and Metabolism (Medical-Surgical Nursing: Middle-Age and Older Adult)

Thinking Exercise 29D-1

Answers

B, C, D, E, F, H

Rationales

Cyclobenzaprine is a muscle relaxant that has anticholinergic effects that can cause drowsiness (Choice D), blurred vision, urinary retention (Choice E), and constipation. The client should not drink alcohol (a depressant) with a drug that can cause drowsiness (Choice B). To prevent constipation, the nurse would teach the client to consume high-fiber foods and incorporate more water into his diet (Choice F). Because cyclobenzaprine can also cause dysrhythmias, the client should report any chest discomfort or palpitations to his primary health care provider as soon as possible (Choice H). Naproxen is an NSAID that can cause bleeding or easy bruising. The nurse would teach the client that if these side effects occur, he should notify his primary health care provider (Choice C).

Cognitive Skill

Take Action

References

Burchum & Rosenthal, 2019, pp. 254–255, 895–896

Thinking Exercise 29D-2

Answers

A. Client's Drugs	B. Drug Class	C. Correct Drug for Drug Class
1 Simvastatin	Anti-epileptic drug	3 Pregabalin
2 Empagliflozin	HMG-CoA reductase inhibitor	1 Simvastatin
3 Pregabalin	5-Alpha-reductase inhibitor	5 Finasteride
4 Glyburide	NSAID	6 Celecoxib
5 Finasteride	SGLT-2 inhibitor	2 Empagliflozin
6 Celecoxib	Sulfonylurea	4 Glyburide

Cognitive Skill

Take Action

References

Burchum & Rosenthal, 2019, pp. 240–241, 579–580, 693, 804, 863–864

Thinking Exercise 29D-3

Answers

Nurses' Notes

7/19/20 1915. Given hydrocodone/acetaminophen as prescribed an hour ago but reports 7/10 lower back pain on a 0 to 10 pain intensity scale. Pulse = 98, B/P = 164/88, which have increased since admission. No obvious blood in stool but sent to lab for occult blood testing. Waiting for lab results for CBC and BMP.

—————————————————— D.L. Morgan, RNC

Rationales

Even though the client was given an analgesic, she continues to have moderately severe pain as evidenced by her subjective report and elevated pulse an blood pressure. Acute pain can cause these changes in vital signs.

Cognitive Skill

Recognize Cues

References

Burchum & Rosenthal, 2019, pp. 285–286, 297–299

Thinking Exercise 29D-4

Answers

The nurse teaches the client that zolpidem is a commonly prescribed hypnotic that promotes sleep but does not reduce pain. Common side effects include drowsiness and dizziness, which could place the client at risk for injury. In addition, some people of all ages perform activities during their sleep that could be dangerous, including sleep driving. Tramadol is a nonopioid analgesic that will help promote comfort and allow the client to rest and sleep.

Cognitive Skill

Take Action

References

Burchum & Rosenthal, 2019, pp. 294, 388–389

Thinking Exercise 29D-5

Answers

The nurse anticipates that the primary health care provider will prescribe a(n) analgesic because the client has acute pain. However, he will continue to receive his fentanyl patches to help control his chronic cancer pain.

Rationales

Although the client is receiving fentanyl for his chronic cancer pain, he sustained a new injury, which he reports is painful. In addition, his pulse and blood pressure are increased, which is common in clients who are in acute pain. The client will require an analgesic to manage his acute pain.

Cognitive Skill

Prioritize Hypotheses

Reference

Ignatavicius et al., 2018, Chapter 4 (Pain)

Exemplar 29E. Drugs That Manage Infection (Medical-Surgical Nursing [Young and Middle-Age Adult]; Pediatric Nursing)

Thinking Exercise 29E-1

Answers

B, F

Rationales

In addition to taking his antibiotic, the child will need an NSAID to control his fever and promote comfort, and should continue his fluticasone propionate and pseudoephedrine (Choice F). The parent should ensure that all doses of amoxicillin are given even if the child's earache improves (Choice B).

Cognitive Skill

Evaluate Outcomes

Reference

Burchum & Rosenthal, 2019, pp. 1035–1038

Thinking Exercise 29E-2

Answers

The nurse will instruct the client that she should not continue taking trimethoprim/sulfamethoxazole because the drug likely caused the skin reaction to sulfa. The nurse will instruct the client that she may not be able to continue taking glipizide because the drug is a sulfonylurea.

Cognitive Skill

Take Action

Reference

Burchum & Rosenthal, 2019, pp. 1068–1070

Thinking Exercise 29E-3

Answers

The nurse teaches the client that he needs to take ethambutol with meals or food to prevent GI upset. The client should take the other prescribed antituberculosis drugs every day on an empty stomach. After the 8-week drug regimen to effectively manage the client's infection, he will likely continue taking some of these drugs for an additional 18 weeks.

Cognitive Skill

Take Action

Reference

Burchum & Rosenthal, 2019, pp. 1081–1093

Thinking Exercise 29E-4

Answers

C, E, F, G

Rationales

Acyclovir is an antiviral drug that can cause kidney damage; therefore the client's kidney function is carefully managed during the time that the client receives it (Choice C). Gabapentin is a psychoactive drug that is being used for this client to reduce nerve pain caused by herpes zoster (Choice F). This drug can cause sleepiness, especially after the first few doses, and can be taken with or without food (Choices E and G).

Cognitive Skill

Take Action

Reference

Burchum & Rosenthal, 2019, pp. 1113–1116

CHAPTER 30 Pharmacology in Management of Complex Health Problems

Answers With Rationales for Thinking Exercises

Exemplar 30A. Drugs That Affect Perfusion and Gas Exchange (Medical-Surgical Nursing: Older Adult; Pediatric Nursing: Adolescent)

Thinking Exercise 30A-1

Answers

The nurse's primary responsibility for the client receiving dopamine will be to monitor her urinary output and titrate the infusion rate of the drug based on agency or primary health care provider protocol. During drug infusion, the nurse would also observe for adverse effects of dopamine including chest pain and dysrhythmias.

Rationales

Dopamine is an adrenergic agonist that activates beta$_1$ receptors in the heart to increase cardiac output and improve organ perfusion. Therefore it is used for clients who are in a shock state. Because urine output depends on renal perfusion, monitoring the client's urinary output indicates whether the client's overall perfusion status is improving. Activating cardiac beta$_1$ receptors, though, can cause chest pain, dysrhythmias, and tachycardia.

Cognitive Skill

Analyze Cues

Reference

Burchum & Rosenthal, 2019, p. 155

Thinking Exercise 30A-2

Answers

If the client feels that she is having problems breathing, she would use albuterol MDI for quick relief. In addition to oxygen therapy, if she has a severe asthma attack, the drugs of choice would most likely include systemic corticosteroids, nebulized formoterol, and nebulized ipratropium.

Rationales

Albuterol MDI is a *short-acting* beta$_2$ agonist that can be used as needed for difficulty breathing for clients who have asthma. For acute severe asthma exacerbations, initial therapy includes oxygen to relieve hypoxemia, systemic corticosteroids to decrease airway inflammation, and nebulized ipratropium and a nebulized long-acting beta$_2$ agonist such as formoterol to reduce airway obstruction.

Cognitive Skill

Generate Solutions

Reference

Burchum & Rosenthal, 2019, pp. 936–942

Thinking Exercise 30A-3

Answers

A, C, D, E, F

Rationales

To prevent further myocardial damage, oxygen therapy helps to improve tissue perfusion (Choice A). Myocardial infarctions occur as a result of coronary vessel obstruction by one or more clots. Therefore, heparin is prescribed as an anticoagulant that prevents further clot formation or any enlargement of clots that are already present (Choice C), and the client will likely be prescribed an anticoagulant or antiplatelet drug when he is discharged (Choice D). Propranolol is a beta-adrenergic blocking agent that decreases chest pain and will likely be prescribed for the client to take at home after hospital discharge (Choices E and F). This drug decreases heart rate rather than increases it, and therefore this is an incorrect choice (Choice G). Nitroglycerin dilates blood vessels rather than constricts them, and therefore this choice is also incorrect (Choice B).

Cognitive Skill

Take Action

Reference

Burchum & Rosenthal, 2019, pp. 634–638

Thinking Exercise 30A-4

Answers

The nurse would question the primary health care provider before administering tamsulosin because it can interact with propranolol and cause severe hypotension.

Rationales

Tamsulosin is a drug to manage benign prostatic hyperplasia and can interact with antihypertensive drugs, such as propranolol, a beta-adrenergic blocking agent, and cause severe hypotension.

Cognitive Skill

Take Action

Reference

Burchum & Rosenthal, 2019, pp. 805–806

Thinking Exercise 30A-5

Answers

Nursing Action	Indicated	Contraindicated	Non-Essential
Teach the client to increase his oral fluid intake, especially water.	X		
Perform a urinary catheterization.		X	
Start an IV infusion of 1000 mL saline.			X
Help the client stand to use the urinal or bathroom.	X		
Run water while the client is trying to void.	X		
Request a diuretic for the client to facilitate voiding.		X	
Review the client's serum electrolyte values.			X

Rationales

The nurse needs to help the client urinate using evidence-based strategies that can help with voiding. Many men have difficulty voiding when lying or sitting in the bed using a urinal. Therefore allow the client to stand using a urinal or bathroom toilet to establish the usual position that men typically use to void. Increasing the client's fluid intake and running water may help facilitate voiding. Performing a urinary catheterization may cause trauma and bleeding in a client who was recently receiving heparin. Urinary catheterization may also contribute to catheter-related urinary tract infection (CAUTI). Starting a saline IV solution and reviewing the client's serum electrolyte levels are not related to the problem the client is having with difficulty voiding.

Cognitive Skill

Generate Solutions

References

Burchum & Rosenthal, 2019, pp. 607–610, 805

Exemplar 30B. Drugs That Affect Immunity (Medical-Surgical Nursing: Young Adult; Middle-Age Adult)

Thinking Exercise 30B-1

Answers

B, C, D, E, F

Rationales

Most drugs given to clients for management of rheumatoid arthritis affect the immune response and can cause infection. Therefore the nurse teaches the client to avoid crowds and people who have infection (Choices B and D). Hydroxychloroquine is an antimalarial drug that helps decrease joint inflammation, but it can cause retinal damage. Therefore the nurse reminds the client to have frequent eye examinations (Choice C). MTX can cause bone marrow suppression and damage to the liver, lungs, and kidneys. Therefore the client needs to follow up on all laboratory testing to monitor for these changes (Choice E). MTX is taken weekly and should be taken on the same day and time each week to maintain serum drug levels (Choice F).

Cognitive Skill

Take Action

Reference

Burchum & Rosenthal, 2019, pp. 883–887

Thinking Exercise 30B-2

Answers

> **Office Progress Note**
>
> 12/20/19 1030 Client reports that she has had increasing episodes of fatigue for the past month and has noticed new inflammation in both wrists. Both wrists are reddened and swollen with right wrist worse than left wrist. Is right-handed. Has a good appetite and is able to function most days without major difficulty. Recently visited her eye doctor and no vision changes noted since she began hydroxychloroquine. Unintentionally lost 5 lb (2.3 kg) since last visit 6 months ago. Says she feels "down" and sad most days about her disease. —————————————————— M.J. Brown, CMA

Rationales

The client is having signs and symptoms consistent with a disease exacerbation ("flare-up") as evidenced by new inflammation in her wrists and unintentional weight loss, a later stage of the disease. In addition, the nurse would be concerned that the client is potentially depressed about how her disease is affecting her as a young woman.

Cognitive Skill

Recognize Cues

Reference

Burchum & Rosenthal, 2019, p. 881

Thinking Exercise 30B-3

Answers

The nurse recognizes that golimumab is a(n) tumor necrosis factor antagonist that works to modify the immune response. The nurse would administer 148 mg of golimumab via IV infusion for the first dose if the client does not have infection.

Rationales

The nurse knows that golimumab is a drug that works to neutralize tumor necrosis factor (TNF), an important immune mediator that causes joint injury in clients with rheumatoid arthritis. As such, the drug modifies the immune response. The client weighs 74 kg (163/2.2) and would need 2 mg of drug per kg of body weight or 148 kg for the first dose if she is free of infection. Clients who take TNF antagonists are at a high risk for serious systematic infection, so having an infection is a contraindication for administering the drug to the client.

Cognitive Skill

Take Action

Reference

Burchum & Rosenthal, 2019, pp. 885–889

Thinking Exercise 30B-4

Answers

B, C, D, E, G

Rationales

Ribavirin is an oral drug and peginterferon alfa is administered subcutaneously, so Choices A and F are not correct responses. Ribavirin can cause hemolytic anemia, which requires regular follow-up laboratory testing, and fetal toxicity that can lead to injury (Choices B and D). Peginterferon alfa commonly causes flulike symptoms and less often can lead to depression (Choices C and E). This drug has antiviral and immunomodulating effects (Choice G).

Cognitive Skill

Take Action

Reference

Burchum & Rosenthal, 2019, pp. 1120–1122

Exemplar 30C. Drugs That Manage Psychoses (Mental Health Nursing: Young Adult)

Thinking Exercise 30C-1

Answers

A 21-year-old male client was recently diagnosed with schizophrenia, for which he has was prescribed chlorpromazine, a first-generation antipsychotic (FGA) drug. After the client was on the drug for several weeks, his mother found the client in the basement having a seizure and called 911. In the emergency department, the nurse documented the following client assessment findings:

Assessment Findings
• Temperature = 104°F (40°C)
• Heart rate = 118 beats/min
• Respirations = 26 breaths/min
• Blood pressure = 174/102 mm Hg
• O_2 saturation = 91% on room air
• Muscle rigidity in all four extremities
• Drowsy at times
• States he is nauseated, but has not vomited
• Has abdominal pain 3/10 (on a 0 to 10 pain intensity scale)

Rationales

The client is demonstrating signs and symptoms associated with a rare but serious complication of first-generation antipsychotic (FGA) drugs. He had a least one seizure and has decreased level of consciousness, muscle rigidity, and abnormal vital signs. The nurse would be concerned about the client's presentation because this complication is potentially fatal.

Cognitive Skill

Recognize Cues

Reference

Burchum & Rosenthal, 2019, pp. 335–336

Thinking Exercise 30C-2

Answers

Based on the nurse's assessment findings, the client mostly likely has neuroleptic malignant syndrome, a rare but potentially fatal complication of first-generation antipsychotic drugs. Management of this complication includes giving the client two major drugs: dantrolene and bromocriptine.

Cognitive Skill

Prioritize Hypotheses

Reference

Burchum & Rosenthal, 2019, pp. 335–336

Thinking Exercise 30C-3

Answers

Signs and Symptoms	Parkinsonism	Acute Dystonia	Anticholinergic Effects
Constipation	X		X
Resting tremors	X		
Urinary hesitancy			X
Blurred vision			X
Facial muscle spasms		X	
Muscle rigidity	X		
Very dry mouth			X

Cognitive Skill

Recognize Cues

Reference

Burchum & Rosenthal, 2019, pp. 334–335

Thinking Exercise 30C-4

Answers

A. Drug Choice	B. Extrapyramidal Symptom (EPS)	C. Drug That May Be Used to Manage EPS
1 Propranolol	Acute dystonia	**2** Benztropine
2 Benztropine	Parkinsonism	**4** Amantadine
3 Clozapine	Akathisia	**1** Propranolol
4 Amantadine	Tardive dyskinesia	**6** Lorazepam
5 Zolpidem		
6 Lorazepam		

Cognitive Skill

Analyze Cues

Reference

Burchum & Rosenthal, 2019, p. 334

Thinking Exercise 30C-5

Answers

C, D, E, F

Rationales

Olanzapine is a second-generation antipsychotic (SGA) drug that causes less serious complications than first-generation antipsychotic (FGA) drugs, so Choice A is incorrect. This drug can cause sleepiness, so insomnia is unlikely (Choice B). Depression is also not a likely side effect of this medication, so Choice G is also not correct. However, olanzapine can cause anticholinergic effects (Choice C) and leukopenia, which would make the client susceptible to infection (Choice D). The nurse would teach the client ways to prevent constipation (an anticholinergic side effect) including adding high-fiber foods and more fluids into the client's diet (Choice F). Unlike FGA drugs, SGA drugs can cause metabolic problems including obesity and diabetes mellitus (Choice E).

Cognitive Skill

Take Action

Reference

Burchum & Rosenthal, 2019, p. 341

Exemplar 30D. Drugs That Manage Emergencies (Medical-Surgical Nursing: Young Adult; Older Adult)

Thinking Exercise 30D-1

Answers

Nursing Action	Indicated	Contraindicated	Non-Essential
Maintain the client's airway and ventilation.	X		
Place the client in a flat supine position.		X	
Establish an IV line immediately and administer a benzodiazepine such as IV lorazepam or diazepam.	X		
Document type and duration of each seizure.	X		
Monitor vital signs, especially temperature and heart rate, and cardiac rhythm.	X		
Draw labs to assess serum electrolyte values.			X
Monitor the client's level of consciousness frequently.	X		

Rationales

Status epilepticus is a medical emergency that can cause loss of consciousness or even death. Therefore the nurse would frequently monitor the client's level of consciousness and vital signs and maintain her airway. IV benzodiazepine is used to control seizure activity, and the client is placed in a semi-Fowler position to promote breathing and prevent airway obstruction by her tongue. The nurse would document all seizure activity including the type, time, and duration of each seizure.

Cognitive Skill

Generate Solutions

Reference

Burchum & Rosenthal, 2019, p. 244

Thinking Exercise 30D-2

Answers

Before administering the drug, the nurse calculates that the hourly rate of the drug infusion should be 750 mcg. During drug administration, the nurse monitors the client's blood pressure, which should decrease, and heart rate, which may increase.

Rationales

The client weighs 110 lb, which is 50 kg; 50 kg × 0.25 mcg × 60 minutes = 750 mcg of the drug should be infused per hour. Fenoldopam is an IV drug indicated for short-term hypertensive emergencies. The drug works to dilate blood vessels and promote sodium and water excretion via the kidneys to decrease blood volume. Therefore the nurse would expect the client's blood pressure to decrease and her heart rate to increase reflexively.

Cognitive Skill

Analyze Cues

Reference

Burchum & Rosenthal, 2019, pp. 524–525

Thinking Exercise 30D-3

Answers

A 78-year-old male client has been diagnosed with diabetes mellitus type 2 and chronic health failure for many years, for which he takes hydrochlorothiazide (HCTZ), digoxin, and metformin. After his wife died last year, his health declined and he was admitted to a local nursing home. For the past 6 months, he has experienced cognitive decline, most likely due to hypoxia and/or multi-infarct dementia. The nurse referred the client to the registered dietitian nutritionist because of a 10-lb (4.5-kg) weight loss in 2 weeks, anorexia, and increasing blood glucose levels. The registered dietitian nutritionist prescribed oral supplemental feedings, and his metformin dose was increased by the primary health care provider. Today the charge nurse receives the client's latest lab work as follows:

Laboratory Test Values

- Blood urea nitrogen (BUN) = 67 mg/dL (23.9 mmol/L)
- Creatinine (Cr) = 1.2 mg/dL (106.08 mmol/L)
- Fasting blood sugar (FBS) = 259 mg/dL (14.4 mmol/L)
- Sodium (Na) = 141 mEq/L (141 mmol/L)
- Potassium (K) = 4.6 mEq/L (4.6 mmol/L)
- Chloride (Cl) = 96 mEq/L (96 mmol/L)
- Calcium (Ca) = 5.0 mEq/L (50 mmol/L)
- Carbon dioxide (CO_2) = 22 mEq/L (22 mmol/L)

Rationales

The client has a high blood glucose and BUN, but his creatinine is within a high normal range. These findings suggest dehydration, especially because the client suddenly and unintentionally lost significant weight and is receiving a daily diuretic.

Cognitive Skill

Recognize Cues

Reference

Burchum & Rosenthal, 2019, p. 704

Thinking Exercise 30D-4

Answers

Based on the physical assessment findings, medical diagnoses, and lab test values, the nurse suspects that the client most likely has hyperglycemic-hyperosmolar state, which requires emergency management with intravenous fluids and IV regular insulin.

Rationales

The client has a diabetic complication known as hyperglycemic-hyperosmolar state (HHS) that can occur as a result of diabetes mellitus type 2. It is different from diabetic ketoacidosis, which occurs as a complication of diabetes mellitus type 1, in that the client does not typically have metabolic acidosis and ketosis. However, the client is very dehydrated owing to serum hyperosmolarity from a high glucose level, which is consistent with HHS. HCTZ is a diuretic that contributes to the client's dehydration as evidenced by significant weight loss (water weight) and a high BUN.

Cognitive Skill

Prioritize Hypotheses

Reference

Burchum & Rosenthal, 2019, p. 704

References

Burchum, J. L. R., & Rosenthal, L. D. (2019). *Lehne's Pharmacology for Nursing Care* (10th ed.). St. Louis: Elsevier.

Halter, M. J. (2018). *Varcarolis' Foundations of Psychiatric-Mental Health Nursing*. (8th ed.). St. Louis: Elsevier.

Hockenberry, M. J., & Wilson, D. (2019). *Wong's Nursing Care of Infants and Children*. (11th ed). St. Louis: Elsevier.

Ignatavicius, D. D., Workman, M. L., & Rebar, C. R. (2018). *Medical-Surgical Nursing: Concepts for Interprofessional Collaborative Care*. (9th ed.). St. Louis: Elsevier.

Lowdermilk, D. L., Perry, S. E., Cashion, M. C., Alden, K. R., & Olshansky, E. (2020). *Maternity and Women's Health*. (12th ed.). St. Louis: Elsevier.

Pagana K.D., & Pagana, T. J. (2018). *Manual of Diagnostic and Laboratory Tests* (6th ed.). St. Louis: Elsevier.

Pagana, K. D., Pagana, T. J., & Pike-MacDonald, S. A. (2019). *Mosby's Canadian Manual of Diagnostic and Laboratory Tests* (2nd ed.). Toronto: Elsevier.